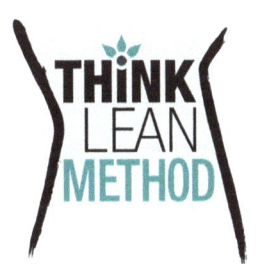

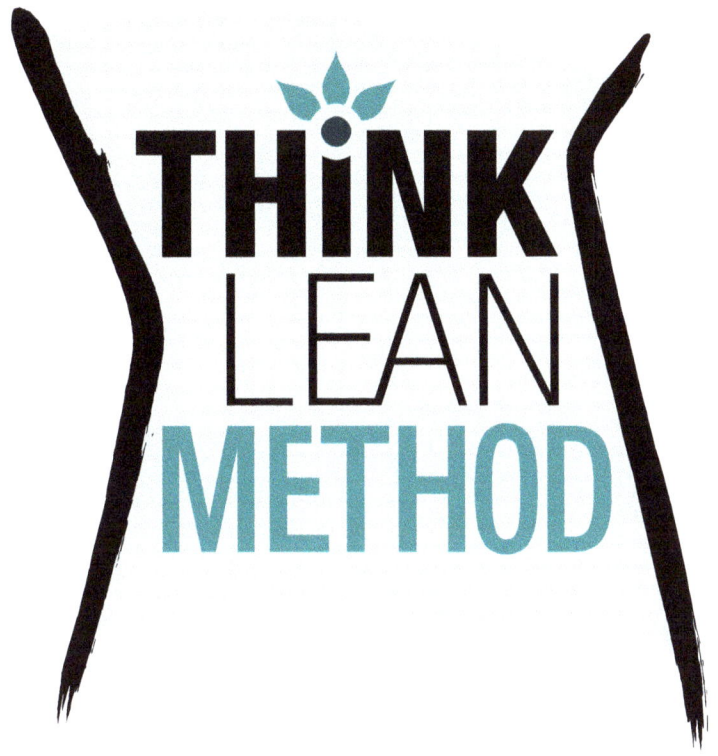

The **whole-brain** guide to get **lean for life**

Jurie G. Rossouw

With Susan D. **Whitmore**

Sydney - Australia

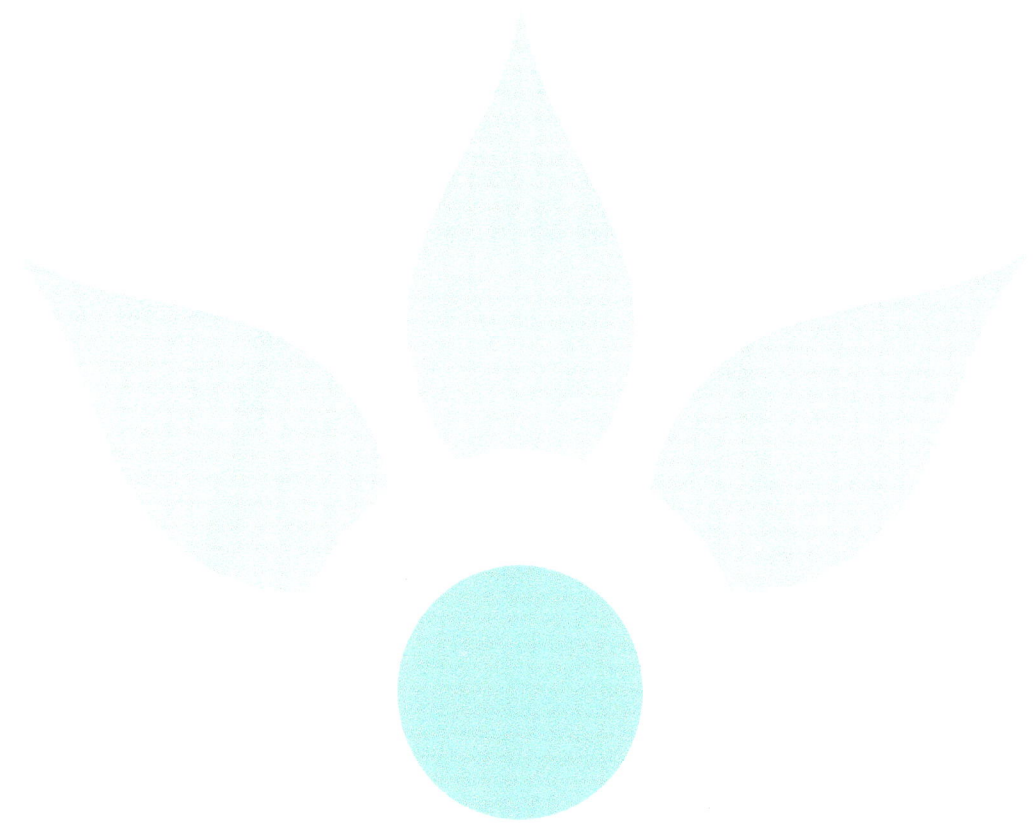

The information in this book is for educational purposes only. It is not intended nor implied to be used as a substitute for professional medical advice. The reader should always consult a healthcare professional to determine the suitability of the information for their own situation or if they have any questions regarding a medical condition or treatment plan. Think Lean Method Pty Ltd, the author and associates are not responsible in any manner whatsoever for any adverse effects directly or indirectly as a result of the information provided in this book.

First printed in 2015

Copyright © Think Lean Method Pty Ltd

All rights reserved. No part of this book may be reproduced or transmitted in any form or by any means whatsoever without express written permission from the author, except in the case of brief quotations embodied in critical articles and reviews. Please refer all pertinent questions to the author.

Author: Jurie G. Rossouw

With: Susan D. Whitmore

Think Lean Method Pty Ltd
Sydney, Australia

ISBN 978-0-99424-120-7

For more information, please contact us through:
www.thinkleanmethod.com

Dedicated to every person that wants to advance.

Contents

Introduction i

1   Fundamental Nutrition 5
   1.1   Macronutrients 5
   1.2   Micronutrients 32

The First Key:

2   Automatic Calorie Management 41
   2.1   The rules of Automatic Calorie Management 42
   2.2   The Think Lean food pyramid 55
   2.3   Exercise 57
   2.4   Busting myths 60

The Second Key:

3   Boost Your Brain 65
   3.1   What is the brain? 66
   3.2   What affects your brain? 78
   3.3   Take action to boost your brain 88

The Final Key:

4   Think Lean 91
   4.1   Personal resilience 95
   4.2   Quality beliefs 116
   4.3   Developing clear goals 127
   4.4   Make it real 146

5   The Think Lean Plan 147
   5.1   Set goals 148
   5.2   Involve others 148
   5.3   Clean up 149
   5.4   Pick a meal plan 150
   5.5   Think Lean and eat clean 159
   5.6   Keep track 159

6   Easy Recipes 166

Appendix A – Vitamins 204
Appendix B – Minerals 215
Appendix C – Foods 223
References: 228

Introduction

Nutrition is easy. You just need to follow a few simple rules to manage your weight and be lean and healthy. Right? So why does it all seem so hard? Truth is, there is so much information out there - in books, on the internet, from people who swear that this or that works for them, advertising, miracle drugs, magazines, the list is endless! – that it's hard to see the **truth** through all the fads! So you set off down a very long road of trial and error which, let's be honest, is mostly error. Trying different things, losing weight for a bit only to pile it back on, plus some. Or wanting to gain muscle weight and **definition** only to find most of the weight gain is fat.

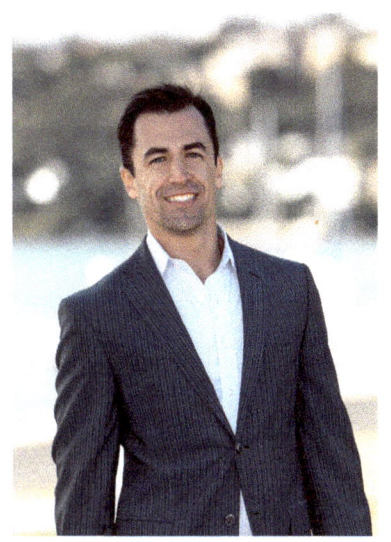

This is the road I found myself trudging along year after year, wanting to get healthy and wanting to achieve my **goal body**, but failing at every turn. I'd try exercising for a bit, switch things around in my diet, drink more water, add more fruit, eat less fat. I tried high-carb, low fat and saw my weight head in the right direction, but not my health. My asthma got worse and I had frequent headaches. Every few weeks I'd come down with something – a cold, 'flu, a runny nose - which was unusual because I never used to get sick, and if I did, it was usually mild and would be gone in a day or two. Now I was getting sick for weeks at a time and worst of all, my health issues affected my **motivation**. So before I knew it, I was back to square one. Unhealthy, unhappy, and unmotivated.

But I learned something very important through the process – **health must come first!** Also, I was so focused on my weight that I had failed to realise the importance of muscle versus body fat. Instead of getting a **lean** and **defined** body, I'd simply been swapping muscle for body fat! Fed up, I decided to approach weight management scientifically, focusing my studies around peer-reviewed scientific research on **healthy nutrition**, which I eventually expanded into nutritional neuroscience, psychology and neuropsychotherapy in search of a healthy mind. I slowly started to understand all the things I was doing wrong – neglecting brain health, not understanding the importance of consistency, or that the grain products I was eating were full of omega-6, resulting in the chronic inflammation that was playing havoc with my body.

I used my research to construct a new healthy eating plan for myself and the results were amazing – I lost body fat, while **muscle mass** improved, I stopped getting sick, I got fewer headaches and even my asthma improved. As my health got better, my motivation came back **stronger** than ever before. But what really astounded me was not how simple it was to make the changes to my lifestyle, but how long it took me to work it out! I realised how unhelpful the information I had been relying on was, the fad diets pushing their tired old myths, the wonder drugs promising me quick results, and the friends who had lost weight but were now off the diet-wagon.

But that's just it - most "diets" or "body transformation plans" focus on achieving short-term body or health goals but provide no support or strategies for maintaining these goals for the rest of your life. And who wants their **goal body** or optimum level of health for only a short period of time? To achieve long term goals, you need to be **consistent**. But that's the hard part, just how do you stay consistent year after year? How do you motivate yourself and overcome the challenges you will face along the way? How can you **think lean for life**?

I spent many years researching and trialling strategies to help me stick to my healthy eating and body goals. Along the way, I learned how nutrition affects the **brain**, how the brain works, and the psychology behind setting and **achieving goals**. Through my work in the field of Resilience, I also realised the importance of **personal resilience** in helping us stay consistent, regardless of all the challenges that life throws our way.

I'll be honest, I'm frustrated that I had to spend so much time and effort to achieve an effective healthy eating plan and the skills to stick to it long term. I wish that someone could have given me what I needed most in the beginning – **this book**! So while I can't get back all the years I spent researching and trialling, I can be that "someone" to you!

This is why I wrote the **Think Lean Method**. I want to help you to become healthy, lean and confident. I want to teach you simple techniques you can use to reach your goals quickly, and to turn healthy living into a **permanent lifestyle**. I want you to experience the **whole life transformation** that I did, and to become the person you've always wanted to be!

I know only too well that we live in a time where information is extremely accessible. Unfortunately, not all information is created equally – some of it is just plain wrong and can be detrimental to your **health** and **wellbeing**. In fact, some of the loudest opinions or most popular diets flatly ignore proven nutritional science and instead tout flawed "miracle cures" with "guaranteed fast results". The Think Lean Method is not a diet – it is a method for achieving long-term physical and mental health using concepts based on proven **scientific research**. I encourage you to start your journey with an open mind and to let the evidence be your guide. By doing this, you will set off on the right path to achieve your goals, for both your **body** and your **mind**.

Jurie G. Rossouw

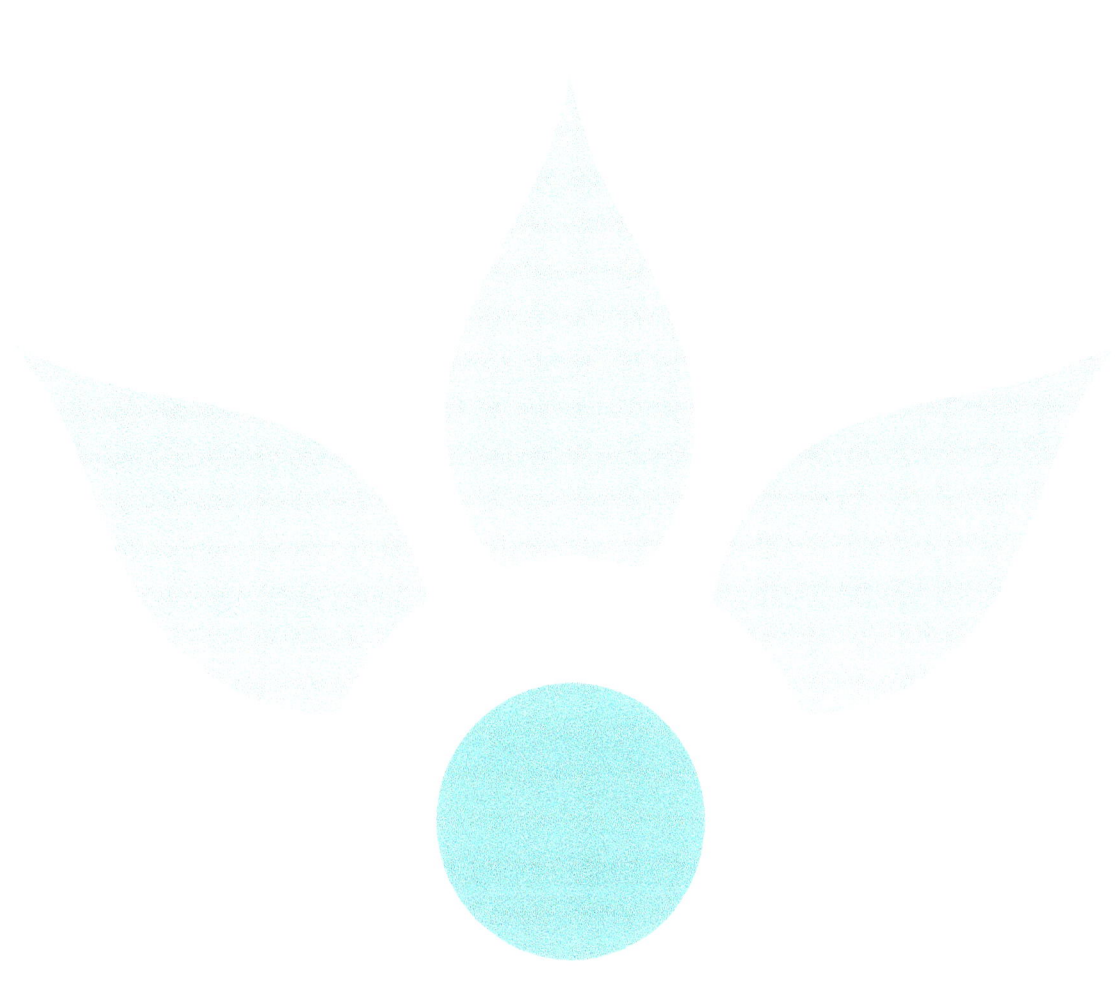

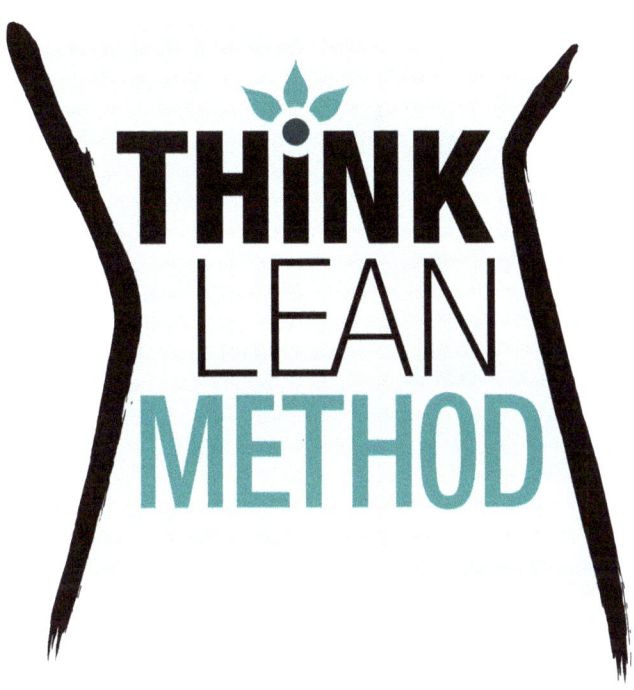

Healthy, lean and confident. This is the very essence of the Think Lean lifestyle. This is something we all want – a lean and healthy body, filled with the confidence to take on and succeed in every aspect of life. Here you will learn how to create your goal body quickly and also experience a fantastic and fulfilling lifestyle change.

For you to put this lifestyle change into action and make it a reality, you need a *transformation*. This is what the **Think Lean Method** is all about – a transformation for your body and your mind – a transformation that can improve your whole life.

Enhanced confidence, healthy and successful habits, relaxed determination and effortless discipline. Think about that for a minute. What would your life be like if you had those qualities? Not just your eating habits, but your relationships, your work, your hobbies. Wouldn't that be amazing? This is what I want to help you achieve.

And it is achievable!

In the first section, **Fundamental Nutrition**, we will work through the essentials of healthy eating to give you a good foundation to build upon. We'll also look at why the method works and the science behind it.

Once we have worked through the fundamentals, we'll move into the **three keys to transforming your life**. These three keys work together to help you achieve a lasting transformation. Together, we will work through each key, to learn how and why they work.

- *The first key:*
  Automatic Calorie Management – No more calorie counting! Start your body transformation by learning the secret of healthy eating that keeps you feeling full while also keeping you lean!

- *The second key:*
  Boost Your Brain – What you eat has a huge impact on your brain and how you feel. Learn from the latest research and feel energised, positive and happy!

- *The final key:*
  Think Lean – The true source of a real transformation. Here you will find the secret to changing your thinking, building your confidence and changing your habits – for good!

These three keys form a complete program. We will work through each key separately to learn how it works and then we will look at the simple steps you need to put them all into action.

We will then move onto **The Think Lean Plan** section, which has meal plans and tracking sheets to keep you on track for achieving your lifestyle transformation, and also provides you with information on cleaning up your social media and involving others in your goals.

The **Easy Recipes** section provides you with tasty recipes to keep you feeling satisfied and full. I created these easy recipes to support you to achieve your goal body. These are simple recipes you can cook every day or you can make extra to last you the entire week.

What could be easier?

The **Think Lean Method** is designed to provide you with everything you need to transform your body and your mind. There are many interacting parts to this book, and skipping some parts may reduce the effectiveness of others. With that said – *you do not have to follow everything in this book to the letter*. In fact, you may end up only adopting a few ideas, or you may follow the entire system and then go on holidays and forgo the nutrition plan for a few weeks as you relax. Well guess what – you can just pick up where you left off and the results will start coming back as quickly as before! If you follow the nutrition plan 90% of the time, you will still get most of the benefits and see results. **This is not an all or nothing diet**.

Reading guide

Depending on what you want to achieve, here are few ways to read this book:

- ### "I want a lasting lifestyle change!"
  Read the whole book! This will give you the knowledge and confidence to stay consistent with healthy eating and each your goals. If you've had trouble sticking to a diet before, then definitely read the entire book.

- ### "Just tell me what to eat to stay lean"
  If you're not too worried about the science behind everything and just want to start eating healthy, skip to **Chapter 2 – Automatic Calorie Management** for eating guidelines and then skip to **Chapter 5 – The Think Lean Plan** for meal plans. Simple!

- ### "I want to know how to stay consistent with my existing diet"
  If you already have a diet that you are happy with and want to be better at sticking to it, then it's all about having a healthy brain and the right mindset. Skip to **Chapter 3 – Boost Your Brain** and **Chapter 4 – Think Lean** to learn how to stay consistent!

Ok! Let's get started with the basics about nutrition to get you up to speed with the fundamentals of what your body needs and how it works!

1 Fundamental Nutrition

*Nutrition is a big topic because our bodies are so complicated! Many of the things we thought were true 20 years ago have significantly changed due to advances in modern science and research methodology. This is why I am so excited about the **Think Lean Method** – you get the benefits from the latest scientific studies and cut out all the myths and outdated research that are working against you!*

Our intake of nutrients can be broken into two main groups – macronutrients and micronutrients. Macronutrients, or macros for short, are the ones that we hear about almost on a daily basis. These are proteins, dietary fats and carbohydrates. Micronutrients, or micros for short, are the various minerals, vitamins, metals, and other assorted nutrients that our bodies need to function well.

Understanding these is crucial to maintaining healthy eating habits. After all, if you know the reasoning behind why you have to eat a certain way, you are much more likely to keep doing it, particularly when you understand how it will help you achieve your goal body! Let's take a closer look at macros for a start.

1.1 Macronutrients

The majority of what you eat is made up by macros - proteins, dietary fats and carbohydrates - along with water. While fibre is not a macro, we will include it in this section to compare to other macros as it is a big part of what we eat. Overall, when we talk about 'macros' we will be referring specifically to protein, dietary fats and carbohydrates. In this section, we will see how some macros are more important than others and how the different types play different roles.

Your body is fantastically adaptive, allowing it to cope with the different amounts and types macros you eat. However, since your body has evolved to react in particular ways to the different nutrients, it does not always do what you want it to. This is especially true for foods that your body is not historically used to consuming. For example, if you eat a lot of refined carbohydrates and little protein, your body will do the best it can to manage the constant spike in blood sugar by storing the excess energy as fat.

Wouldn't it be fantastic if your body could understand that times have changed and that you can now get food whenever you want from the supermarket or fast-food outlet? That it could understand you don't need it to store additional fat for times of famine? While your brain has figured this out, your body still acts like it did 50,000 years ago, desperately hunting for food. This is why when the body gets a lot of nutrients, it stores as much as it can as fat because, from its perspective, the abundance can stop at any moment and it will need those reserves to survive!

Of course the good news is that if you work with your body by eating the right way, it will give you the body you want and will make you feel great too.

Macros are the main players in weight and body composition (muscle vs body fat), so understanding the importance of macros and making sure that we eat the right types and amounts are crucial for us to reach our goals! Foods can contain one, two, or all three macros in varying ratios. Before we delve into the detail of each, have a look at the table below which provides a quick overview of the different types of macros. The table looks at a few different aspects such as: the different types, where you find them, what the body uses them for, why they are necessary for sustaining life, and how many calories are in each.

	Protein	Carbohydrates	Dietary Fat	Fibre
Calorie count	4 calories per gram	4 calories per gram	9 calories per gram	0 calories per gram
Main sources	Beef, chicken, fish, dairy, whey, nuts, soy	Vegetables, grains, breads, pasta, rice, fruits, berries, sugars	Oils, butter, fatty meats, some from vegetables, grains	Vegetables, legumes, nuts, seeds, fruits, grains
Necessity	We can't live without protein, all cells need it	Not essential for survival[1,2]	Crucial for the brain and cell function, including vitamin absorption	Fibre isn't a macro and is not necessary for survival
What are they	Chains of amino acids	Varying compounds consisting of hydrogen, carbon and oxygen	Triglycerides, including omega-3 and omega-6	Indigestible parts of plants
Types	• 22 different amino acids in total • 13 that the body can create • 9 essential amino acids that the body can't create	• Simple carbohydrates • Complex carbohydrates • All have different effects on blood sugar, measured on the Glycaemic Index	• Monounsaturated • Polyunsaturated, includes Essential Fatty Acids • Saturated • Trans-fats	• Soluble fibre • Insoluble fibre
Function	• All cells need protein as building blocks • Muscle maintenance and growth • Feeling full after meals	• Mainly used to provide energy • Has varying effects on blood sugar levels, measured on the Glycaemic Index	• Primarily an energy source • Essential fatty acids protect against heart disease, cancers and inflammatory diseases	• Helps us feel full • Reduces calorie density of meals • Can be prebiotic • Regulate blood sugar and lower cholesterol

There is still a lot of confusion and misconceptions around proteins, carbohydrates, dietary fats and fibre, while micros like vitamins are fairly well accepted and understood to be important. Therefore, to give you a more detailed view into the reasoning behind the nutrition plan, we will spend a good deal of time in this section going over the fundamentals of macros.

As for the three main macros themselves, you might notice from the table that carbohydrates are the only macro that is not essential to life[3,4]. This is interesting, given just how large a portion of our diet tend to be carbohydrates! The reality is that there are cultures such as the Inuit that live mainly without carbohydrates. They live in the frozen arctic where they can only hunt animals, yet they still live healthy lives. In fact, on their traditional meat and fat-heavy

> **Note on calories**
>
> By now, nearly everyone is familiar with the word 'calorie', and that protein and carbohydrates have four calories per gram, while dietary fats have nine. Fibres have zero calories since they cannot be absorbed. To some extent, our metabolism allows us to eat a certain amount of calories each day and if we go over that amount with the wrong foods (without any additional exercise), we will start to put on weight.
>
> Don't worry though, we will set up a healthy eating plan where you will not have to count calories, but for now it's useful to know the difference between them.

diets, they have a lower risk of heart disease than people on western diets[5]! We'll find out why this is the case in the next few sections, so read on to learn more about macros.

At the end of each section we will condense the information into key points to remember. The nutrition plan follows the information in each section, so you'll have a highly effective nutrition plan by the end of the book. So, you can relax as you read because you can always refer back to the key points at the end of each section any time for a quick refresher!

1.1.1 Protein

Proteins are an essential component of every living cell and are a source of energy for your body. They are chains of amino acids that are crucial for the normal functioning of your body. Proteins differ in their type of amino acid profile, depending on which amino acids the particular protein contains. Human bodies can produce 13 of the 22 different types of amino acids itself, but the other 9 need to be ingested and are therefore called 'essential amino acids'.

Nearly all cells within your body need protein to function, and since the body cannot manufacture all these amino acids itself, it is crucial to have an adequate intake of protein. This is why it is a key component of healthy eating. That's right - protein is not just for men who want to build muscle! Protein is needed by every single person as part of their everyday healthy eating. Inadequate protein intake can result in one of the three forms of protein-energy malnutrition (Kwashiorkor, Marasmus & Marasmic Kwashiorkor) found mainly in developing countries. However, these specific conditions are rare in developed countries[6]. To get a sense of just how important adequate protein intake is, just look at the effects of a protein deficiency during pregnancy, which can result in reduced brain size[7], learning difficulties[8], increased obesity[9], and more.

Essential Amino Acids	Non-essential Amino Acids
Histidine	Alanine
Isoleucine	Arginine
Leucine	Asparagine
Lysine	Aspartic acid
Methionine	Cysteine
Phenylalanine	Glutamic acid
Threonine	Glutamine
Tryptophan	Glycine
Valine	Ornithine
	Proline
	Selenocysteine
	Serine
	Tyrosine

It is interesting to note that the negative effects of a diet deficient in protein is much worse than a diet deficient in fats, while carbohydrates can be completely removed from the diet without any real negative effects. For example, the traditional Inuit diet which was high in protein and very low in carbohydrate resulted in low rates of heart disease, although once introduced to a western-style carbohydrate rich diet, Inuit develop heart disease at similar rates[10]. This shows just how important protein is in your diet!

Your body needs protein to maintain and improve muscle mass so that you can achieve and maintain long term health. Without protein, your muscles deteriorate and your body loses its tone and strength. Losing muscle also lowers your metabolic rate which means that your body burns fewer calories when you are not exercising. This means that having more muscle increases your metabolic rate and allows you to eat more without putting on weight[11,12]!

1.1.1.1 Quality protein

It is important to know that all proteins are not equal. There are two factors that distinguish between a high and low quality protein:

1. **Completeness** – A protein with all essential amino acids is a 'complete protein', while one without is an 'incomplete protein'. Proteins have different amounts of each amino acids. The more it has, the more there is for the body to use

2. **Digestibility** – Some proteins are more digestible than others, resulting in the body being able to use different percentages of proteins depending on their digestibility

We should eat high quality protein because our bodies need protein for vital functions. We need high quality proteins to maintain our muscle mass, which in turn keeps us looking good, our metabolism high and our weight well managed.

The World Health Organisation recognised that the difference between high and low quality proteins is important, and adopted a rating method to measure both completeness and digestibility as a single score.

This score is call a Protein Digestibility Corrected Amino Acid Score, or PDCAAS for short[13] (there is a push to replace this with a new system called DIAAS[14], but little data is available so far, so PDCAAS will do the job for now!). We can use this score to guide us when choosing sources of protein to eat.

The chart below helps us to select good sources of protein by indicating the PDCAAS[15] (the higher on the chart is better) and the percentage of protein per 100g of the source (larger bubbles to the right means more protein per 100g).

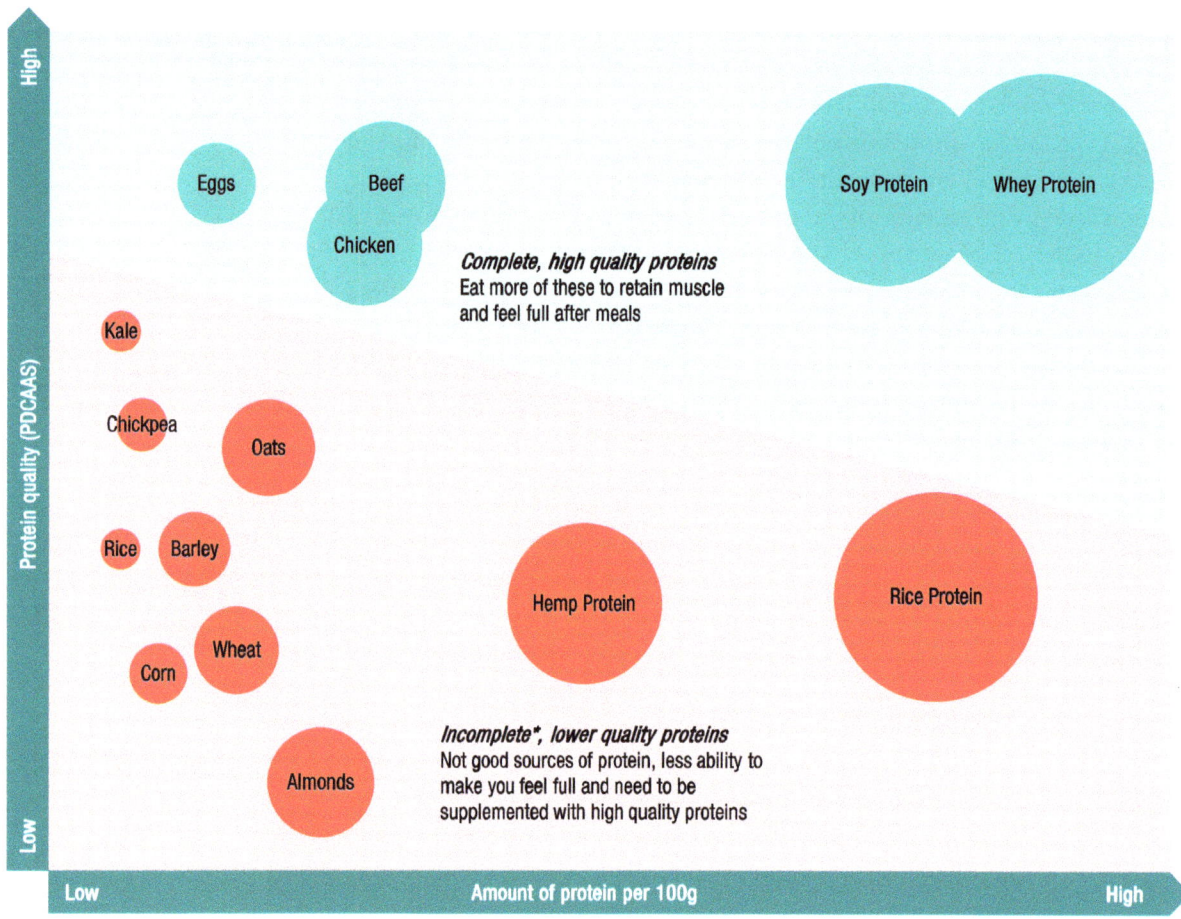

From the chart we can see that animal sources of protein are generally higher quality than other sources, and are often the only complete sources of protein. Interestingly, almonds and nuts generally are low in terms of protein quality. Towards the right we have protein powders, with soy and whey (milk) protein powder in the top right provide high-quality protein in a powdered form, which is easy and quick to consume.

You'll notice grains are low on the graph, showing both a low amount of protein and a lower quality of protein. This means that they are not as useful for us in maintaining muscle mass, or in feeling full after meals. They are also more often associated with calorie-dense foods, such as bread, pastries, biscuits, and more, which is why grains are not useful when we are trying to achieve our weight loss goals.

Protein makes us feel full

High quality proteins make us feel full[16,17], regulate body composition, keep our bones healthy, help with our gastrointestinal function, and so much more[18]. Its role in helping us feel full has been widely researched, and these studies have shown that this is because eating protein affects

the key peptides that regulate our sense of hunger and feeling of fullness more than eating carbohydrates[19]. Even more significantly, these peptides are still higher four hours later, and participants in the study ate less in their next meal as well[16,17].

The key peptides identified in these studies are:

- **Glucagon-like Peptide-1 (GLP-1)** – released by the ileal cells and inhibits the secretion of stomach acids, signalling the brain that it is full
- **Peptide Tyrosine Tyrosine (PYY)** – released by the ileum and colon after eating and is associated with reduced appetite
- **Glucagon** – secreted by the pancreas and raises blood sugar. Signals the brain via the vagus nerve that enough food has been ingested
- **Ghrelin** – produced by the stomach. A higher presence increases hunger

We will continue to learn about and explore the benefits of protein as we work through the book so that we can compare it to other food sources. This way, we can see exactly how protein benefits us and why we should include more in our diets!

> **What to remember:**
> - Protein is crucial for healthy bodies and to maintain muscle and keep our metabolism high
> - Quality protein is proven to make us feel full faster
> - Not all proteins are equal, so eat high-quality, complete proteins like meats, eggs and whey protein shakes

1.1.2 Carbohydrates

Around 5,000 years ago, when our ancestors really got into agriculture, carbohydrates became a bigger and more important part of our diets[10]. This is because our ancestors were able to start growing crops, such as wheat, which provided a cheap and reliable source of food. From an evolutionary perspective, 5,000 years is not a long time, and in that time carbohydrates have evolved from unrefined to refined products, such as white bread, cakes and pasta. It therefore comes as no surprise that the rise of refined carbohydrates in the last few hundred years has caught our bodies by surprise!

Our bodies mainly use carbohydrates to fuel the body. In fact, carbohydrates are so good at providing energy that the body will use carbohydrates for energy first, then burn dietary fat and only after that will it burn protein. This is because carbohydrates consist of simple sugar molecules that are easily absorbed by the body. For example, glucose is a simple carbohydrate that is directly absorbed into the bloodstream and is readily used by cells as an energy source.

From a technical standpoint, there are two main classifications of carbohydrates – simple carbohydrates and complex carbohydrates. These can be measured on a Glycaemic Index (GI), which we will look at in more detail later in the book.

For a macro which is not an essential nutrient, carbohydrates is still a very a big topic. So let's start with simple carbohydrates which include sugars - which hopefully we all know to avoid!

1.1.2.1 Simple carbohydrates

Simple carbohydrates are combinations of small numbers of sugar molecules. When it is just a single sugar molecule, it is called a **monosaccharide**. When there are two sugar molecules, it is a **disaccharide**. The one thing that sugars have in common is that they produce a sharp spike in blood sugar since they are absorbed so quickly into the bloodstream.

Monosaccharide includes the basic sugars that we know more generally, such as:

- **Glucose** (dextrose) – found in plants, grains, fruits, dairy
- **Fructose** – fruits, sugar cane, honey
- **Galactose** – dairy, beets, plant gums

Disaccharides include other forms:

- **Sucrose** – common tables sugar. Consists of glucose and fructose
- **Maltose** – part of malt, found in beer, beverages, cereal, pasta and potatoes. Consists of two units of glucose
- **Lactose** – mainly found in milk. Consists of glucose and galactose

These sugars are usually what you would find in chocolate, sweets, cakes, sugary drinks, jam, biscuits, breads and cereals. Ever wondered why it is so hard to stop eating something sweet once you start? Turns out it is not just the taste that keeps you going back for more, but also the fact that sugar reduces the presence of a key hormone that lets your brain know that you are full.

How sugar makes you eat more:

1. Studies have shown that ingesting sugar drastically reduces the suppression of the hormone **ghrelin**[20] (refer to the protein section above). This means that there is more of the hormone in the bloodstream, making you feel like eating more of that sugary snack!

2. Sugar, particularly fructose, also affects the hormone **leptin**, which normally helps you feel full. Sugar interferes with the transport of leptin, making you feel like you need to keep eating[20,21]. Fructose also does not appear to dampen appetite as it doesn't trigger the normal mechanisms to make us feel full. This link has even been proven through brain scans, where a study was performed to determine the differences in brain states when eating glucose as opposed to eating fructose. The results showed that eating fructose activates regions in the brain that make us eat more[22]

3. **Dopamine** is a 'feel good' chemical that plays a big role in motivating you to perform certain actions. Sugar has been shown to influence dopamine in a similar way as drugs like cocaine and meth. Like drugs, over time you get less pleasure from eating sugar so you eat more of it to get another dopamine hit[23]. More recent research indicates that sugar can be even *more* rewarding than cocaine, possibly due to how we have evolved to actively seek sugar due to how scarce it used to be[24]

The influence of sugar on dopamine is important, as this not only drives you to eat more in the moment, but also causes addictive behaviour where you start to crave it. You want that next sugar hit, but the more you eat it, the less satisfying it becomes, so you need to eat more and more. Afterwards, this type of binge eating tends to be followed by feelings such as being embarrassed by how much you ate, guilt, depression and shame[25,26].

Thinking about it from an evolutionary perspective, it is easy to see why we crave it so much. In prehistoric times, sugar was hard to come by, and was mainly available to us as fruit or honey. Fruits were only available for a few months each year, and honey was guarded by bees. This meant that when we did manage to get our hands on some, our brains told us to get as much as we could.

Back then, we were not at risk of developing addictive behaviour, simply because it was not accessible enough. Now, however, sugar is in almost all of the foods we eat and is available everywhere. Our bodies still crave it, but being so available, it is hard for us to control our intake. The more sugar we eat, the more sugar we want to eat, creating a vicious circle. Interestingly, artificial sweeteners have been shown not to have any effect on feeling full, meaning it does not promote overeating as shown by research comparing it to normal sugar[27,28]. This closely links to the difference between 'pleasure-eating' and 'hunger-eating'.

Sugar and insulin

Eating sugar increases blood sugar levels, which can be dangerous if it goes unchecked. High blood sugar levels can cause blindness and a loss of consciousness, while low levels are even more dangerous, and can result in permanent brain damage and death. **Insulin**, along with its counterpart **glucagon**, is secreted by the pancreas and plays the key role of regulating blood sugar levels. Insulin lowers blood sugar, while glucagon raises it.

The dance between these two is important as it keeps your blood sugar at the right level so that your body and your brain get just the right amount to keep functioning effectively. Insulin can reduce blood sugar by sending it to the muscles if they need it, or otherwise, *store it as body fat*.

It is this role that causes insulin to get a lot of bad press, but in reality it is a hormone that we cannot live without! It is doing the best it can to prevent your blood sugar levels from getting too high or too low:

Let's picture insulin in action – insulin is hanging around, not doing much, when suddenly a massive amount of sugar enters the bloodstream (somewhere in the world, a cake is missing a slice!). Insulin jumps into action and starts to go through its checklist:

1. *Do any muscles need sugar? No, we're all good from breakfast and we haven't done any exercise*
2. *Does the brain need any more sugar? No, not much thinking going on right now*
3. *Well, we have to do something with it, so* **store it as body fat***!*

You can see that insulin is not a bad hormone, it just has limited options available when you decide to eat. In fact, if you exhaust your insulin-producing capabilities, then you can develop a dangerous condition called *insulin resistance*. This is more commonly known as Type 2 Diabetes (Type 1 Diabetes is mainly genetic), which is when your pancreas no longer produces enough insulin or when cells in your body become unresponsive to insulin.

This is a very dangerous condition which can result in chronic high blood sugar levels as your body can no longer lower your blood sugar levels. The onset of Type 2 Diabetes has been clearly linked to the intake of sugars, especially via sugary drinks[29], and even other foods higher on the Glycaemic Index such as white rice[30]. It has been shown that **fructose** plays a big role in developing insulin resistance, and what is particularly scary, is that a continuous high intake of fructose can result in insulin resistance *in as little as one week*[31]!

Sugar, insulin and body fat

Insulin is one of the key players in storing excess energy as body fat. This is why it is essential for us to avoid sugars in our quest to reach and maintain our goal bodies. The only time that insulin does not store a big sugar spike as body fat, is right after a big workout where the muscle glycogen stores have been depleted. In this case, insulin pumps the excess energy directly into the muscles.

This means that for the rest of the time (which, let's face it, is most of the time), insulin will take the only option available to it – and that is to store the excess energy as body fat. Later, when we look at the Glycaemic Index, we'll look at how different foods increase blood sugar at different rates. The slower blood sugar levels rise, the less insulin needs to be released resulting in less energy being stored as body fat. This is one of the key ways we can control our body fat stores and slim down our waists!

Even when insulin is functioning well without any insulin resistance, a diet high in sugar is usually a diet that has a high intake of calories. In this case, all that insulin can do is to store each day's excess as a bit more body fat!

And if all that isn't bad enough, a high intake of sugar, especially sucrose and fructose, has been shown to increase triacylglycerol concentrations which lead to clogged arteries and an increased risk of a heart attack[32]. Recent research has revealed that a high intake of sugar causes the accumulation of glucose 6-phosphate in the heart which causes significant damage to the heart, further increasing the risk of a heart attack[33].

Overall, let's recap some facts about sugar:

- Can cause diabetes
- Makes you want to eat more
- Leads to obesity
- Increases risk of heart attacks

The evidence is clear – **avoid sugar!**

1.1.2.2 Complex carbohydrates

Complex carbohydrates are simple carbohydrates that are linked together in a way that takes the body longer to break down and digest them. Complex carbohydrates are found in vegetables, grains, nuts, seeds and legumes. These are called **polysaccharides** and their structure means that they do not increase blood sugar as quickly as simple carbohydrates do, although the speed at which they raise blood sugar varies widely.

The main types of polysaccharides include:

- **Starch** – the main way plants store glucose
- **Glycogen** – the animal version of starch which is the secondary energy storage system of the body (the first system being body fat)
- **Cellulose** – the structural component of plants (found in stems, leaves and all areas of plants) which is critical to helping them keep their shape

Starch is a polysaccharide that is mainly found in potatoes, wheat, maize and rice. Even though starch is a complex carbohydrate, it breaks down very quickly to release the simple sugars that it consists of. This is because starch is the way that plants store glucose and they need to be able to easily break the starch down to simple sugars when they need it, which is also why white potatoes aren't as good for us – they are a rich source of starch which our bodies break down to sugar all too easily.

> **What about cellulose?**
> Cellulose is a dietary fibre that comes from many different sources. It is interesting that cellulose is also composed of simple sugars, but we do not have any bacteria in our gut that can break the beta bonds in cellulose, resulting in cellulose passing through us without any nutritional value. Termites, on the other hand, do have bacteria that can break down the beta bonds, allowing them to release the sugars from wood so they can feast on all the stuff that we can't digest!

There used to be a school of thought that we should avoid simple carbohydrates and focus on eating complex carbohydrates, though further research found that this distinction is not useful from a nutritional perspective. It was later determined that the speed at which blood sugar increases after eating different types of carbohydrates vary a lot between simple and complex carbohydrates. Contrary to the thinking at the time, some simple carbohydrates raised blood sugar slowly, while some complex carbohydrates raised it quickly. For example, starches (not to be confused with fibre) found in potatoes and grains are chains of glucose that breaks down very quickly, even though it is a complex carbohydrate.

Early research showed the importance of recognizing the difference in speed of blood sugar increase[34], as well as the resulting insulin spikes which can lead to additional fat storage and even insulin resistance and diabetes[35]. This is what resulted in the creation of the **Glycaemic Index**.

1.1.2.3 Glycaemic Index

The Glycaemic Index (or GI) is simply a score given to foods based on how quickly they raise blood sugar levels. In simple terms, the faster your blood sugar rises, the more insulin is released and the more fat tends to be stored. Fat storage tends to happen when your body is not in desperate need for more energy. For example, when you've had a big breakfast that fully satisfies your energy needs and shortly after you have a white baguette for lunch. The spike in blood sugar sends a quick surge of energy that is not needed by the body, so insulin stores the excess energy as fat. However, if instead of the white baguette you ate something that slowly released energy such as a chicken breast and salad. Your body would be able to use the energy as it was released, and there would be no excess to be stored as fat. The difference between these two scenarios is how quickly glucose is released into the bloodstream after you eat food – the faster blood sugar rises, the greater the chance it will be stored as fat. We use GI scores to understand how quickly a particular food will raise our blood sugar, with a score of zero as the slowest and 100 the fastest.

Put simply, if you eat lower GI foods, your body will have less excess energy to store as fat.

The charts below show groups of foods ranked by their GI score on the vertical axis and by the average amount of carbohydrate per serve on the horizontal axis (which is also illustrated by the size of the bubble[36]). If a food source is higher and more to the right, it means that it spikes your blood sugar and is more calorie-dense, resulting in your body storing more body fat. Food groups below the line show us which release energy slowly and contain fewer carbohydrates.

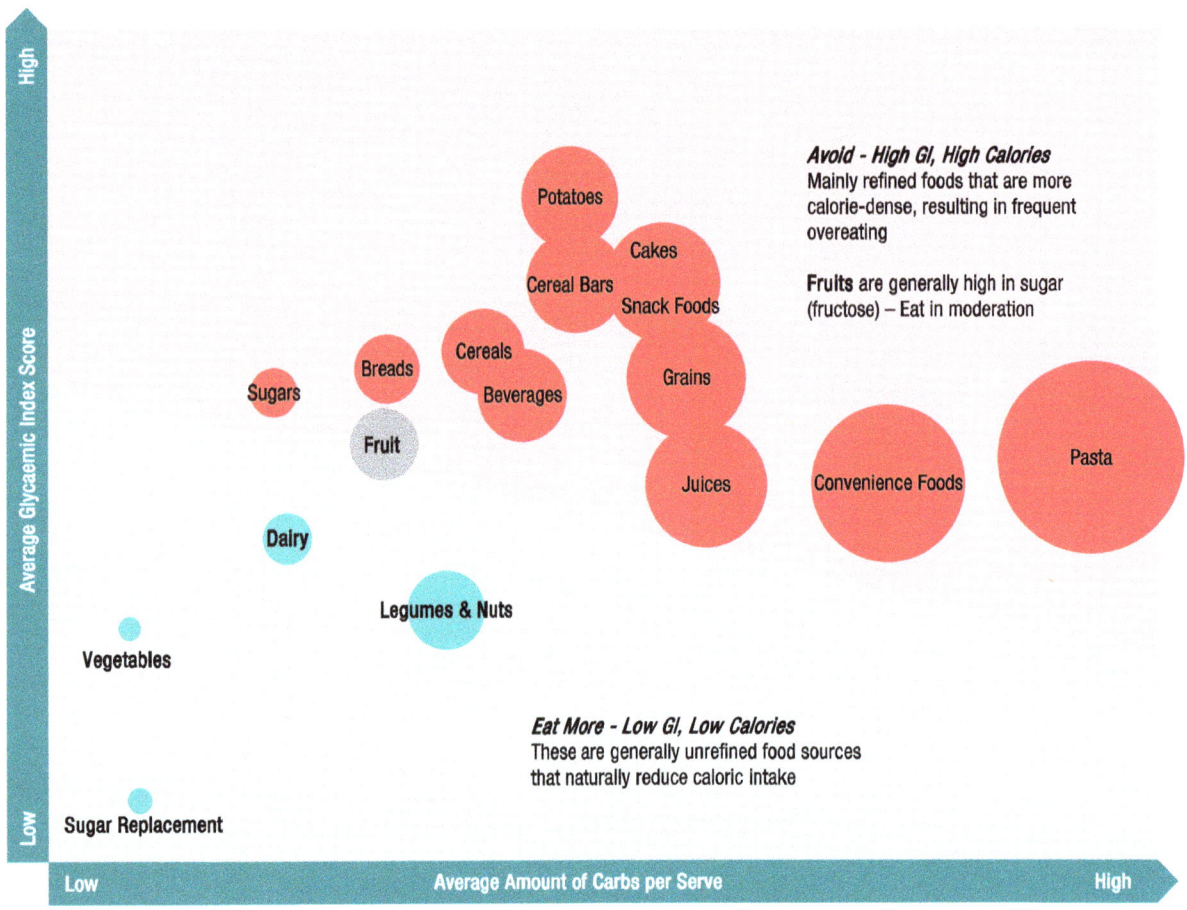

It's not hard to guess why vegetables, dairy and nut sources are the preferred choices as these are mainly natural and unrefined food sources. As you look higher and to the right of the chart, you generally see more refined foods which are more calorie-dense. This is why refined foods are such a big contributor to gaining weight – they are packed with calories, and they spike blood sugar levels which leads to storing excess energy as fat.

Two exceptions here are fruits and potatoes:

- **White potatoes spike blood sugar levels very quickly and are fairly calorie-dense**. For this reason, you should generally avoid eating potatoes as a regular part of your diet, especially crisps and fries!

- **Fruits generally contain high amounts of fructose which can work against your goals if eaten regularly.** Let's be honest, they taste great, and that is very much because they are loaded with sugar. As you can see, they are just on the border of healthy foods, but if you are serious about weight loss, minimise your intake of fruit. Once you have reached your goal, you can eat them more regularly but in small quantities so that you don't find weight creeping on again!

GI scores of foods help us identify foods that help us to achieve our goals, and also those that work against us.

The table below shows the GI scores of popular food items[36], grouped into the same categories shown in chart above. The sources highlighted in green are natural foods that help us reach our goals, while the sources highlighted in red works against us. Fruits are not coloured as they are an 'in-between' category. As mentioned above, keep intake low if you have a very ambitious weight loss goal.

Popular foods and GI Scores							
Vegetables		Pears	33	**Cereals**		Scones	92
Lettuce	15*	Apple	38	All-Bran	42	**Convenience Foods**	
Spinach	15*	Plums	39	Special K	54	Lean Cuisine	36
Celery	15*	Oranges	42	Oat Bran	55	Fish Fingers	38
Broccoli	15*	Peaches	42	Natural Muesli	57	Beef Pies	45
Cucumber	15*	Grapes	43	Froot Loops	69	Chicken Nuggets, Frozen	46
Asparagus	15*	Mango	51	Weet-Bix	70	Spaghetti Bolognaise	52
Kale	15*	Banana	52	Coco Pops	77	Pizza	60
Carrots	32	Kiwi	53	Cornflakes	77	**Pasta**	
Sweet Potato	44	Apricots	57	**Cereal Bars**		Fettuccine	40
Sweet Corn	47	Pineapple	59	Rice Bubble Treat Bar	63	Rice Noodles	40
Green peas	48	Lychee	79	Crunchy Nut Bar	72	Instant Noodles	47
Dairy		Dates, Dried	103	K-Time Just Right Bar	72	Macaroni	47
Full Fat Milk	27	**Breads**		Fibre Plus Bar	78	Gluten-free Pasta	54
Skim Milk	32	Rye-kernel Bread	41	**Grains**		Gnocchi	68
Yogurt	36	Wheat Bread	52	Wheat	48	**Snack Foods**	
Ice-cream, High Fat	37	Whole-meal Bread	67	Corn	53	Potato Chips	54
Soy Milk	44	Gluten Free Bread	79	Brown Rice	55	Corn chips	63
Ice-cream, Regular	61	White Bread	80	Couscous	61	Mars Bar	65
Legumes		**Beverages**		White Rice	64	Popcorn	72
Soya Beans	18	Banana Smoothie	34	Rolled Barley	66	Jelly Beans	78
Chickpeas	28	Coca Cola	53	Cornmeal	68	Pretzels	83
Kidney Beans	28	Orange Cordial	66	**Cakes**		Roll-Ups, Fruit Bars	99
Lentils	30	Gatorade	78	Sponge cake, plain	46	**Potatoes**	
Butter Beans	31	**Juices**		Blueberry Muffin	59	Baked Potato	60
Baked Beans	48	Apple Juice	39	Croissant	67	French Fries	75
Fruit		Pineapple Juice	46	Waffles	76	Mashed Potato	91
Cherries	22	Orange Juice	53	Lamingtons	87	Boiled Potato	101

Estimated scores

The easiest thing to remember here is which food groups to include in your eating plan. This will save you from having to remember a bunch of numbers! It's interesting to note that the GI scores of some vegetables are estimated as it is not possible to perform the test to determine the real score. This is because to perform the test, at least 50g of carbohydrates from the source must be ingested, which means someone would need to eat 1.5kg of cucumber to test it! This does highlight that we should separate starchy and non-starchy vegetables and take a deeper look.

Separating vegetables

Some vegetables, like white potatoes, raise blood sugar much faster than others and also are higher in carbohydrates than others. This combination of high-GI and high-carbohydrate content makes it work against us as it results in excess energy that causes insulin to store more fat.

To get a clear idea of which vegetables are best for weight loss, we should take a look at the numbers to see what we can eat in large quantities, without gaining weight! We will separate these out as 'starchy' and 'non-starchy' vegetables. Keep in mind that essentially all vegetables have starch in them, since that is how plants store energy. This is why there is no official list of 'starchy' and 'non-starchy' vegetables, so we will define our own list. When we call a vegetable 'starchy', we are basically saying a vegetable has a bit too much starch. For this, we need to look at the combined effect of carbohydrate content per 100g and the GI score for each vegetable:

- A combination of **low carbohydrates and low GI** makes the best weight loss vegetables
- Either **higher carbohydrates or around medium GI** makes it a veggie that is better for when you have an active lifestyle and need extra energy to fuel gym sessions and muscle building
- A combination of **high carbohydrates and high GI** makes it bad for weight maintenance overall, and should be avoided altogether

The table to the right shows the result.

Low-GI, non-starchy vegetables – The best weight loss vegetables are listed in the left and middle columns, next to their carbohydrate content for a 100g serve. Lucky for us, the majority of vegetables are low-carbohydrate and also so low in GI that they don't officially have GI scores (other than carrots at 35), so they are not listed in the table.

Low-GI, non-starchy vegetables Best for weight loss				Starchy vegetables For an active lifestyle		
Veggies - 100g	Carbs	Veggies - 100g	Carbs	Veggies - 100g	Carbs	GI
Watercress	1	Peppers	4	Pumpkin	6	75
Alfalfa seeds	2	Rhubarb	4	Beets	9	64
Chinese-cabbage	2	Swiss chard	4	Green peas	15	48
Asparagus	3	Tomatoes	4	Sweet corn	17	47
Celery	3	Cabbage	5	Sweet potato	20	44
Chinese Broccoli	3	Green onions	5	Chickpeas	28	28
Cucumber	3	Turnips	5	Yam	28	37
Lettuce	3	Brussels sprouts	6	Plantains	28	38
Mushrooms	3	Shallots	6	Lentils	60	30
Radishes	3	Fennel	7	Kidney beans	61	28
Spinach	3	Leeks	7	**High-GI, starchy vegetables** **Exclude from diet overall**		
Zucchini	3	Eggplant	8			
Broccoli	4	Onions	9	Cassava	39	46
Cauliflower	4	Squash	9	Taro	35	55
Chicory	4	Carrots	9	White potato	21	60
Okra	4	Artichoke	11	Parsnips	16	97

Starchy vegetables – On the top right we have starchy vegetables with either higher carbohydrates or a mid-level GI score. Next to them are listed their carbohydrate content per 100g serve and their GI scores. These are best for when you need additional fuel for exercise or a generally active lifestyle. If you notice your waistline is not decreasing, then cut out these until you reach your goal.

High-GI starchy carbohydrates – At the bottom right of the table we have vegetables that are too high in both carbohydrate content and GI score. This means they increase fat storage and work against us, so they are not part of healthy eating, regardless of how active you are.

Cassava, taro and parsnip are not the most common foods, so white potato is the notable exception here. Out of the starchy vegetables, potatoes raise blood sugar very fast as the starches are quickly broken down into sugars. As we learned, the sugar spikes cause insulin to turn excess energy into body fat, adding to our thighs. Especially dangerous are the processed forms of potatoes, such as fries and chips, which include a dangerous combination of starchy sugars and fats from all the oil it is prepared in which very quickly turns into body fat.

1.1.2.4 Grains

You would likely have seen book after book come out in recent years talking about taking extreme caution with grains and how gluten is a 'silent killer', slowly destroying your health and eating away at your mind. Let's take a look at the science behind these claims and see if it is really that bad.

Generally, I like to get away from the hype and sensationalism and focus on the facts, then make decisions from there. So let's look at grains and gluten, and their place in our diets.

Grains can effectively be split into two categories:

- **Cereals and pseudocereals** such as maize (corn), barley, oats, rice, rye, wheat, buckwheat and quinoa
- **Legumes** such as chickpeas, beans, lentils, peanuts and soybeans

Cereals and pseudocereals (let's call them both 'cereals' for short), are what we have seen in the GI graph above to have higher GI scores and are also more nutrient-dense. These also include wheat, barley and rye which contain gluten. Below we will have a look at gluten and its effects on people with coeliac and gluten sensitivity. Knowing the blood sugar spiking nature of cereals and how calorie-dense it is, suggests we should remove it from our diets.

Legumes, on the other hand, tend to have lower GI scores and are slightly less calorie-dense. This makes them a better food source for our bodies as they do not play as much havoc with our blood sugar and we are less likely to overeat when we eat legumes. For our purposes, they are essentially so different from cereals that we remove them from our definition of 'grains'. So, it seems that legumes may still be ok, but how about grains?

From a GI perspective, grains and foods based on grains are generally high-GI, giving us a good reason not to eat them.

1.1.2.5 Gluten

There is a lot of focus on **gluten**, so what exactly is it? Essentially, it is a compound found in wheat, barley and rye grains, and it helps breads to rise and keep its shape. It has been increasingly recognised that many people are gluten intolerant or sensitive[37,38,39,41]. Gluten intolerance is called coeliac disease, which is an autoimmune disorder that can result in pain, constipation, diarrhoea, tiredness, bloating, and more.

Quick facts about gluten	
What is Gluten?	◆ A compound found in wheat, barley and rye
What does it do?	◆ It makes bread rise and keep its shape
What does it do to humans?	◆ 1% of people have coeliac disease[37,38] ◆ 6% to 7% have gluten sensitivity[39] ◆ Can result in bloating, water retention, abdominal pain, diarrhoea, constipation and tiredness
What else?	◆ It marks a food group that is very calorie-dense and generally has a high GI score
Why remove it?	◆ Reduce bloating and other effects related to coeliac and gluten sensitivity, and also results in reduced calorie intake
How can this affect my brain?	◆ Can result in cognitive decline if you have coeliac and continue to eat gluten[40]

Coeliac is mainly a genetic disease that affects around 1% of people[37,38] and is a reaction to gliadin, mainly found in wheat, barley and rye. Beyond those that have coeliac, new studies have shown that there is an even larger problem, known as 'gluten sensitivity'[41] that has been estimated by Dr. Fasano, a leading researcher in the field, to affect 6% to 7% of people[39].

If you do have coeliac or gluten sensitivity, you may notice less bloating and abdominal pain along with a decrease in other common symptoms once you remove gluten from your diet. Coeliac is often mistakenly diagnosed as Irritable Bowel Syndrome (IBS), so if you have been diagnosed with IBS, you might find some relief as well.

Another thing is that if you have coeliac and you continue to eat gluten, you can do long-term damage to your brain! A study has shown a link between coeliac and cognitive impairment[40] and that symptoms improve once gluten was removed from the patients' diets. If you are feeling a bit of a 'brain fog', it could be related to gluten. Cut out grains and you might notice some significant health improvements!

Even if you tolerate gluten very well, there is still one more big reason to cut gluten from your regular meals – it's part of grain-based foods (breads, pasta, biscuits, pastries) that are very calorie-dense and generally have a higher GI score. Simply, this means these are the kind of foods that, even in smaller amounts, will still result in fat storage in your body.

What to remember:
- Avoid grains - They come with the negative effect of gluten and are also very calorie-dense
- Avoid sugar which causes us to overeat, leading to obesity, diabetes and heart disease
- Focus on slow energy-releasing carbohydrate sources such as vegetables, legumes and nuts, with small amounts of fruit

1.1.3 Dietary fat

We need to make an important distinction before we start talking about fat. This distinction is between **body fat** and **dietary fat**. When we usually talk about being overweight, we use the word 'fat', and when we talk about the nutritional fat content of food, we also use the word 'fat'. Effectively, we use the same word to refer both to what makes bellies flabby and the main ingredient in butter.

This causes a lot of confusion, as they are actually different and the mechanics of these two are not as closely related as people would think. Therefore, we need to break these down as follows:

- *Body fat* is the adipose tissue that we find in our hips and bellies (among other places)
- *Dietary fat* is what we find in food and take in through our diet

With that clarified, we need to remember one important thing – **body fat is not the same as dietary fat!**

Eating dietary fat is not automatically going to result in you building up body fat. Instead, the same rules apply as you still need to overeat on a consistent basis for the body to store excess energy as body fat. Just consider this – *even though our average intake of dietary fat has decreased over the last three decades, obesity has increased!* So clearly dietary fat is not the main cause of obesity[42]!

There have been many low-fat diets that have been shown to help people lose fat, just like there are many low-carbohydrate diets that work as well. The reality is that they both work for weight loss, though increasingly the science is pointing out that there are more health benefits to going low carbohydrate, than going low fat[43,44]. You saw in the carbohydrate section that there are many negative health effects from carbohydrates, especially high-GI sources like sugar, as well as the effects of gluten.

On top of that, carbohydrates are not an essential nutrient, meaning our bodies can function just fine without eating any carbohydrates at all. Dietary fat, on the other hand, is an essential nutrient because humans do not have the desaturase enzyme to produce key fatty acids. Dietary fats perform vital functions within our bodies, and are also used as a form of fuel that is safer than carbohydrates as it does not promote overeating and does not produce an insulin response.

The types of dietary fats are:

- **Monounsaturated** fat
- **Polyunsaturated** fat, which includes the following two Essential Fatty Acids (EFAs):
    - **Omega-3** (Alpha-linolenic acid)
    - **Omega-6** (Linoleic acid)
- **Saturated** fat
- **Trans** fat

The dietary fats are all slightly different and have different health effects, sources, and some are even more stable than others. The table below shows a breakdown of each of the types of dietary fat for comparison.

Fundamental Nutrition - Dietary Fat

	Mono-unsaturated fat	Polyunsaturated fat			Saturated fat	Trans fat
		Omega-3	Omega-6	All others		
What are they	Fatty acids with a single double bond	Fatty acids with more than one double bond			Fatty acids with no double bonds	Fatty acids with a double bond in a trans configuration
Class	Natural, non-essential	**Natural, essential fatty acid**	**Natural, essential fatty acid**	Natural, non-essential	Natural, non-essential	**Man-made, non-essential and harmful**
Found in	Milk products, red meat, nuts, avocados, olives, egg yolk	EPA and DHA - herring, salmon, tuna, trout, fish oil, ALA – vegetable oils, flaxseed oil, berry oil, hemp oil	Poultry, eggs, flaxseed oil, vegetable oils, sunflower oil, nuts, wheat, cereals, avocado, coconut	Walnuts, sunflower seeds, sesame seeds, peanuts, olive oil, seaweed	Beef, poultry, milk products, butter, coconut oil, chocolate	Snack foods, fast foods, fried foods, baked goods
Stability	Somewhat unstable, can become rancid through heating	Unstable, becomes rancid easily, especially when exposed to heat or the sun, creating free radicals that cause oxidative damage			Very stable	Stable, designed to increase product shelf life
Effect on health	Linked to lower risk of heart disease[45], can help to reduce blood clots[46]	Reduces inflammation, risk of heart disease[47], cancer, arthritis[48]. Balance intake with Omega-6[49]. Linked to lower rates of depression and can help prevent neurodegenerative diseases[50]	Necessary for health, but overconsumption increases inflammation that is the basis of many diseases. Needs to be balanced with Omega-3[49]	Some types can increase satiety (feeling full), reduce heart disease risk and help the immune system[51]	Theories linking saturated fat to heart disease have been disproved, leaving it as a healthy fuel source[52,53]	Strongly linked to heart disease[54,55] and can cause systematic inflammation[56]
Guide	Include for health and as a fuel source	Include in diet for health	Include in diet, but limit and balance	Include for health and as a fuel source	Include as a fuel source	**Always avoid**

Looking across the types of fat in the table, we can see that all of the fats, except for trans fats, are part of normal, healthy eating. That also includes saturated fat! This can seem like quite a departure from the messages we've been getting for a long time – that saturated fat is bad and clogs our arteries. In the Busting Myths section we'll go into more detail around why saturated fat is actually healthy, but long story short, there was never any real science proving it was bad, and studies since 1950 have continually shown that saturated fat doesn't increase mortality. The end result – we can eat saturated fat without feeling like we are sabotaging our health[57]!

Trans fats are the only fats that are man-made, usually on an industrial scale through a process of hydrogenating unsaturated fatty acids via a catalyst. Trans fats are made because they are very stable and can last a long time in products on the shelf, making them great for biscuits, potato chips and other snack foods. The use of a catalyst, such as a nickel, platinum or palladium plate, is necessary as otherwise a very high temperature would be necessary to develop a trans fat.

In fact, without a catalyst you would need to heat up your stove to over 500°C (930°F) to start turning an unsaturated fat into a trans fat. Given that the average stove only goes up to about 250°C (480°F), you wouldn't be able to accidentally turn a fat into a trans fat at home, so just avoid the ones found in snack foods. Just to confirm that point – you cannot make trans fat at home. **It is a myth that normal cooking oils can turn into trans fats at home.** Trans fats simply do not work that way.

That means that all the natural forms of fat are actually healthy additions to our diet. This is something that many people are catching on to, helped on by all the interest in coconut oil (because it seems to have some small health benefits) which consists almost entirely of saturated fat.

There's an important story around fats, particularly two groups of polyunsaturated fats called omega-3 and omega-6. These are the two fats that are essential for our bodies, and have a huge impact on our health. Let's delve into these in more detail.

1.1.3.1 Omega-3 and omega-6

These two are the Essential Fatty Acids (EFAs) that we need to take in through our diet because our bodies cannot synthesize them. What is interesting about omega-3 and omega-6 is that it is not so much about the amount of each that we get, but more so about the *ratio* in which we eat them.

By ratio, we mean how many of one compared to the other. Research shows that around a few hundred thousand years ago, the ratio of omega-3 and omega-6 in our diet was around 1:1[58]. That is to say that we ate roughly the same amount of each due to a diet rich in fish and animal meats. Through the introduction of agriculture and changes in food production, current dietary intake ratios of omega-6 to omega-3 are around 15:1 to 20:1[59]. This is a massive change from where we used to be, and actually comes with serious health implications.

You see, even though omega-6 and omega-3 are both essential nutrients, they are not equal in their effects on health. The differences were briefly mentioned in the table above, so let's break it down in more detail.

Omega-3 includes three fats: ALA, EPA and DHA

- **ALA** (alpha linolenic acid) is found in vegetable oils and it has been shown that supplementation reduces anxiety, improves sleep and lowers cortisol levels[60]. ALA must be converted into EPA and DHA for the body to be able to use it, however our bodies are inefficient in conversion, with as little as 5% of ALA converted successfully[61]

- **EPA** (eicosapentaenoic acid) naturally occurs mainly in fish sources and is also found in breast milk. The body is much better at absorbing EPA through dietary sources than converting ALA into EPA. This fatty acid has been shown to have neuroprotective abilities, with studies showing that low levels of EPA are linked to suicide attempts[62] and that EPA can assist with treatment of depression, schizophrenia and Alzheimer's disease[63]

- **DHA** (docosahexaenoic acid) is an essential component of skin, nerve, brain and eye tissue. It is also mainly found in fish (with some in breast milk), originating mainly from algae that fish eat. DHA is a crucial component of the brain and is associated with inhibiting cancer[64], assisting with memory, slowing the progression of Alzheimer's disease[65], help with heart disease[66] and possibly help with managing attention deficit hyperactivity disorder (ADHD)[67]

Omega-6 includes one main essential fatty acid: LA

- **LA** (Linoleic acid) is an essential fat, meaning that we have to ingest it for proper health and is found in nearly all foods, especially grains. Not getting enough of it can result in scaly skin and hair loss[68], though is extremely unlikely to have a deficiency of LA due to the amount contained in modern food sources. In fact as mentioned above, it is just the opposite – we generally get way too much of it. Getting too much LA and omega-6 in general results in systemic and chronic inflammation. This kind of inflammation is at the heart of many diseases, so we absolutely have to avoid it!

There is a misconception that omega-3 has an anti-inflammatory effect, but this is not accurate[48,49]. In reality, the omega-3 fatty acids mentioned above are still slightly inflammatory, but they are far less inflammatory than omega-6 fatty acids. It would be more accurate to say that omega-6 is inflammatory, while omega-3 is more neutral. Because of this neutral effect and how it competes with omega-6 for resources, higher levels of omega-3 effectively reduce the chance for omega-6 to cause inflammation, thereby reducing inflammation and increasing our overall health.

What is inflammation, and why is it important to limit it?

The one kind of inflammation we are most familiar with is acute inflammation, such as when we bump into something, like stubbing a toe and the toe swells up, starts to feel warm, hurts, and goes red. This inflammation is caused by the body trying to help repair the damaged tissue.

On the other side we have chronic and systemic inflammation, which involves ongoing inflammation that underlies a large number of diseases and conditions[69,70] such as:

- Cardiovascular/heart disease (atherosclerosis) which is now understood to be very strongly linked to inflammation at all stages[71]
- Diabetes
- Cancer
- Obesity
- Asthma
- Arthritis
- Autoimmune disorders
- Joint pain

There's a lot of research and knowledge about the mechanics of how inflammation works through **eicosanoids**, specifically that the rate of synthesis of eicosanoids needs to be balanced with the rate of eicosanoid metabolism. The rate of synthesis from omega-6 is much higher than omega-3, while the eicosanoids from omega-6 is also much more inflammatory than omega-3. Eicosanoids control key functions within the body, meaning that too many eicosanoids from omega-6 causes issues with heart health, triglycerides, blood pressure and arthritis.

Interestingly, this function is well known in the pharmaceutical industry, as is seen through the mechanism of anti-inflammatory medication such as aspirin, ibuprofen and naproxen (Disprin, Nurofen, Aleve, etc.). These drugs work by downregulating eicosanoid synthesis. In fact, this class of drugs are called **NSAIDs** – *non-steroidal anti-inflammatory drugs*[49,72]. They work by doing exactly what more omega-3 would do – prevent omega-6 eicosanoid synthesis.

Of course, it is not in the interest of the pharmaceutical industry to tell you to cut out grains and eat more fish, so you won't hear that message from them! But effectively you can perform the same treatment on yourself as these drugs do, but in a natural, healthy and consistent way, reducing the need for drugs.

Fundamental Nutrition - **Dietary fat**

PS – this doesn't mean that you can now just eat some salmon when you have a headache. It takes a while for the imbalance to even out, which is why it is important to maintain healthy eating for the long term. That way you get more and more benefits down the track by living healthy!

The ratio of one to the other is important because omega-3 and omega-6 competes for conversion, meaning that if you take more omega-6, then there is less chance for omega-3 (especially ALA) to get converted into useful compounds. For example, one study has shown that a diet rich in omega-6 can reduce ALA conversion by 40% to 50%[61] on top of ALA conversion already being low! This is why it is key to balance the ratio between omega-3 and omega-6 intake. Get the right ratio and you will get more health-promoting EPA and DHA in your body.

1.1.3.2 Sources of omega

The table to the right shows some common sources of omega-3 and omega-6[73]. Here you'll see how much omega-3s (DHA, EPA and ALA) are in each food, along with how much omega-6 (LA), and also the ratio between omega-3 and omega-6.

The numbers show how many grams of omega there are per 100g of the food, with smaller amounts marked as milligrams. For ratios, we are looking for ratios that have more omega-3 than omega-6, so the number on the left should preferably be higher than the number on the right (e.g. 2:1 is better than 1:2).

Each list goes from best at the top to worst at the bottom. Using our usual colour scheme, good sources of omega-3 are highlighted in green, bad ones in red, and neutral foods uncoloured in the middle. The uncoloured foods are not essentially bad, but don't really help either, so we must balance them with good foods. Let's

Sources of omega-3 and omega-6
Ranked from best to worst. Values show grams per 100g

Oils	Omega 3 DHA	EPA	ALA	Ω6 LA	Ratio Ω3:Ω6
Fish oil - Salmon	18.2	13.0	1.1	1.5	21:1
Fish oil - Cod liver	11.0	6.9	0.9	0.9	20:1
Flaxseed oil	-	-	53.3	12.7	4:1
Coconut oil	-	-	-	1.8	-
Olive oil	-	-	0.7	9.7	1:13
Canola oil	-	-	9.1	18.6	1:2
Corn oil	-	-	5.8	23.0	1:4
Soy oil	-	-	6.9	51.2	1:7
Sunflower oil	-	-	0.2	39.8	1:199
Grapeseed oil	-	-	0.1	69.6	1:696
Safflower oil	-	-	-	74.6	-

Animal sources	DHA	EPA	ALA	LA	Ω3:Ω6
Caviar	3.8	2.7	-	0.1	81:1
Mackerel	3.0	1.6	0.2	0.4	13:1
Salmon - Coho	1.4	0.5	0.1	0.1	22:1
Salmon - Atlantic	1.1	0.3	0.3	0.2	10:1
Herring	0.9	0.7	0.1	0.1	13:1
Trout	0.5	0.5	0.2	0.3	4:1
Tuna	0.9	0.3	-	0.1	22:1
Salmon - Farmed	1.1	0.9	-	0.9	2:1
Quail	-	-	0.4	2.3	1:5
Beef - grass-fed	16mg	-	70mg	0.4	1:5
Beef - grain-fed	-	-	50mg	0.3	1:6
Chicken breast	10mg	10mg	-	0.6	1:12
Chicken thigh	30mg	10mg	0.1	1.9	1:15
Egg - Whole	40mg	-	0.1	2.4	1:14

Plant sources	DHA	EPA	ALA	LA	Ω3:Ω6
Flax seeds	-	-	22.8	5.9	4:1
Chia seeds	-	-	17.6	5.8	3:1
Spinach	-	-	0.4	-	-
Chinese broccoli	-	-	0.3	0.1	3:1
Cauliflower	-	-	0.2	0.1	3:1
Broccoli	-	-	0.1	-	3:1
Lettuce	-	-	0.1	-	2:1
Green peppers	-	-	0.8	5.1	1:7
Raspberries	-	-	0.1	0.2	1:2
Blackberries	-	-	0.1	0.2	1:2
Strawberries	-	-	0.1	0.1	1:1
Blueberries	-	-	0.1	0.2	1:1
Walnuts	-	-	9.1	38.1	1:4
Tofu	-	-	1.3	10.0	1:7
Wheat germ	-	-	0.7	5.3	1:7
Quinoa	-	-	0.3	3.0	1:10
Oat flour	-	-	0.1	3.2	1:22

Refined foods	DHA	EPA	ALA	LA	Ω3:Ω6
Mayonnaise	-	-	5.0	40.6	1:8
Noodles - Chow mein	-	-	2.0	15.4	1:8
Muffins - Blueberry	-	-	1.2	8.5	1:7
Crackers	-	-	0.9	11.5	1:12
Special K	-	-	0.6	4.8	1:8
Cake - Vanilla	-	-	0.3	4.8	1:14
Bread - Whole wheat	-	-	0.3	2.9	1:8
Spaghetti	-	-	-	0.5	1:23
Rice - White	-	-	10mg	41mg	1:5

step through each of the lists:

Oils
- Fish oils win out overall since they have more DHA and EPA. Flax oil has more ALA in total, but since our bodies are inefficient at converting ALA to DHA and EPA, it is not as beneficial for us as fish oils. Preferably stick to eating fish rather than taking fish oil supplementation. More on this later
- Coconut oil gets a pass since it is very low in LA (omega-6) compared to other vegetable oils
- Vegetable oils overall are on the naughty list because they are just loaded with omega-6. Grapeseed oil has 700 times as much omega-6 as omega-3! They contain much more omega-6 than fish oils have omega-3, so you can see how easy it is for us to overdose on omega-6 in a 'normal' diet, especially with all those oils covering our salads!

Overall the trend here is to get more fish and flax oils, and avoid vegetable oils.

Animal sources
- Turns out them rich folk have been a step ahead all along, given that caviar is a fantastic source of omega-3 coming in at an awesome ratio of 81:1. Still, you'd be hard-pressed to eat 100g of it, so the other fish sources, especially salmon, are a great choice to supplement for health
- Interestingly, farmed salmon has much higher omega-6, likely due to the feed they are given, making them a less healthy choice than wild salmon
- Poultry and beef are in themselves not good sources of omega-3, but do not contain that much omega-6 either, making them more neutral foods. You can see in the chart that grass-fed is better than grain-fed, though it still doesn't come near the omega-3 levels of fish, so we can't substitute fish with grass-fed beef

Overall even if your particular choice of fish isn't listed here, it is likely to be a good source of omega-3. Our diets should therefore include a good amount of fish to supplement other meats.

Plant sources
- Vegetables contain lower amounts of omega-3 and omega-6, but in themselves are balanced sources, so they are good to include – even in large amounts
- Fruits generally don't have significant quantities of fat in them, so don't really contain either omega-3 or omega-6
- Not all grains are listed here, but you can see that grain products are loaded with omega-6, making them a very unhealthy choice. A diet rich in grains quickly results in an overload of omega-6, with all the associated negative effects of systemic inflammation

Eat as much and as many different types of vegetables as you like, but stay away from grains.

Refined foods
- No surprise here, they are all loaded with omega-6. Most of them are refined forms of grains with added sugars. There are no two ways about it – they are bad for your health and your weight, so focus on healthy natural foods instead!

Overall avoid refined foods and grains – build your healthy eating habits on good, whole foods.

1.1.3.3 Omega-3 in ancient diets

At this stage you might be wondering – if omega-3 mainly comes from fish, how is it that ancient humans living inland managed to eat omega-3 and omega-6 in equal ratios? It's a good question with an interesting answer. What was different back then is that wild animals ate grass and the leaves of wild plants which are a richer source of omega-3, resulting in the meat of those animals being high in omega-3. This meant that land animals *used* to be as good an omega-3 source as fish.

To give you an idea of how much better the meat from land animals used to be, wild Alaskan moose meat contains around 800mg of omega-3 in a 100g serving, which is as high as some fish sources[74]. This is because they forage in the wild for plants and leaves, and are therefore not grain-fed like farm-raised animals. Beef and poultry would be up there as well if they were still consuming their ancient diets, but modern farming techniques pump them full of grains, and even grass-fed beef are often only finished on grass, meaning that they still eat a lot of grains throughout their lives.

Modern meat farming techniques (especially grain-fed sources) results in much less omega-3 in land meat sources. This is why grass-fed meat is so much better for your health! Feeding grains to cows mean that they also have an imbalance of having much more omega-6 than omega-3 in their systems. This means that the meat itself is also less balanced, which is then transferred into our bodies when we eat it, resulting in a further imbalance in our own ratios.

1.1.3.4 Effects of dietary fat

We've learned a lot here about the effects of Essential Fatty Acids on the body and the brain, and about the role of omega-6 in causing inflammation and omega-3 in reducing it. But what other effects do dietary fat have?

Dietary fat does not promote overeating like carbohydrates do

We learned earlier how carbohydrates negatively affect the peptides ghrelin and leptin, resulting in us not feeling full and wanting to eat more. Some of the latest research into dietary fats shows that it positively affects **PYY** (the same peptide that is positively affected by protein) to help you feel full faster[75]. This is particularly true for saturated fat, which is more filling than unsaturated fats.

Dietary fats are higher in energy than carbohydrates, coming in at nine calories per gram, versus four calories per gram of carbohydrate. This can make us feel a bit wary about including dietary fat in our diets. From what we've seen, there is a much bigger problem with carbohydrates, given how carbohydrate-rich foods tend to be much more energy dense overall. For example:

- 100g of bread has around 300 calories – nearly all from carbohydrates
- 100g of fillet steak has around 190 calories – mainly from protein, around 36% from fat

The two options above show a simple choice where the same size meal (100g) provides over 50% more calories if bread is chosen. Also, the high GI nature of bread creates an insulin spike, affecting mood[76], and inhibits peptides that produce satiety[20,23,21] and increases fat storage[77]. The steak, on the other hand, produces no insulin spike, provides the body with essential nutrients, is proven to make us feel full and is less calorie-dense. It's also unlikely that we'd eat bread on its own, so we'd have to factor in other condiments such as butter, jam or Nutella.

It quickly becomes clear that a similar sized steak is a much healthier option than bread, despite what we have been led to believe. In the same way, it is simply not as easy to overeat dietary fats as it is with carbohydrates for the simple reason that dietary fats by themselves are not as appetising (plus they make you feel full too fast). We could easily eat a packet of sweets or cookies, but it's unlikely you'd be eating a stick of butter, or 100g of animal fat by itself. Sweets make you want to eat more, but the mere thought of eating dietary fat by itself makes you feel full already!

What to remember:
- Body fat is different from dietary fat
- All dietary fats are good as a fuel source and for health, except for trans-fat which must be avoided
- Balance omega-3 with omega-6 by including fish in the diet and removing grains
- Dietary fats, especially saturated fats are proven to help you feel fuller for longer

1.1.4 Fibre

Dietary fibre is the indigestible parts of plant foods. It is one of the most common compounds in nature and is only found in plants. Even though it is listed here as a macronutrient, it yields zero calories and doesn't actually provide any direct nutrition to your body like protein, carbohydrates and fats do. Instead it has other benefits that still make it a fantastic addition to a healthy eating. The table below provides an explanation of the two main types of fibre.

	Characteristics	Sources
Soluble fibre	• Dissolves in water and becomes soft and gelatinous as it ferments • The fermentation process is important for the growth of healthy bacteria in the intestines • Soluble fibre can also help to slow emptying of the stomach • Helps us to feel full and reduce the calorie density of meals	Broccoli, carrots, sweet potatoes, onions, legumes, oats, fruits, psyllium husks and almonds
Insoluble fibre	• Does not dissolve in water and can provide bulking and/or help gut flora through fermentation • Helps to regulate blood sugar, lowering the intensity of insulin spikes • It helps to speed transit time of food through the digestive system, helping with constipation and regularity • Helps us to feel full and reduce the calorie density of meals	Green beans, celery, cauliflower, zucchini, nuts, seeds, wheat, corn, and the skins of tomatoes and grapes

The ability of soluble fibre to absorb water means that a high-fibre diet can result in constipation if not enough water is taken through the day. A lot of research has been done about fibre and the mechanisms of how it works in the body, resulting in health benefits from fibre to be well understood. Let's have a look and see just why fibre is so beneficial.

Fibre helps you feel full and reduces meal energy density

When you've eaten a meal, ideally you want to feel full and not hungry anymore. This effect is called *satiation*, as mentioned before in the protein and carbohydrate sections. We saw there that carbohydrates, especially sugars, make you feel less full, while protein makes you feel more full, helping with satiety. Feeling full after meals means you will not crave snacks and overall you will eat less, making it easier for you to maintain your goal body.

Like protein, fibre also helps with feeling full, and does so in different ways[78]:

- Fibre adds bulk, resulting in the same size meal having a lower energy density
- Fibre requires more chewing before you swallow, increasing a feeling of satiety
- Fibre swells in the stomach as it absorbs water, creating a physical feeling of fullness
- Soluble fibre slows stomach emptying, meaning you feel fuller for longer
- Fibre can slow the movement of foods through the intestinal tract, allowing more time for macros to interact with the mechanism that produce satiety

As you can see, there are a lot of ways that fibre helps us to feel full! This is a key reason why we should include it in our diet – it helps us to feel fuller for longer, reducing the likelihood that we will snack on other foods in-between meals. This lowers our overall caloric intake, which is what we need to do if we want to lose those flabby bits. Foods which contain the kind of fibre that has been proven to help with satiety naturally include good old vegetables and fruits.

In addition to this satiating effect, fibre is also proven to *lower the digestibility of fats and protein*[79] allowing us to eat the same size meals as before, but absorb less of the macros, resulting in reduced calorie intake and less excess energy that can be turned into fat.

Fibre lowers cholesterol and risk of some diseases

Small dense LDL (low-density lipoprotein) particles are what clog our arteries and can result in heart attacks. Fibre has been shown to decrease these LDL particles[80] by preventing bile salts from being reabsorbed, and also through reducing the insulin response from eating foods[81].

This reduction of the insulin response is also helpful from a weight loss perspective as it reduces the chance that food will be stored as fat. Fibre also helps to produce short chain fatty acids which have been shown to reduce the risk of some gastrointestinal disorders[82]. High colonic pH has been shown to increase the risk of colonic cancer. Fibre helps to balance colonic pH by releasing more short chain fatty acids through fermentation[83].

Fibre regulates blood sugar

By slowing down the rate at which the stomach empties into the intestines[33], the nutrients in foods take longer to be adsorbed by the body and therefore slows the overall release of glucose into the body. Combine this with the effect of fibres shielding carbohydrates from absorption when soluble fibre swells with water, and you have lower spikes in blood sugar.

As you would know by now, this results in a lower insulin response which means less excess energy is stored as fat, a more gradual release of nutrients and less of an energy rollercoaster ride for you!

Fibre can be prebiotic

Prebiotics help with the growth of healthy bacteria in the digestive system through fermentation and can help the immune system to resist infections in the digestive system[86]. There are two forms of fibre that have been proven to be prebiotic[87]:

- **Inulin**, found in onion, garlic, agave, banana, chicory, and other plant sources
- **Galactooligosaccharide**, found in some specialised milk products

Interestingly, it is not important how much of a prebiotic substance you eat to get a benefit from it. A small amount can still stimulate the whole population of the particular bacteria that it benefits[87].

> **A note on fibre and constipation**
>
> There has been much talk in the past about treating constipation with fibre, with many doctors prescribing it as the best way to treat this affliction. Recent research has shown that constipation is better treated with increased liquid intake[84] (score another one for water!) and that increasing fibre intake does not reduce any symptoms. Sometimes even reducing fibre intake may help to alleviate serious constipation[85].

1.1.4.1 Sources of fibre

Let's look at what foods are good sources of fibre. The table below shows a list of common sources of fibre[88]. The colour coding follows our classification used in the GI table.

Source	Serving	Fibre	Source	Serving	Fibre
Vegetables			**Fruits**		
Artichoke, cooked	1 medium	10.3	Raspberries	1 cup	8
Green peas, cooked	1 cup	8.8	Pear, with skin	1 medium	5.5
Broccoli, boiled	1 cup	5.1	Apple, with skin	1 medium	4.4
Turnip greens, boiled	1 cup	5	Banana	1 medium	3.1
Brussels sprouts, cooked	1 cup	4.1	Orange	1 medium	3.1
Sweet corn, cooked	1 cup	4	Strawberries (halves)	1 cup	3
Sweet potato, with skin, baked	1 cup	4	Figs, dried	2 medium	1.6
Tomato paste	1/4 cup	2.7	Raisins	30 grams	1
Carrot, raw	1 medium	1.7	**Grains, cereal & pasta**		
Legumes, nuts and seeds			Spaghetti, whole-wheat	1 cup	6.3
Split peas, cooked	1 cup	16.3	Barley, pearled, cooked	1 cup	6
Lentils, cooked	1 cup	15.6	Bran flakes	3/4 cup	5.3
Black beans, cooked	1 cup	15	Oat bran muffin	1 medium	5.2
Lima beans, cooked	1 cup	13.2	Oatmeal, instant, cooked	1 cup	4
Baked beans, cooked	1 cup	10.4	Popcorn, air-popped	3 cups	3.5
Sunflower seed kernels	1/4 cup	3.9	Brown rice, cooked	1 cup	3.5
Almonds	30 grams	3.5	Bread, rye	1 slice	1.9
Pistachio nuts	30 grams	2.9	Bread, whole-wheat	1 slice	1.9

- **Vegetables and legumes** highlighted in green are the best sources of fibre as they are also less calorie-dense and have lower GI values. Eat most of these!

- **Fruits** are again an in-between source, as the fructose in them means they have higher GI values, though they are usually less calorie-dense, making them a *sometimes* treat

- **Grains** in red have decent amounts of fibre, but their calorie-dense nature and higher GI values means that they do not support weight loss. Avoid these

It's clear that fibre provides a lot of health benefits which makes it an important part of healthy eating. It helps us feel full, adds bulk to our meals, reduces caloric density of meals, regulates blood sugar, and even helps preventing some diseases!

What to remember:
- Fibre helps you to feel full after meals, reducing cravings for more food
- As we have seen, there are many proven health benefits provided by fibre, so make sure there are plenty of vegetables in your diet

1.1.5 Macronutrient metabolism

Before we head into the micronutrients, it's useful to know how the different macros are used by our metabolism. When we talk about metabolism, we are talking about how our bodies use foods for energy. There has also been a lot of talk in the media and diet books about 'increasing your metabolism' to burn foods faster and lose weight, so let's take a look and see what is really happening and what actually works!

The rate at which you burn calories is generally called '24 Hour Energy Expenditure'. This is the total amount of energy that you burn during a full 24 hour day, and consists of a few different types that make up your total amount of energy used. These are:

1. **Basal metabolic rate** – how much energy the body uses in a resting state, which can be around 70%[11] of your total energy used. The main factors that influence your base rate include:

    a. **Muscle mass** – more muscle requires more energy to maintain

    b. **Body surface area** – more body surface results in greater heat release, requiring more energy to maintain body temperature

    c. **Body temperature** – higher temperatures, especially due to exercise, require more energy to maintain

    d. **Age** – as you age, metabolism slows down naturally, though healthy eating and exercise can curb this

    e. **Nutrition** – if the body isn't getting enough nutrients, it can go into starvation mode, drastically reducing metabolism

2. **Thermic effect of food** – this is essentially how much energy the body expend digesting and absorbing different types of nutrients, and it makes up about 10% of our 24 hour energy expenditure. Some foods have a higher thermic effect, taking more energy to break them down into energy to be used. The list below shows how much energy is needed to process nutrients[12]:

    a. **Carbohydrates** – 6% to 8%

    b. **Fats** – 2% to 3%

    c. **Proteins** – 25% to 30%. You can see that a much higher percentage of energy is needed to use protein. This effectively means that 100g of carbohydrate is equivalent to around 140g of protein, making protein a fantastic weight-loss component of your diet

    d. **Fibre** – 0%. Fibre doesn't make a real difference to the thermic effect of food[89], but it is still useful to add bulk and make you feel full, particularly in combination with protein[16,17]

3. **Activity** – physical activity, including exercise can vary a great deal through the day. The more active your lifestyle is, and the more you exercise, the more energy the body burns.

Note: To clarify the thermic effect of food, the body does not burn 25% to 30% of the protein you just ate to digest it; instead, it will still get absorbed while other energy sources are used for digestion.

What can you do to increase metabolism?

There are a few practical things we can do to increase our metabolic rate:

- **Eat more protein** – as you saw above, protein has a higher thermic effect, meaning if you eat more protein, your body will spend more energy metabolising it. This is a great benefit of a high-protein diet – it naturally increases your metabolism while keeping you full, as well as help you to maintain and build more muscle mass

- **Improve muscle mass** - the more muscle mass you have, the more energy you burn, even while you sleep. Low protein diets tend to result in you losing muscle mass, meaning you see results on the scale, but this doesn't help you in the long term as you feel weak and your metabolism slows. Low protein diets also mean less muscle definition, meaning you don't get that fantastic lean look. Eating more protein will help you to maintain muscle mass if you don't exercise, and increase muscle definition if you do exercise. Either way, having more muscle will boost your metabolism!

- **Drink coffee** – a factor that has been proven to increase metabolism is caffeine[90]. We have to be careful with this one, as too much caffeine can have negative effects, such as anxiety and insomnia[91]. Therefore we need to keep overall caffeine intake at a reasonable level so we get a benefit without the negative side effects. Stick to one cup in the morning if are you focusing on health. Note this does not mean coffee is a 'magic weight loss cure' – you still need to eat healthy. Also, the metabolism-increasing effects of caffeine increases as you get leaner!

What to remember:
- Eating protein and building muscle mass are proven ways of increasing your metabolism
- Drink a cup of coffee in the morning to improve metabolism your, but focus on healthy eating as the main way to lose weight!

1.2 Micronutrients

In addition to macros, there is another essential element to healthy eating called **micronutrients** (or 'micros' for short). They are called this because they appear in much smaller quantities than the more abundant macros. They are needed for a wide variety of functions within our bodies, and since our bodies can't manufacture most of them, it is crucial to include these in your diet to ensure your body is working well and you are feeling great.

Micros include **vitamins** and **minerals**. There is a vast amount of science behind how these interact with our bodies to keep us healthy and feeling good. We all probably feel like we generally understand vitamins and minerals which is why many diet books don't provide much information about them. I feel it is useful to have a refresher on why they are important to us, and what they do. Understanding their roles also makes it easier for us to recognise if we have a deficiency and need to improve our eating habits.

In this section, we will go through the vitamins and minerals to see how they fit into healthy eating and how they help our bodies and minds. While we are looking at the individual micros, we won't be focusing on which individual foods are the best sources.

"Why not call them out as we talk about them?"

Mainly because when it comes to vitamins and minerals, you often hear things like *"Spinach is a good source of vitamin A"* and *"Beef is a good source of iron"*. This is technically correct, but as you'll see, both spinach and beef are good sources of a whole lot of other vitamins and minerals too!

The tendency of the industry to single out individual characteristics of foods without comparing them to other foods ends up making us feel stressed. We start worrying about things like not getting enough vitamin A because we are not eating enough spinach even though, in reality, we can get vitamin A from a lot of other sources. This thinking creates a mindset where we try to construct meal plans with all these different types of food that we heard about that are 'good' and this ends up being impossible since we'd have to eat at least 30 different types of food in a day!

Instead of continuing the tradition of singling out specific points about individual foods, we will take an overview of different foods in context of others, looking at all vitamins and minerals at once. Getting this overview will show you how many foods are great sources of nearly all vitamins and minerals and you'll realise it is not that hard to create a balanced healthy eating plan, once you know what the right food groups are.

The great benefit of this approach is that it removes the stress and worry about which foods to include for a 'balanced diet'. This means we can relax and enjoy our meals knowing we are eating right, nourishing out bodies and minds, and we can use our energy to think about more constructive things! In the appendix we go through each vitamin and mineral in detail and provide a short table of food groups with the percentage of the recommended daily intake so you can easily see which sources are the best for multiple vitamins and minerals.

To keep things moving along, we will focus on the key vitamins and minerals that we commonly don't get enough of.

1.2.1 Vitamins

The multivitamin commercials on television over the years have been very successful in drumming into our heads how important vitamins are for us. Still, it is useful to get back to the basics about what vitamins are, why they are important and whether we really need to take a supplement.

Vitamins are organic compounds that we need in small amounts because our bodies cannot manufacture them itself. This is why we need healthy gut bacteria to manufacture some, while other vitamins need to be ingested. Vitamins are classed by their function, and not their structure. This is why when you delve deeper, you will often find a number of different compounds that are classed within a single vitamin.

Vitamins need a certain amount of balance, so you can have too much as well as too little. For many vitamins, there are health conditions relating to having too much of them, just as there are conditions for having too few. Naturally, this is something that most vitamin distributors don't highlight in their advertisements when they try to convince us we need more! Overdosing is also influenced by whether or not the vitamin is water soluble or fat soluble:

- **Water soluble** vitamins (B and C) dissolve easily in water and are more easily excreted by the body. This makes it easier for the body to control the amount of the vitamin in the body and therefore there is less chance to overdose on them

- **Fat soluble** vitamins (A, D, E and K) are absorbed in the intestinal tract through fats, which mean they are more likely to accumulate in the body

To help us get the right balance of vitamins, countries release charts with the Recommended Daily Intake (RDI) of both vitamins and minerals as well as Upper Limits (UL). The table to the right shows the RDI for adult women[92]. Male RDI's are usually around 10-20% higher.

Vitamin	Solubility	RDI	Upper Limit
Vitamin A	Fat	700 mcg	3000 mcg
Vitamin B1	Water	1.1 mg	N/A
Vitamin B2	Water	1.1 mg	N/A
Vitamin B3	Water	14 mg	35 mg
Vitamin B5	Water	4 mg	N/A
Vitamin B6	Water	2.4 mg	50 mg
Choline	Water	425 mg	3500 mg
Vitamin B9	Water	400 mcg	1000 mcg
Vitamin B12	Water	2.4 mcg	N/A
Vitamin C	Water	45 mg	N/A
Vitamin D	Fat	5 mg	80 mg
Vitamin E	Fat	7 mg	300 mg
Vitamin K	Fat	60 mcg	N/A

The guidelines are published in countries by health authorities such as:

- The Australian Government's *Department of Health and Ageing, National Health and Medical Research Council* as the *Nutrient Reference Values for Australia and New Zealand*

- In the United States of America, these are published by the *National Academy of Sciences, Institute of Medicine, Food and Nutrition Board* as the *Dietary Reference Intakes: Recommended Intakes for Individuals*

The Australian version is well documented and contains sources for claims throughout. If you are interested in further reading into any particular vitamin or mineral, it is a good place to start. Since most of the claims are generally accepted, we will focus our citations on newer research and health claims beyond what is mentioned in the guidelines.

If you'd like to read more detail on each of the vitamins we covered above, have a look through Appendix A at the end of the book which covers each vitamin, what they do and the effects of having too much or too little in your diet.

Fundamental Nutrition - **Micronutrients**

1.2.1.1 Vitamin summary

The table below shows vitamins mapped against different food groups. Each box shows the percentage of our RDI we would generally find within that food group. These percentages are corrected for portion sizes to make the percentage realistic in terms of how much we generally eat.

The percentages themselves are in coloured boxes, with darker colours meaning more RDI than other food sources. For example, on average 100g of red meat and poultry have around 22% of our RDI for choline. Since it has more than any other food source, the 22% is in a darker coloured box.

What we can quickly see from this is that meat products overall provide the best sources of vitamins. Fish is the standout, coming out on top as the best source of vitamins. It does have a few gaps though, which vegetables and a bit of sunshine fill in nicely.

We see that fruits are actually fairly low in vitamins overall, with even vegetables having more vitamin C than fruit. Grains have the most vitamin B9, but this is due to mandatory supplementation in grain products[93]. Overall grains are not as good as a source of vitamins as meat products, and lack key vitamins such as A, C and B12.

Vitamin sources Average % RDI for Vitamins in Food Sources	Red meat & poultry	Fish	Dairy products	Legumes & nuts	Vegetables	Fruit	Grains	Sweets
Serving size (g)	100	100	50	30	100	100	100	100
Vitamin A	4%	10%	9%	-	122%	4%	-	-
Vitamin B1	8%	17%	-	18%	6%	3%	28%	-
Vitamin B2	23%	27%	9%	4%	8%	4%	15%	-
Vitamin B3	43%	44%	-	4%	4%	5%	17%	-
Vitamin B5	23%	36%	3%	6%	8%	8%	10%	-
Vitamin B6	16%	17%	-	4%	6%	5%	5%	-
Choline	22%	7%	2%	2%	3%	2%	6%	-
Vitamin B9	3%	4%	1%	13%	16%	6%	17%	-
Vitamin B12	45%	415%	10%	-	-	-	1%	-
Vitamin C	2%	-	-	1%	103%	50%	-	-
Vitamin D	3%	54%	3%	-	-	-	-	-
Vitamin E	6%	13%	5%	2%	9%	10%	18%	-
Vitamin K	3%	1%	2%	5%	135%	13%	17%	-

Sugary candy live up to their stigma as being 'empty calories', since they do not contain a single vitamin.

Effect of too little or too much

The table below consolidates the effects of vitamin deficiencies and the effects of taking too much. Naturally there is much more information that could be added so this is in no way a complete list of side effects, though it gives us a sense of the kind of effects we might experience with an imbalance.

Vitamin	Deficiency symptoms	Overdose symptoms
Vitamin A	Night blindness, impaired immune function	Nausea, irritability, headaches, hair loss, drowsiness
Vitamin B1	Tiredness, depression, confusion, loss of coordination	-
Vitamin B2	Cracked lips and mouth corners, scaly skin	-
Vitamin B3	Poor concentration, delirium, skin sensitivity, slow metabolism	Skin flushing, liver damage
Vitamin B5	Fatigue, irritability, cramps, restlessness	-
Vitamin B6	Neural damage, confusion, drowsiness, skin conditions	Neural damage, pain in extremities
Choline	Liver damage, heart disease, neural damage, muscle damage	Sweating, fishy body odour, diarrhoea, vomiting
Vitamin B9	Weakness, fatigue, irritability, palpitations	Neurological issues when B12 deficiency is present
Vitamin B12	Mania, psychosis, weakness, fatigue, depression	-
Vitamin C	Fatigue, bone pain, rough skin, bruising, loose teeth	Indigestion
Vitamin D	Muscle aches and weakness, muscle twitching, fragile bones	Dehydration, decreased appetite, irritability, muscle weakness
Vitamin E	Nerve damage, neuromuscular disorders, red blood cell destruction	Bleeding, vitamin K deficiency
Vitamin K	Bruising, excessive bleeding, stomach pains, cartilage calcification	-

Looking at these, we can see some major themes emerge:

- **Tiredness and fatigue** – these are the most common symptoms that appear from a vitamin deficiency, presenting in almost half of the vitamins. Note that it doesn't mean that if you experience tiredness it is mainly caused by vitamin deficiency as it can also be caused by many other things, such as stress and not sleeping enough. Still, we want to make sure that we keep our vitamins balanced so that we can work out what else we need to improve

- **Brain function** – nearly all the B vitamins and some of the others are involved in effective brain function. Depression, confusion and irritability are common symptoms of vitamin deficiency, highlighting just how important it is to have proper nutrition to keep our brains healthy

- **Immune function** – a number of vitamins combine to help keep our immune systems working well, reminding us that if we are getting sick often, we might have to look at what we are eating

Of course, this only shows half the picture – we also need to bring in minerals to complete it. Once we bring in the average scores of calories, proteins, carbohydrates and dietary fats, you'll easily see the reasons supporting the Think Lean Method, and why it works.

1.2.2 Minerals

So far we have looked at macros and vitamins, which are both chemical compounds made up of a number of different chemical elements. Dietary minerals, on the other hand, are mainly individual elements by themselves that are needed by the body to perform chemical processes.

As with vitamins, government authorities provide recommended daily intake values for minerals, along with upper limits where they have been shown to be toxic at high levels. The table to the right shows these values along with the minerals that we'll have a look through in more detail below.

Mineral	RDI		Upper Limit	
Calcium	1000	mg	2500	mg
Iron	8	mg	45	mg
Magnesium	400	mg	350*	mg
Phosphorus	1000	mg	4000	mg
Potassium	3800	mg	NP	mg
Sodium	690	mg	2300	mg
Zinc	8	mg	40	mg
Copper	1.2	mg	25	mg
Manganese	5	mg	NP	mg
Selenium	60	mcg	400	mcg

*Upper limit for magnesium applies only to supplementation

1.2.2.1 Mineral summary

Let's take a look at mineral sources and side effects from having too much or too little. We'll do a quick overview, then combine the vitamin and mineral tables, along with calorie information, to see what the real story is in terms of what is good for us and what isn't.

Sources

The table to the right uses the same formatting as the vitamin tables, with higher mineral values shown in darker colour boxes to make it easy to spot which are the highest sources. Looking at which sources are rich in minerals, we see that fish come out on top for about half the minerals we have listed. Grains also have a few top scores, though one of these is for

Mineral sources Average % RDI for Minerals in Food Sources	Red meat & poultry	Fish*	Dairy products	Legumes & nuts	Vegetables	Fruit	Grains	Sweets
Serving size (g)	100	100	50	30	100	100	100	100
Calcium	2%	7%	13%	5%	4%	2%	4%	-
Iron	12%	14%	-	8%	4%	2%	15%	1%
Magnesium	6%	24%	2%	15%	7%	5%	19%	-
Phosphorus	20%	25%	9%	15%	4%	2%	21%	-
Potassium	8%	12%	2%	7%	10%	7%	7%	-
Sodium	13%	9%	13%	-	5%	-	34%	4%
Zinc	34%	8%	7%	13%	3%	3%	18%	-
Copper	13%	11%	-	23%	5%	7%	18%	-
Manganese	-	-	-	12%	5%	5%	26%	-
Selenium	35%	62%	5%	5%	1%	-	42%	1%

*Excludes caviar which contains high amounts of sodium

sodium and we don't need too much of this.

To make the table more intuitive, it has been adjusted for serving sizes, particularly for dairy and nut products, which are usually eaten in smaller quantities. The fact that they are adjusted conceals the fact that nuts and legumes actually have the most minerals per 100 grams. Cashews are one of the overall best sources (and a personal favourite snack), with cheese also being a great source of calcium, which is usually lacking in other sources.

Some of these values are a little skewed because specific foods in the groups shown have very high values, so if you are interested in specific foods, check Appendix B for the full tables.

Effect of too little or too much

Minerals are involved in a large number of body functions and processes, including keeping your immune system, bones, blood and skin healthy. Because minerals are such a fundamental part of keeping our bodies in top shape, it's no surprise that there are a lot of symptoms that present when we have too much or too little.

The table below consolidates the effects of mineral deficiencies and the effects of taking too much. Naturally there is much more information that could be added so this is in no way a complete list of side effects, though it gives us a sense of the kind of effects we might experience with an imbalance.

Minerals	Deficiency symptoms	Overdose symptoms
Calcium	Skin spots, tingling, hyperactive reflexes, hand contractions	Kidney stones
Iron	Fatigue, tiredness, apathy, anaemia	Liver damage, heart damage
Magnesium	Irritability, dizziness, muscle spasms, fatigue, nausea	Breathing difficulty, fatigue, nausea, vomiting
Phosphorus	Muscle weakness, bone pain, anaemia, rickets	Calcium deficiency
Potassium	High blood pressure, cramps, weakness, irritability, insomnia	-
Sodium	Headaches, confusion, irritability, fatigue, nausea, seizures, unconsciousness, coma	High blood pressure if salt sensitive
Zinc	Slowed growth, diarrhoea, hair loss, eye and skin conditions	Decreased immune function, vomiting, nausea
Copper	Anaemia, difficulty walking, spinal degeneration, eye problems	Muscle pain, joint pain, liver disease, abnormal kidney function
Manganese	Skin conditions, joint pain, inflammation, nausea	Neurological damage
Selenium	Heart enlargement, heart failure, arrhythmia	Skin rash, hair loss, fatigue, irritability, brittle nails

Too much mineral intake can result in varied symptoms. One of the most common themes you'll see in the information in the appendix is that as long as you eat natural, whole foods and don't overdo the supplements, you are very unlikely to suffer from an imbalance. This might not be a ground-breaking idea, but it's good to see that the evidence supports the idea of consuming more natural and whole foods as the source of healthy eating.

Fundamental Nutrition - **Micronutrients**

1.2.3 Best sources for healthy eating

Now let's bring it all together! Using the tables that we've used so far, we can produce an overview of the food groups to see which food groups contain the highest amounts of vitamins and minerals.

The combined table has a new section at the bottom which shows the average amount of calories, carbohydrates, dietary fat and protein in each food group.

Given what we learned before about macros, we want to avoid high amounts of calories and carbohydrates. Protein and dietary fats help us feel full, while carbohydrates, especially high-GI carbohydrates, and sugars make us want to eat more.

Looking through these figures, the following becomes clear:

Red meat, poultry and fish
The foods in this group are an excellent source of vitamins and minerals. On top of that, they contain lower calories in general and are high in protein, which makes us feel full after meals and helps lean muscle mass to increase our metabolism. Looking at this summarised view, it's quite impressive to see how rich in vitamins and minerals these are, particularly as we don't always think of them this way, with all the time the media spends saying how bad red meat is for us.

Even though there is some dietary fat in meat, if you eat vegetables with meat, you won't have the blood sugar spike that turns the dietary fat into body fat. Instead, your body will slowly use the low GI carbohydrates from the vegetables and burn the dietary fat for energy instead.

Dairy products
Dairy is mainly good for calcium, coming out as the top source even when eaten in lower serving sizes. Cheese is overall the best source of calcium, and since it is mainly protein and fat with little carbohydrate, it's actually a decent addition to healthy eating!

Average % RDI for Vitamins and Minerals in Food Sources	Red meat & poultry	Fish	Dairy products	Legumes & nuts	Vegetables	Fruit	Grains	Sweets
Serving size (g)	100	100	50	30	100	100	100	100
Vitamin A	4%	10%	9%	-	122%	4%	-	-
Vitamin B1	8%	17%	-	18%	6%	3%	28%	-
Vitamin B2	23%	27%	9%	4%	8%	4%	15%	-
Vitamin B3	43%	44%	-	4%	4%	5%	17%	-
Vitamin B5	23%	36%	3%	6%	8%	8%	10%	-
Vitamin B6	16%	17%	-	4%	6%	5%	5%	-
Choline	22%	7%	2%	2%	3%	2%	6%	-
Vitamin B9	3%	4%	1%	13%	16%	6%	17%	-
Vitamin B12	45%	415%	10%	-	-	-	1%	-
Vitamin C	2%	-	-	1%	103%	50%	-	-
Vitamin D	3%	54%	3%	-	-	-	-	-
Vitamin E	6%	13%	5%	2%	9%	10%	18%	-
Vitamin K	3%	1%	2%	5%	135%	13%	17%	-
Calcium	2%	7%	13%	5%	4%	2%	4%	-
Iron	12%	14%	-	8%	4%	2%	15%	1%
Magnesium	6%	24%	2%	15%	7%	5%	19%	-
Phosphorus	20%	25%	9%	15%	4%	2%	21%	-
Potassium	8%	12%	2%	7%	10%	7%	7%	-
Sodium	13%	9%	13%	-	5%	-	34%	4%
Zinc	34%	8%	7%	13%	3%	3%	18%	-
Copper	13%	11%	-	23%	5%	7%	18%	-
Manganese	-	-	-	12%	5%	5%	26%	-
Selenium	35%	62%	5%	5%	1%	-	42%	1%

Average Macronutrient Profiles (does not indicate RDI)

Calories	193	179	159	135	43	63	374	393
Carbohydrate (g)	-	-	3	11	6	11	60	98
Dietary Fat (g)	11	9	14	8	2	2	11	-
Protein (g)	22	23	4	5	1	1	9	-

Legumes and Nuts

Even though legumes are usually classed with grains, they actually have very similar vitamin and mineral profiles to nuts. Generally we don't eat legumes in the same amounts as we can eat breads, and they are lower in GI scores as well, so it makes sense to group them together with nuts instead. Nuts and legumes are good for snack foods and additions into meals (cashew chicken, maybe?).

Overall they are high in minerals, though they can be high in omega-6, so we won't be adding in too many in our eating plans. Personally I eat cashews and macadamias as a snack food, and the omega-6 from small amounts is not enough to put it out of balance, so we can keep it in there!

Vegetables

Meats still leave a little bit of a gap in some vitamins, such as vitamin B9, E and K. This is where vegetables come in. Vegetables are a great source of many vitamins and minerals, beating out fruits in nearly every category. Vegetables are also low in calories overall, and where they do have carbohydrates, it is mostly low GI (except for starchy vegetables like potato). This means we can eat loads of vegetables without having to worry about putting on weight!

Vegetables combined with meat and sunshine for vitamin D give us everything we need – *a healthy eating plan that keeps us feeling full, bodies and brains that are nourished and healthy, and consistent energy to be successful in every area of life!*

Fruit

We are always told to eat fruits to get our vitamins. Well, no. This does not seem to be correct, at all. In fact, fruit is pretty much low in everything. Even vitamin C, which we are told fruit is great for, is more easily found in vegetables. A big reason is that fruits are mostly water, so do not have the density of other foods to have more vitamins and minerals.

Even blueberries, touted as an amazing super fruit, if you look at the detailed tables in the appendix, you'll see that it is only relatively high in vitamin K, with much less antioxidants than it is said to have. What about the phytochemicals and anthocyanins that blueberries contain that is supposed to prevent heart disease, cancer, and help your brain? Well, these were only shown to have an effect

---

Get confident!

Of course, we are covering a lot of ground that you are probably familiar with. Much of what we are saying here is stuff you probably know already, have heard of, seen in an article somewhere, and so on.

If you are well researched in nutrition, there probably wouldn't have been anything new here so far, and that is great! As we aim to have an evidence-based healthy eating plan, the ideas here are those with real concrete evidence behind it.

So if you already knew this stuff, what was the point of all these pages so far? One big reason:

Confidence.

There is a big difference between knowing *that* healthy eating works, and knowing *how* it works. If you only know *that* it works:

- It is hard to defend it when you are challenged by people (especially those on fad diets with little evidence)
- It is hard to stick to when difficult situations come up
- You won't know where you can bend the rules, and what the effects are of bending them, making it seem rigid and hard to maintain

On the other hand, if you know *how* healthy eating works, it starts to build the right beliefs in your mind, and it gives you confidence to deal with situations:

- Having seen the evidence here, even if you don't remember it, gives you confidence because you know there is science behind it. If someone challenges your eating habits, you can always point them to these pages
- You'll know much more about why the rules are the way they are, and therefore where you can bend them in different situations. This makes healthy eating easier to maintain long term and makes it stress free. This is crucial to make it into a lifestyle!

Having seen the evidence and the detail behind healthy eating makes it easier to have confidence in it. Having confidence in what you are doing is really important to help you follow it in the long term and make it a lifestyle. Confidence helps you stick to it when life throws tough times at you. Confidence gives you conviction – the kind that can flow into other areas of your life, helping you have more confidence at work, with your family, in your relationships, in your hobbies.

And importantly, knowing the reasons behind healthy eating will protect you from the whiplash of the latest fad that shows up in the media. The media is very prone to misinterpret scientific findings, and are all too quick to sensationalise something to make snazzy headlines and draw readers. This can cause havoc with your diet if you try to follow the latest news. Instead, stick to the Think Lean Method, and it will give you confidence to stay consistent and get real, lasting results.

in animals, with studies showing that digestion prevents them from having any significant effect[94]. Sure, the hype is great for blueberry farmers, but the evidence shows otherwise, so don't eat it and expect miracles. You'll be better off eating more meat and vegetables.

Combine this with fruits being higher in sugar, and it becomes clear why it is not part of the good foods (meat, dairy, legumes, nuts, vegetables), but it is also not a bad food (grains and sweets). Fruits stay in the grey zone as a 'sometimes' food.

Grains

Even though grains contain a decent amount of minerals, they are not the best vitamin sources, are second highest in calories (after sweets), and are loaded with carbohydrates. Per 100g, they generally contain about **twice the calories** of meat, fish and dairy products. Compared to vegetables, grain products have more than **eight times the calories** for the same weight! This is what we mean by calorie-dense foods. Grain products are densely packed with calories, so even if you eat a small amount, you are still consuming a lot of calories.

> **What are antioxidants?**
>
> Oxidation is a natural process that happens in our bodies every day. Sometimes though, these reactions can become damaging by producing free radicals that cause chain reactions.
>
> Antioxidants are oxidised themselves and therefore help to stop free radicals. Of course, the body does actually need free radicals for a bunch of chemical processes, so they are not inherently bad. It is only when we have too many that it becomes a problem and we need more antioxidants.

In fact, their average carbohydrate content is about **six times higher** than whole foods (remember that breads, pasta, etc. are processed, therefore not whole foods) and the carbohydrates contained in grains are generally high GI, meaning they spike blood sugar and raise insulin levels. Since grains contain both carbohydrate and dietary fat, the insulin spike quickly stores the excess energy and dietary fats as body fat, resulting in our waistlines increasing. That is why grains are marked in red as a food group to avoid.

Sweets

Living up to their reputation, candies are simply empty calories. They have zero vitamins, and almost no minerals either. You can see that all other food sources have a large range of vitamins and minerals, except for sweets.

> **What to remember:**
> - Many food sources contain nearly all vitamins and minerals, so don't worry about eating specific foods to get specific vitamins
> - Fish is overall the best source of vitamins, followed by beef and poultry, with vegetables and sunshine filling in the gaps
> - Grains and sweets are too calorie dense and are not needed for healthy eating
> - Fish, meat, legumes and nuts are our preferred sources of minerals

The First Key:

2 Automatic Calorie Management

Imagine being able to eat as much as you like, not having to count calories, and still being able to achieve your ideal body! This is what Automatic Calorie Management, or **ACM** for short, is all about. By following this method, you can achieve a new level of freedom in managing weight. This idea is not just another fad – it is a fact recognised by research, even stating that with this approach *"...caloric restriction is not imposed but appears to be an inevitable outcome..."*[95]. Doesn't that sound fantastic? No need to count calories or stop eating when you are still hungry!

What we covered in the first section has given us the foundation and the scientific evidence to support ACM which we'll cover in detail here. In short, it works through these factors:

- *Controlling your appetite through protein and dietary fats that keep you feeling full*
- *Burning calories faster by eating more protein to boost your metabolism*
- *Reducing calories by eating nutritious foods such as vegetables which are less calorie-dense*
- *Creating consistent energy and blood sugar levels by going grain-free and sugar-free*

Why do we say 'automatic'? Because it actually becomes difficult to eat too much! Since proteins, dietary fats and fibre make you feel full, you tend to stop eating sooner. Even if you eat more, the low calorie-density nature of vegetables mean you can eat a lot without adding weight.

What does Automatic Calorie Management give me?
- Eat larger portions and feel full after meals
- Lose body fat and get lean, even without exercise
- Maintain lean muscle mass to boost metabolism
- Get healthy and heal your body

In the first section, you saw for yourself why healthy eating works – how peptides produced by protein, dietary fat and fibre make you feel full, that sugar and high-GI carbohydrates make you crave more, how low-GI carbohydrates give you consistent energy, the negative effects of gluten, the importance of the omega-3 to omega-6 ratio, and how proteins take much more energy to absorb through the thermic effect of food, allowing you to eat more without gaining weight.

This is how managing the amount of calories you eat becomes 'Automatic'. No need to count calories since these eating habits will automatically result in you eating fewer calories, helping you to maintain your ideal weight without having to spend a lot of time measuring out portion sizes.

That's it. There's no magic, just pure, proven science. It works for me, and it will work for you. In fact, it works for a lot of people. In September 2013, health authorities in Sweden finished a review of 16,000 studies and concluded that this type of diet is the most efficient for weight loss, specifically in getting results quickly[43,44].

A very recent study also showed that low carbohydrate diets are more effective for weight loss and improves cardiovascular health in the process[57]. All this recognises that high protein and low carbohydrate diets are healthy, and as we've seen, whole, natural foods provide us with all the vitamins and minerals we need to keep our bodies super healthy. The real diet dangers are found in grains and sugars. Cut out these, and everything becomes easier!

So we've seen the research and why this way of eating is so healthy. But for us to use this method, we need to get it down to a few simple rules. This will help get ACM working for you so you can easily get your ideal body!

2.1 The rules of Automatic Calorie Management

There are five simple rules which will set you free from a life of counting calories. These rules provide the key food groups which form the foundations of healthy eating, along with guidelines to apply to all your meals. Follow these easy rules and you can achieve effortless weight loss, without feeling hungry:

- Rule 1 – **Quality protein with every meal**
- Rule 2 – **Low-GI carbohydrates**
- Rule 3 – **Whole foods**
- Rule 4 – **Mix it up**
- Rule 5 – **Slow down**

Simple! Of course it means there are some foods that we need to set ourselves free from, especially calorie-dense foods that are high in inflammation-causing omega-6.

As we go through these rules, you also need to look at your lifestyle and adapt the rules based on how much exercise you do:

- *Core ACM* – designed for if you are exercising three days a week or less. Core ACM is named so because it is made up of the core staple foods in healthy eating, and can be depended on to give you the body you want. Core ACM is the main approach to go on to lose weight and get your goal body, and is also one you can stay on in the long term for maintenance and overall health. It is the fall-back approach as well if you try new things and notice you are picking up weight or bulging in the wrong places. We are all different, so you might find you gain weight while on Complete ACM even though you are exercising. In that case, fall back to Core ACM to get results. Though do keep an eye on measurements, as muscle gain would result in good weight gain since muscle weighs more than body fat

- *Complete ACM* – for an active lifestyle of intense exercise four or more days a week. For that you need extra calories to keep the muscles going. Complete ACM includes all the Core ACM foods, though has more calories than Core ACM as it is designed for regular gym goers, athletes and people who have a hard time putting on weight (yes, people like that exist!)

We'll clearly set these out later when we put together **a whole new food pyramid**, and finally do away with the old, out-dated food pyramid that's been driving and sabotaging our diets for decades!

Let's go over the rules first, and then look at the other foods and factors that help support ACM.

Rule 1 – Quality protein with every meal

We saw the filling effect of protein, how crucial it is for our bodies, how it helps to maintain our muscle mass which in turn keeps our metabolism high. Protein is the most important part of healthy eating. That's why we want to have protein with every meal.

But not only do we want to have protein with every meal, we want to have **quality protein**. You may remember we talked about the quality of proteins in the macronutrient section. This means we want most of our protein from sources such as red meat, poultry, fish and eggs which contain all the amino acids we need.

▶ Lean meats – Core ACM and Complete ACM

If you are not doing any exercise (or very little), we want to stay with lean meats. It is difficult to specify exactly which cuts of meats are 'lean', as they vary greatly even within the same cut of meat, so here is a simple way for you to determine if it is lean or not – **if you can see visible strips or pieces of dietary fat (the white bits), then it is a fatty meat (not lean)**. If you can cut it all off with very little visible fat remaining, then you can turn it into a 'lean' meat, though this is not possible for meats where it is very marbled (thin strips of dietary fats within the meat itself), such as ribeye steak.

Core ACM	Complete ACM
Lean meats	Fatty meats
Best for weight loss	For an active lifestyle
Guidance	**Guidance**
No or very little visible fat. Trim fat before you cook (except fish)	Visible fat Marbled cut
Examples	**Examples**
Chicken breast	Chicken thighs
Sirloin	Porterhouse steak
Tenderloin	Ribeye steak
Round steak	T-bone steak
95% lean ground beef	Wagyu
Fish	Ribs

If you do try to turn fatty meat into a lean meat by cutting off visible dietary fats, make sure you cut it off before you cook it - otherwise a lot of it will melt into the meat and will still be higher in calories, even if you cut it off afterwards.

Fish with visible dietary fats, like salmon with skin on, is actually very healthy as we saw before, since it contains a lot of omega-3. Because it is so good for you, **we count fish as a 'lean meat'** (though avoid high mercury fish like swordfish, shark and orange roughy). Sure, it has more dietary fats than other lean meats, but the fat on it is so good for you that we want to eat it regularly, even as part of Core ACM. So when eating fish, don't trim any fat on it – in fact, when buying fish, get it with the skin on so you can get more omega-3!

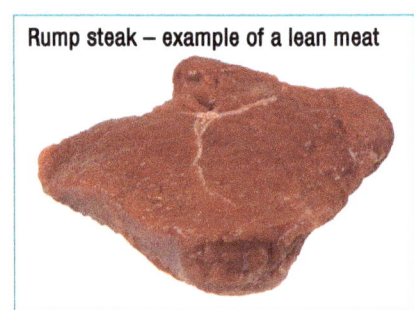
Rump steak – example of a lean meat

In Australia, you can look in stores for 'Heart Smart' marked meat. These usually have around five grams of dietary fat or less per 100g. Of course, we've learned that there is more to heart disease than saturated fats, so it isn't necessarily better for your heart, but you can still use the label to identify lean meats.

Core ACM works even if you do not do any exercise at all. That's right - **you can lose weight on Core ACM even if you do not go to the gym**. That's why we keep the foods within Core ACM very lean, so that you can eat a lot of it and feel full, while still losing weight.

Fatty meats – Complete ACM only
Fatty meats have visible dietary fat, like rib eye steak and chicken thighs. The additional dietary fat makes it easier to have more calories, which is why they are reserved for Complete ACM when you are doing a lot of gym work or training.

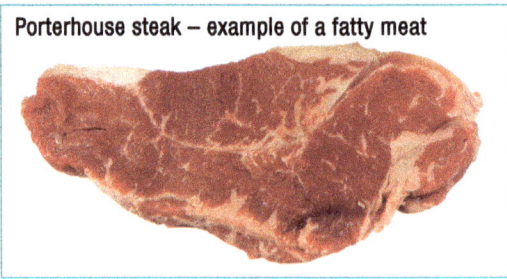
Porterhouse steak – example of a fatty meat

Protein powders – Core ACM and Complete ACM
A good way of getting extra protein in your diet is through protein powders. You can have it both with Core ACM and Complete ACM. Protein shakes can help save a lot of time when we are in a rush and we still want to get a decent amount of macros in our day. Protein is also great to mix with vegetables and other foods to efficiently deliver a complete meal. Keep in mind that a protein shake is not going to make you feel as full as an actual meal as it lacks the bulk of real food, so try to stick to whole foods if your goal is to lose weight. This makes it more useful if your goal is to get toned or build muscle mass.

There are many types of protein powders available, though the most common is whey protein which is made from milk as a by-product of cheese production. Whey protein is what you would usually see on supermarket and supplement store shelves, often alongside the abbreviations WPC, WPI or WPH.

- **WPC (Whey Protein Concentrate)** – this is the cheapest and lowest quality form of protein and generally contains more carbohydrates and dietary fats in the powder, giving it a lower overall protein content. This is what is mostly used in protein bars and other foods as it is cheaper for the manufacturer than higher quality protein

- **WPI (Whey Protein Isolate)** – this is a higher quality protein which has been processed to remove carbohydrates and dietary fats, leaving the powder with 90% or more protein per weight. This makes it a purer source of protein, even though it is little bit more expensive than WPC. WPI provides much better quality protein which also has higher bioavailability levels.

Bioavailability refers to the body's ability to absorb a nutrient – the more available it is, the better it can absorb it

- **WPH (Whey Protein Hydrolysate)** – this is partially hydrolysed so that it is digested and absorbed faster than WPC or WPI. Whether or not this is actually useful is arguable, and may only be relevant for competitive level body builders. For the most part, this is too expensive to justify any possible additional benefits

There are also many other forms of protein powder available, like soy protein and rice protein. These are alternatives for if you are lactose intolerant and really want to include protein powder into your diet. If you are not lactose intolerant, stick with whey protein – particularly WPI.

Keep an eye on the nutritional value of the powders, as many are flavoured with sugar. We need to avoid sugar, even in protein powders, so rather look for artificially flavoured powders, preferably with a natural sweetener like erythritol and/or stevia. Always look for protein powders that are above 90% pure.

> **Meal replacement powders**
> Meal replacement powders are usually protein powers with added ingredients such as carbohydrates and dietary fats. Avoid these as they are specifically designed as 'mass gain' products. In other words, you buy them if you are trying to gain weight and are struggling to get enough calories through real food.

Protein powders remain one of the cheapest sources of protein – one you can even use as a low calorie snack between other meals. If you do make a shake with other foods, remember to follow the ACM rules and stay away from sugar, no grains and limit fruits. Even a banana every day in a protein shake can end up adding a lot of sugar to your diet over time, so stick to low-GI vegetables for protein shakes and smoothies.

Overall

Eating protein with every meal means that we will feel full after eating and reduce cravings later on for snacks. And because protein has a much higher thermic effect of food (around 30% is burned in metabolising it), you can eat more of it without adding to your waistline!

Eating plenty of protein is also crucial if you are doing exercise, as it helps you to build and maintain muscle, giving a nice lean and toned look, leaving you feeling strong and looking great. Diets low in protein result in muscle wasting, leaving you feeling weak and slowing your metabolism. When you have a low protein diet, part of your weight loss is actually from muscle loss, rather than from body fat.

Protein sources include **dairy products** such as milk, cheese and yoghurt. Since these often have a higher dietary fat content, we need to make sure they are low sugar, as sugar combined with dietary fat results in your body storing more fat. For this reason, steer clear of cream cheeses, flavoured milk and sweetened yogurts and stick to hard cheeses, natural milk and unsweetened yoghurt.

A high protein approach to your diet means you can get toned while focusing your weight loss on body fat only. This means you can slim your waistline while keeping a healthy high metabolism, because more muscle means you can eat more without gaining weight!

Rule 2 – Low-GI carbohydrates

Back in the macronutrient section, we learned about the Glycaemic Index (GI) and how low-GI foods give us a consistent release of energy by keeping blood sugar level, helping to protect us against diseases such as diabetes.

Vegetables are the best source of low-GI carbohydrates, as other sources, such as grains, are generally higher in the GI index and more calorie-dense. This means you can eat a lot more without expanding your waistline. This helps add bulk to your diet, keeping your plate and stomach full, helping you to achieve your goal body. And, as we have already learned, vegetables are an excellent source of key vitamins and minerals, which helps keep your body healthy and in great condition.

Low-GI, non-starchy vegetables – Core ACM and Complete ACM

You might remember the table below from the Carbohydrate section, showing **32 low-GI, non-starchy vegetables** that are the best for weight loss. These are mostly water-based vegetables, making them less calorie-dense and ideal for feeling full while losing weight.

Nuts are included as they are a source of good carbohydrates. Even though they are more calorie-dense, they contain proteins and fats which make you feel full, and their carbohydrates are low-GI. Legumes are excluded from Core ACM as they contain more carbohydrate (some legumes are high GI) than protein or fat, making them less filling.

Low-GI, starchy vegetables – Complete ACM only

Complete ACM includes all the Core ACM vegetables but with the addition of starchy vegetables as well. We include starchy vegetables as they contain more carbohydrates overall than non-starchy vegetables, which will provide energy for your gym sessions and replenish muscle glycogen after a good workout. They also provide your body with energy to help protein synthesis in the muscles, so that they heal faster and you can exercise more!

Core ACM				Complete ACM		
Low-GI, non-starchy vegetables Best for weight loss				Starchy vegetables For an active lifestyle		
Veggies - 100g	Carbs	Veggies - 100g	Carbs	Veggies - 100g	Carbs	GI
Watercress	1	Peppers	4	Pumpkin	6	75
Alfalfa seeds	2	Rhubarb	4	Beets	9	64
Chinese cabbage	2	Swiss chard	4	Green peas	15	48
Asparagus	3	Tomatoes	4	Sweet corn	17	47
Celery	3	Cabbage	5	Sweet potato	20	44
Chinese broccoli	3	Green onions	5	Chickpeas	28	28
Cucumber	3	Turnips	5	Yam	28	37
Lettuce	3	Brussels sprouts	6	Plantains	28	38
Mushrooms	3	Scallions	6	Lentils	60	30
Radishes	3	Fennel	7	Kidney beans	61	28
Spinach	3	Leeks	7	High-GI, starchy vegetables Exclude from diet overall		
Zucchini	3	Eggplant	8			
Broccoli	4	Onions	9	Cassava	39	46
Cauliflower	4	Squash	9	Taro	35	55
Chicory	4	Carrots	9	White potato	21	60
Okra	4	Artichoke	11	Parsnips	16	97

Remember that we always exclude the high-GI starchy vegetables like cassava, taro, parsnips, and the really big one, white potatoes. White potatoes raise blood sugar too fast, and many of the forms it comes in (hash browns, chips, fries) are cooked in oil, making it a great cocktail for putting on body fat. So it is time to go white potato-free!

We also include **legumes** in Complete ACM. While legumes are technically grains that can have higher amounts of calories and omega-6, they are often not that bad once cooked and contain a lot of other vitamins and minerals. When eating in its natural form (*Whole Foods* is one of our rules!), we are less likely to binge on them and have too many.

Still, they are often high in carbohydrates, so they are excluded from Core ACM. If you are keeping active (regular gym sessions, etc.), then you can include them if you need additional calories. However if you notice you are gaining weight, go back to Core ACM.

When we went through the vitamins and minerals for different foods, we grouped legumes together with nuts because they have very similar micronutrient profiles. If you look at the detailed sheets in the appendix though, you'll notice that legumes tend to have quite a bit more carbohydrates than nuts, while nuts tend to have more dietary fats instead. That is why we split them up and end up with nuts going into Core ACM, and legumes going into Complete ACM.

Fruit – one piece per day at most with Core ACM and Complete ACM

In most of the charts and tables so far, fruit ends up in a grey area as a neutral 'sometimes' food. It is a natural food containing vitamins and minerals, but it tends to be higher in sugar (fructose). This means it's not great to have a lot of it, despite what we get told in the media.

Based on all we've seen, fruit is a 'sometimes' food – something to eat in moderation and preferably not daily. You'll even see in the diets of many fitness models that they tend to stay away from fruit for the most part. The reason is not so much the amount of calories in fruit, but more that they are a source of sugar, and we want to stay free of sugar as far as we can. Limit your fruit intake to a maximum of one piece per day for both Core ACM and Complete ACM.

Chocolate – dark (85% cocoa) or sugar-free chocolate with Core ACM or Complete ACM

Most chocolate comes loaded with sugars, making them something to avoid. Essentially, they break two rules:

- **Low-GI carbohydrates** – chocolate is usually loaded with sugar
- **Whole foods only** – chocolate is refined food

This means that chocolate is not an ACM food, so not part of your everyday food. Still, that doesn't mean you need to cut out chocolate altogether – you can still enjoy some dark chocolate from time to time. From a weight loss perspective, going for a sugar-free dark chocolate bar would be the best choice as it only contains some fat and fibre.

Sugar-free chocolate is not to everyone's taste, so if you want to have a chocolate bar, go for at least 85% dark chocolate. This means there is still 15 grams of sugar for a 100g bar, but it's better than a normal bar which would contain 50 grams of sugar! Try to eat only one or two pieces to enjoy the taste, then stop and keep the rest for the next day.

Chocolate is not going to help with your weight loss goals, but if you can't live without it, you at least have options. If you do want to lose weight as fast as possible, look for ways to reduce your consumption by going for artificially sweetened chocolate or try to find ways to cut it out, such as keeping chewing gum handy to overcome cravings.

Sugar-free

Yes, we are setting ourselves free of sugar! We saw earlier that sugar works against us in pretty much every way. It is extremely calorie-dense, it actively makes us crave and want to eat more of it, it has zero nutritional value, all working towards expanding our waistlines and causing diseases such as diabetes and heart disease! Even honey, which strangely is allowed in many diets, is still just sugar in a different form. From both a health and weight loss perspective, natural sweeteners like Stevia and others are better for us (more on this later).

There is nearly nothing that is good about it, so we need to cut it out from every part of our diets. This can be tough if you are not eating whole foods, since sugar hides in nearly all processed foods:

- Coffee or tea with sugar
- Sugary soft drinks (a big source of sugar!)
- Most sauces and salad dressings
- Breads, cakes, cookies and most baked goods
- Peanut butter, Nutella
- Yoghurt
- Cream
- Some cheeses
- Breakfast cereal
- Fruit juice
- Canned vegetables and fruit
- Chocolate, fruit bars, breakfast bars, nut bars
- Most fast food add extra sugar for taste
- Restaurant food
- Dried fruit
- Sweets

That's a lot of food sources with sugar in them. Is it even possible to avoid sugar at all? Of course it is! Stick to the five rules and you can be sugar free in no time. If you are used to eating a lot of sugar, you may have brought onto yourself a little bit of an 'addiction'. As we saw in the research before, sugar has addictive properties, affecting your brain in the same way that cocaine and meth does[23], and that it can be even more 'rewarding' than cocaine[24]!

What happens is that your brain becomes used to having high amounts of sugar every now and then, which is followed by a sugar crash, which then prompts the need for another sugar high. Your genes are also programmed to make you want more, so once you start getting more, the neural pathways become stronger as you eat more sugar, and you are more likely to act on a craving. A cycle forms when you constantly want the next sugar rush, craving one high after the next.

The good news is that it is totally possible to go sugar free, and after a while, you no longer crave sugar as your blood sugar levels even out and the neural pathways become used to eating healthy food. So while quitting sugar can be challenging initially, all you need to do is stick with it for a few weeks while you get into your new habit, and soon you will no longer want sugar! If you do need some help, one study has shown that chewing sugar-free gum a few times a day drastically helps to reduce snacking[96].

As you go on this plan, you will start to reprogram your body and your brain to no longer want sugar. In the beginning, your brain will still want the highs. This is where you have to steer clear and stay sugar free. As you keep going, the cravings do go away and it becomes a lot easier to stay focused on your new healthy lifestyle.

Grain-free

Summarising what we went through before, there are four reasons why we need to cut out all grains from our diet:

1. **They are calorie-dense** – too many calories cause us to gain weight. Cut out grains and we remove a big source of calories

2. **They are high-GI** – high GI scores spike our blood sugar, causing insulin to store excess energy as body fat. Most grain products are also refined (bread, pasta, etc.) and the carbohydrates affect peptides and hormones that motivate you to eat more

3. **They are high in omega-6** – this kind of omega causes inflammation and needs to be balanced with omega-3. Grain products are so high in omega-6 that it is near impossible to take enough omega-3 to balance it out

4. **They have gluten** – gluten can have many negative effects on your health and your brain (this only applies if you have coeliac or are gluten sensitive)

These are all things we need to avoid, and simply makes grain products in general bad for our weight and bad for our health. It can be hard to accept that breads and baked goods are bad for us, but the evidence is overwhelming and can't be ignored.

You'll see in many books and articles what the original story was for why grains formed the largest part of the old food pyramid. Long story short, it was a commercial decision because there were so many grain producers in America. So really, it was more about profit than health, and we were raised on that being called a 'healthy diet'.

Fortunately, now the reality of the evidence is getting more accepted and it is becoming clear that we need to cut out grains to achieve a greater level of health and wellbeing. If you've been eating a lot of grains, on this you'll feel better than ever!

> **Regularly including grains**
>
> If you are focused on gaining muscle, you might find it necessary to include grains to be able to get enough carbohydrate for better protein synthesis.
>
> In that case, if you can go through each of the reasons and confirm that they do not apply, then you can eat grains more regularly. For example, here are the four reasons along with potential answers:
>
> 1. **They are calorie-dense** – Maybe you want more calories because you are on a bulking diet, or you are disciplined with portion control and can avoid eating too much
> 2. **They are high-GI** – You can stick to lower GI grains, like quinoa, brown rice and oats (they are whole foods, and have a GI around 50, so not that low, but at least not that high)
> 3. **They are high in omega-6** – If you are having smaller portions, you can still balance the omega-6 by regularly eating fish
> 4. **They have gluten** – If you tolerate gluten very well, then this is not an issue for you
>
> Keep an eye on your goals. If this is helping you progress towards them and you do not feel any ill effects, then you can continue to include grains on a regular basis.

Rule 3 – Whole foods

This is key and applies to rules one and two – eat whole foods, as close to their original state as possible. Whole, natural foods are what our bodies are used to, as our ancestors ate whole foods for hundreds of thousands of years. This means our bodies are very well adapted to eating whole foods, keeping us lean and full of energy.

The more foods are refined, the more calorie-dense and less nutritious they become. We saw this in particular with sweets that are highly refined and contain almost no vitamins or minerals! Breads and grain foods are generally refined as well and are usually calorie-dense, high-GI and loaded with omega-6 – all things we need to avoid!

A recent study showed that eating more whole vegetables and fruit help people live longer. In a 7.7 year study of over 60,000 people, it was evident that people who ate most vegetables are about half less likely to die from any cause (including cancer and heart disease) than those who ate the least amount per day[97]. In addition, eating processed foods like canned fruit actually increased the chance of death[97]! The study also showed that vegetables are four times better than fruits at protecting us. **It is clear that if you want to live longer, eat at least seven portions of whole vegetables a day**[97].

Keep it clean and eat whole foods. Protein sources are usually whole, although avoid foods like pâtés and processed meats which are not close to their original forms, are calorie-dense and loaded with additives like sugars and trans fats.

Dairy products are one exception as processing milk into products such as butter, cheese and yoghurt doesn't always make it unhealthy and can still be very natural. The problem is when there are all sorts of sugars and flavouring added. Stick to sugar free, natural dairy products to maintain automatic calorie management.

Water – drink more water for both Core ACM and Complete ACM

Water is really important to be successful in maintaining your goal body, not so much because of the health benefits, but more because of *what it replaces*. Instead of sodas and other flavoured drinks, drink water! You'll be amazed at how much sugar you can cut out of your diet if you drink water instead of all those popular drinks.

If you are not a regular water drinker, then this is your chance to make it your drink of choice. Keep a water bottle handy for any time you get thirsty to prevent the temptation of going for a soda or juice. Cultivating a desire to drink water instead of other drinks will be a massive help throughout your life.

Water itself is a crucial substance that is absolutely needed by our bodies. As we all know, we simply can't live without water. Water makes up most of our bodies, and is used in nearly every chemical process happening inside us. Clean water is simply one of the healthiest things we can ingest! I personally actually drink quite a lot of water – probably around two to three litres a day. From personal experience, too little water often results in headaches and feeling tired.

But how much water do we actually need? You might be surprised to learn that there is no evidence that we need a lot of water, or that more water has any health benefits. In fact, the common advice to drink eight glasses a day is not supported by evidence at all[98]. Turns out, the water in foods, coffees, and even some alcohol like beer all add towards your total water intake, and really, your body knows when it needs water, which is when you feel thirsty.

This is how you really know if you need to hydrate – if your body tells you it is thirsty, then drink some water. If you feel thirsty, it does not mean you are already dehydrated. Dehydration follows much, much later after initial thirst. Of course, if you are exercising a lot, sweating a lot, or in a very hot environment, then you need more water. Keep that water bottle close so you don't turn to something else!

> **Take an honest look...**
>
> Sugary drinks are one of the biggest causes of obesity as they are so good at pumping us full of sugar throughout the day. It can actually be hard to recognise that you are drinking a lot of sugary drinks, as many of them try to look like healthy drinks with labels saying things like "organic" or "all natural". Meanwhile they are still loaded with sugar!
>
> Take a good look at what drinks you buy – at work and at home. Look at what you drink and what is in it. Is there sugar? Then it needs to go out!
>
> By far the easiest way to eliminate all the sugary drinks it to swap it with plain tap water. Get a water bottle and keep it close. Fill it up with tap water and keep drinking from that when you are thirsty. Soon you'll only want water and your goals will be so much easier to reach!

Oils and fats – coconut oil and butter is best for cooking for both Core ACM and Complete ACM

As you saw in the Dietary Fat section, most plant oils are very high in omega-6, which is what we are trying to avoid. This actually makes them unhealthy, as they work against us in reaching a healthy omega-3 to omega-6 balance. When our balance is out, it results in systemic inflammation, causing headaches, joint pain, asthma, heart disease, and a number of other diseases.

An alternative to vegetable oils is coconut oil, which is mainly saturated fats and thus has almost no omega-6. For cooking purposes, you can always also use butter, ghee or tallow as healthy alternatives to vegetable oils.

▶ Coffee and caffeine – limit to one cup in the morning for both Core ACM and Complete ACM

What's the deal with coffee – is it good or bad? At the end of the day, caffeine is a psychoactive drug, meaning it crosses into the brain and affects your mood and behaviour. While a lot of it can be bad for your health, a bit can be helpful too. Again, it is about balance.

We will talk more about coffee in the Boost Your Brain section, but for now, the main advice is to keep it to one cup a day in the morning. Avoid coffee (or any caffeinated drink) in the afternoons and evenings, especially if you have trouble sleeping. Remember that we are keeping away from sugar, so don't add sugar. Later we will go into more detail about the science behind coffee and how it affects us.

▶ Herbs and spices – use as much as you like with both Core ACM and Complete ACM

If you don't love these already, it is time to start discovering the all the amazing and delicious herbs and spices available to you! Not only do they taste great, but they also provide micros, so eating a variety of herbs and spices is a great way of getting more vital nutrients into your diet while also keeping meals tasty and interesting.

▶ Sweeteners – limit and use instead of sugar for both Core ACM and Complete ACM

While many diets will tell you to stay away from sweeteners, the Think Lean Method is an *evidence-based healthy eating plan* which means we go where the evidence goes. And unfortunately for the common opinion, there doesn't appear to be real evidence that sweeteners are dangerous.

Aspartame is generally considered to be the worst of the lot, but there is no credible evidence to prove it is bad for us[99]. Some would point to animal studies that caused tumours in rats, but even then the rats were fed huge amounts of aspartame. For humans, this would be on the order of seven litres of sweetened soda per day, every day. At those levels, just about anything is poisonous. After all, even lemons, onions and broccoli contain cancer-causing substances[100]. You could even die from a water overdose! In reality, if there was any conclusive evidence that sweeteners are bad for us in *normal amounts*, they would have been pulled from the market ages ago.

Compare that with actual sugar that is *proven* to be dangerous even in moderate amounts as shown in the Carbohydrates section. We know it causes diabetes, it causes overeating and obesity. This growing evidence that real sugar is bad for us is increasing the call for sugar to be regulated like alcohol and tobacco[101]. Compare sugar to sweeteners and it becomes clear that if you really want something sweet, sweeteners are a much better choice.

If you are looking for something to do cooking with, sweeteners like stevia, xylitol or erythritol can be good options. Xylitol does actually have calories in it – around half that of usual sugar, but it is much lower on the Glycaemic Index, meaning it has less of an effect on blood-sugar. Xylitol is natural, and is even good for your teeth[102]. Erythritol is emerging as a good substitute overall as it has zero calories, is very safe[103] and is completely absorbed by the body, meaning it does not get the chance like other sweeteners to cause gastric distress[104]. New sweeteners combine erythritol and stevia to be more sugar-like.

I know, after all the fear mongering about sweeteners, it can be difficult to accept that sweeteners are not evil. But look at it this way – it means you can use sweeteners in recipes, coffee, and even eat candy and chocolate that contain sweeteners as a weight-safe treat. Try to avoid sweet foods, but if you really want something sweet, this is a better way to go.

Alcohol – avoid for faster results
"Is alcohol part of Automatic Calorie Management?"

Generally, the answer is *"No"*. ACM is about *Automatic Calorie Management*, while alcohol is more like *Automatically Consume More*. ACM does not need a lot of self-control, as the foods are less calorie-dense and promote you feeling full faster. To keep alcohol intake at a moderate level takes a lot of self-control.

Also, alcohol breaks a few of our ACM rules:

- **No sugar** – Most alcoholic drinks are loaded with carbohydrates, especially sugar. Drinks like mixers are basically sugary soft drinks with alcohol in it
- **No grains** – Beers are usually made from grains
- **Whole foods** – Alcoholic drinks are refined and very distant from their original whole forms, often containing many other chemicals to get the desired taste

"Can I still lose weight while drinking alcohol?"

It is possible, but again it takes self-discipline and moderation. Caffeine is a stimulant that could actually help you with weight loss. Alcohol is not like that. Alcohol slows you down, adds refined calories to your diet, and is usually consumed in a setting with carbohydrate-rich foods like potato wedges.

Regularly drinking alcohol can quickly sabotage your results. The carbohydrates and sugars in drinks quickly add up during the night, leading into the next day with a hangover while you crave fatty carbohydrate-rich foods to get over it.

Comparing drinks in the table to the right shows how many of them come with a lot of carbohydrates and calories. Let's go from best to worst (from a carbohydrate-weight loss perspective):

- **Spirits** are the lowest in carbohydrates, but you'd have to do them straight up, as pretty much any cocktail or mix comes with a whole lot of sugar. Also it can be

Alcoholic drinks	% Alcohol	Serving Size	Calories per Serve	Carbs per Serve
Spirits				
Absolut Vodka	40%	30 ml	65	0
Bacardi Gold Rum	40%	30 ml	65	0
Crown Royal Canadian Whiskey	40%	30 ml	64	0
Smirnoff Vodka	40%	30 ml	64	0
Jack Daniel's Whiskey	40%	30 ml	65	0
Jose Cuervo Gold Tequila	40%	30 ml	64	0
Seagram's Gin	40%	30 ml	80	0
Red wine				
Shiraz	15%	150 ml	142	1
Pinot Noir	13%	150 ml	121	3
Cabernet Sauvignon	11.8%	150 ml	104	4
Merlot	12.5%	150 ml	115	5
Tawny Port	17%	60 ml	167	22
White wine				
Champagne	12.5%	150 ml	132	2
Chardonnay	13.9%	150 ml	104	3
Riesling	8%	150 ml	108	8
Silvaner	10%	150 ml	158	15
Sherry	17%	60 ml	160	20
Beer and flavoured drinks				
Bud Light	4.2%	375 ml	110	7
Budweiser	5%	375 ml	145	11
Guinness	4.2%	375 ml	128	11
Heineken	5%	375 ml	150	12
Corona Extra	4.6%	375 ml	148	14
Smirnoff Ice	5%	375 ml	241	38

very hard to only drink one or two shots for a night, so there is a strong tendency to keep drinking. Still, if you want to get smashed and not gain weight, this is the way to go

- **Red wine** comes in second after spirits from a weight loss perspective. Stay away from the dessert wines like port, which are loaded with sugar. Red and white wines are usually associated with eating at restaurants or the like where you can have food alongside the wine and you may drink less than out at a party or club. A glass of red wine from time to time can actually be healthy

- **White wine** often contains quite a bit more preservatives and can be higher in sugar than red wine. It also contains less of the healthy compounds found in red wine. Again, stay away from the sweet wines. Champagne is actually not a bad choice for a night out

- **Beers and flavoured drinks** are generally too high in carbohydrates and quickly end up sabotaging our results. Mixers like Smirnoff Ice come in with a lot of sugar. After all, that is how they get them to taste so good! Definitely stay away from these if you trying to reach body goals

If you really want to have a drink, go with red wine or champagne. Stick to only one or two glasses and don't drink more than twice a week, but know that this doesn't support healthy eating and is not part of ACM. If you do it only once or twice a week, you can probably still lose weight. Still, if you notice yourself not losing weight, cut more alcohol and see if that helps!

Rule 4 – Mix it up

This is a general rule that also applies to rules one and two. Get some variety and mix it up! This is particularly important for nutrition because you need variety to be healthy. Mix it up means:

- **Eat different foods** – foods have different vitamins and minerals. Eating the same thing over and over is likely to result in a vitamin or mineral imbalance

- **Use different cooking methods** – boiling, baking, frying, steaming and microwaving can have different effects on vitamins and minerals. Use different methods and mix it up!

A quick note on microwaving – it is often thought that cooking food in a microwave destroys nutrients. This is a myth. You can still cook healthy meals in a microwave. For example, broccoli actually keeps more nutrients when you microwave it, than if you boiled it on a stove[105]. As long as you don't overcook in a microwave (same goes for any other method), then you can preserve nutrients.

Apart from the nutritional aspect, mixing it up keeps us from getting bored with eating the same foods over and over. This is something to recognise within yourself early on – if you know you get bored with foods quickly, prepare for that so that you start eating different foods to keep it interesting.

Rule 5 – Slow down

Of course, we can all act like champion competitive eaters and finish off a kilogram steak and still have space for dessert, but we need to start training ourselves to recognise when we are full by **stopping when we start to feel full**. Sure, you can probably speed through a dish and finish it before you even start to feel that you are full.

This is why you need to remember is that it takes a bit of time for your stomach to let you know that you are getting full. The best way to allow yourself to reach the feeling of being full is to **slow down.**

In the Protein Section we learned how new research has shown that protein increases the release of specific peptides that determine if we are full from eating. We saw that eating protein releases more of these peptides than carbohydrates, and so makes us feel full faster. This is all well and good, but here is an important point – *if you are chewing the next mouthful before the previous mouthful have even reached your stomach, then the peptides are not going to be able to release in time to let you know that you are full and shouldn't be eating more!*

There is a simple message here - eat slowly to give your body the time to respond to your food intake. Here are some practical ways to slow down eating.

1. **Have meals with family, friends or colleagues and talk throughout the meal**. This will force breaks in-between bites and extend mealtime, giving your body time to signal when you are full!

2. **Chew thoroughly and enjoy the flavour of the food.** We tend to have this strange urge to take the next bite to taste more food, but really it's not going to taste any different from the current bite, so enjoy the bite you're with!

3. **Take a break between bites and drink plenty of water**. This trick is especially effective because it builds a habit – take a bottle of water along to every meal and take a sip after two or three bites. This helps in two key ways:

    i. It forces you to put down your utensils or food and take a sip, increasing the length of a meal

    ii. The water adds to the volume in your stomach, making you feel full faster

By following these simple tricks, you will start to work *with* your body, giving it the time to tell you when you are full, leaving your feeling satisfied and happy that you didn't eat more than you needed.

If you have had a 'pleasure-eating' habit for a long time, then you might not feel full as soon as you should. In instances like this, you will start to break down the pleasure-eating habit by not going for seconds when your plate is empty by reaching for more whole and healthy foods like vegetables, proteins or drinking more water. Eventually, the pleasure-eating habit will get weaker and weaker, and it will get easier and easier for you to stop eating when you are full. The key is acting consistently, and also, thinking consistently!

Remember – it's not a competition! And don't be afraid to throw away the leftovers if you are scared you might eat more than you are hungry for – and be happy when you are full before your plate is empty! Another trick is to pack the leftovers away in the fridge before you eat them so that you are not tempted to refill your plate!

What to remember – the five rules:
- Quality protein with every meal
- Low-GI carbohydrates
- Whole foods
- Mix it up
- Slow down

2.2 The Think Lean food pyramid

Now that we have our rules ready and know which foods fit in, we can map them out on a *brand new food pyramid* which replaces the old, outdated pyramid that has held us back from reaching our goals. Our new food pyramid shows which foods are proven to help us stay healthy and achieve our body weight goals.

As we talked through the main food sources, we split them between:

1. **Core ACM** where you can eat as much as you like of specific food groups and lose weight, even with little or no exercise
2. **Complete ACM** where you can eat as much as you like from a wider group of foods provided you are living an active lifestyle with regular gym/exercise sessions each week

So, let's put it all together! Here is the Think Lean food pyramid!

How it works:

Each section of the pyramid roughly represents the amount of calories you should be getting from a certain food group.

The dark coloured-in sections shows the foods to eat for **Core ACM**:

- Most calories come from **lean meats**, poultry, fish and eggs. Eat around two servings (150g / 5 ounces) with every meal

- The second-most calories should come from **low-GI, non-starchy vegetables**. Since vegetables are less calorie-dense, a good rule of thumb is to have twice as many vegetables as meat on your plate. Eat around three servings (200g / 7 ounces) with every meal

- **Nuts and oils** are part of healthy eating, including products like almond meal and coconut products. Though stay away from other plant oils because they are high in omega-6. Remember that we want most of our calories to come from lean meats and vegetables, so keep nuts and oils to around one serving (about 30g / 1 ounce) a day

- **Dairy products** with no added sugar can be a regular part of healthy eating too, like milk and hard cheeses (yes, we are excluding ice cream and cream cheeses). Same as with nuts and oils, keep dairy products to around one serving (about 30g / 1 ounce) a day so that we can get the benefits of generous meat and vegetable servings

The light coloured-in sections show the foods to eat for **Complete ACM** in addition to the Core ACM foods:

- It includes all the **Core ACM foods**
- Eat two servings (150g, 5 ounces) of **fatty meats** for one meal a day to get more fuel from dietary fats. Eat lean meats or eggs for the other meals
- Include two or three servings of (max 200g / 7 ounces) **starchy vegetables** (except white potatoes) for one meal a day for more low-GI carbohydrates. Eat non-starchy vegetables for the other meals
- Add in a serving of **legumes** as another carbohydrate and protein source. We still want most of our calories to come from meats and vegetables, so keep this to one serving (uncooked about 45g / 1.5 ounces) a day

At the top of the pyramid is fruit, which is a '**sometimes food**' to be had in moderation in both Core ACM and the Complete ACM. Preferably less than a serving a day. If you regularly eat fruit and are not getting results, cut back and see if that helps.

Remember to **exclude sugar and grains**. They are bad for both your health and your waistline!

It's that simple. Think of Core ACM and Complete ACM as two sides of the pyramid:

- If you need to lose a lot of weight and keep it off with little exercise, stay focused on the Core ACM side of the pyramid
- If you need more calories to support you working out a lot, then you can look at both sides of the pyramid. For those looking to build a lot of lean muscle mass, you can add additional Complete ACM meals (up to six meals in total) as required to get enough carbohydrates and protein

> In the **Think Lean Plan** section, we will put together a list of foods, including herbs, spices, oils and more so you have a good guide for shopping and what to eat. We will also show you practical steps to implement and start following your healthy eating plan, to get real, lasting results!
>
> Want more options? Not everyone's goals are the same, so visit www.thinkleanmethod.com for additional food pyramids designed for different goals. All the food pyramids are based on the research in the Fundamental Nutrition section to provide brain-optimised healthy eating plans.

What to remember:
- Follow Core ACM if you are not exercising
- Follow Complete ACM if you are exercising regularly
- Use the Think Lean Pyramid to guide your eating habits!

2.3 Exercise

So we've mentioned an 'active lifestyle' a few times now, but how does exercise really fit into this plan? A simple rule that is often repeated is that 80% of losing weight is healthy eating, while 20% is exercise.

This is not entirely correct as you can 100% achieve your weight target simply through your eating plan. If you want to weigh less, then you can stick to healthier eating. If you want to weigh more, then you can include more calorie-dense foods. *You have full control over your weight simply through what you eat.* You can even ask any champion fitness model or body builder how they get their well-defined 6-pack abs, and they will tell you: *"Abs are made in the kitchen."*

But if that's true, what's the point of exercising? Apart from all the health benefits for your brain and metabolism, it is simple – **exercise affects body composition**.

Body composition is a term we use to refer to the amount of muscle vs body fat. The more muscle and less body fat you have, the more defined and muscly you will appear. Reality is, even though you can get the weight you want through eating alone, you may want a different body composition to what you will get that way. If you want a strong and lean body, then you have to exercise. You can't become strong through eating alone.

The table below shows a few examples of how different body compositions affect appearance. Of course, body composition varies so widely and different people have different preferences, so the examples below are really just to give you an idea of what kind of types there are out there.

If you do not exercise, then you'll have very little muscle mass. Consistently eating healthy while not exercising will eventually give you a *slim* body. If you want to be *lean*, *toned*, *athletic* or more, you'll need to exercise!

Body composition		
Muscle	**Body fat**	**Body**
Very little muscle	Very low body fat	**Thin** – not necessarily healthy
Little muscle	Low body fat	**Slim** – fashion model look
Little muscle	Med-high body fat	**Overweight** – can be unhealthy
Some muscle	Low body fat	**Lean/Toned** – bikini model look
More muscle	Low body fat	**Athletic** – fitness model look
Large muscles	Low body fat	**Bodybuilder** – bulky look*

* A balanced, competitive physique can take years to develop

How does exercise and weight loss work? To make a long story short:

- Exercise makes muscles ready to grow
- Plenty of protein is needed to grow muscles
- Calorie restriction through healthy eating is needed to reduce body fat
- Endurance or High Intensity Interval Training sessions help to burn body fat

A lot of women are afraid that working out means they will get bulky, so let's dispel that myth right here – it takes massive amounts of effort to develop a bulky, bodybuilder physique. These women put in years of extreme dedication, gorging on healthy meals and spending tons of time lifting very heavy weights to get those bodies. There is **no** chance that you will 'accidentally' get a bulky body like that!

Instead, working out, even with heavy weights, will only make you lean, or at best athletic if you put in a lot of effort. It's important to know that different types of exercise give different kinds of muscles:

- **Light weights with high repetitions** (lifting 5kg a hundred times) make smaller muscles – *imagine a marathon runner who exercises a lot, but has a very slim body*

- **Heavy weights with low repetitions** (lifting 50kg eight times and less) develops larger muscles
  – *imagine a sprinter who runs a short distance and develops bulky muscles*

This is because we have two basic kinds of muscles – **fast and slow twitch muscles**.

- **Fast twitch muscles** are used by sprinters to run fast. They need to be exercised with heavy weights, and grow when there is a large amount of protein in the diet. They also run out of energy quickly, which is why sprinters can only run that fast for short distances. They use glycogen stored within the muscle for energy
- **Slow twitch muscles** need to be exercised with low weights and high repetitions. They can be used for a long time, using oxygen and also body fat (after about 45 minutes)

Now you can start to see that you will need to do different kinds of workouts depending on your goal. **Not doing any exercise means you are working towards a goal of a 'slim' body,** as you will not get much in terms of muscle definition.

The good news is that both sides of the Think Lean food pyramid are great for exercise. If you do any exercise when on this healthy eating plan, you will see great results as you will be getting lots of protein for lean muscles, while getting low calories to keep body fat low. Even if you do not exercise, the higher protein intake will help prevent muscle loss and you'll lose more body fat instead.

Depending on the kind of body you want and how fast you want it, here is a comparison of exercise routines, the target body to get from it, and which part of the pyramid is best to follow for it:

Type and amount of exercise	Target body composition	Speed of results	Diet
No exercise, walking	**Slim** Little to no muscle definition Low body fat	Slow and easy	Core ACM
Some sports, outdoors activities, High Intensity Interval Training (HIIT) (1-3 days a week)	**Slim** Little muscle definition Low body fat	Moderate	Core ACM
Weights or HIIT (3-4 days a week)	**Lean / Toned** Some muscle definition Low body fat	Moderate	Core ACM or Complete ACM
Weights or HIIT (5-6 days a week)	**Lean / Toned** Good muscle definition Low body fat	Fast	Complete ACM
Heavy free weights (4-5 days a week)	**Athletic** Great muscle definition Low body fat	Fast	Complete ACM
Heavy free weights (4 days a week) and Intense HIIT sessions (2 days a week)	**Athletic** Great muscle definition Very low body fat – clear 6 pack!	Very Fast	Complete ACM
Heavy free weights (5-6 days a week) Additional cardio sessions Very high protein intake, very clean diet	**Bodybuilder** *Excellent* muscle definition Very low body fat – clear 6 pack!	Very Fast*	Complete ACM, Core ACM for competition prep
Heavy free weights (5-6 days a week) Additional cardio sessions Very high protein intake, very clean diet Extensive supplementation (*expert supervision recommended*)	**Bodybuilder** *Extreme* muscle definition and bulky muscles Very low body fat – clear 6 pack!	Very fast*, do with supervision	Complete ACM, Core ACM for competition prep

* A balanced, competitive physique can take years to develop

Keep in mind, that the above guidelines are simply that – guidelines. Listen to your body and see what works for you. If you are on Complete ACM, but not losing weight (if that's your goal), then swap to Core ACM. If you are doing a lot of exercise and want a super lean body, you could stay on Core ACM. Or if you want more muscle definition and you're not getting it on Core ACM, then swap to Complete ACM.

There is no one-size-fits-all, as we all have different bodies and different goals. So listen to your body and work with it! Also check in with us online for exercise plans. In the **Think Lean Plan** section, we'll talk more about how to keep yourself on track to get consistent results.

What to remember:
- You can reach 100% of your target weight through healthy eating alone, but exercise is still important!
- Exercise affects body composition which is the ratio of muscle to body fat
- Do different exercises depending on your target body

2.4 Busting myths

Now that we have talked through Automatic Calorie Management, let's put it in context with some common myths that seem to pop up around diets. Let's face it – there is so much misinformation out there about nutrition that even the experts end up disagreeing with each other!

Everyone has an opinion - something they heard, something they read. One friend is doing this, another is doing that, this worked for that person, that worked for another, anecdote after anecdote. How do we get some order to all this and clear up the **facts**?

Simple – let's use scientific research to clear up some myths and show you what has and hasn't been proven. Next time someone brings up a diet myth, you'll have the knowledge to set them straight!

> **The plural of 'anecdote' is not 'data'**
>
> Anecdotes – those little snippets of information.
>
> *"Oh this worked for me"*
> *"I've been doing that and it's great"*
>
> The problem with anecdotes is that they are extremely unreliable. Often the person giving the anecdote doesn't know what really gave the result, but instead attributes the result to what they think it must have come from. This is why we trust in 'data'. Specifically, *scientific data* that has been proven and peer reviewed. Proven data shows us what we can rely on to work for us, as it has been scientifically proven to work for many others.

2.4.1 Myth: It's all about energy in vs. energy out

The basis of a great myth is a hint of truth, which is what has made this myth so pervasive. You'll often hear from trainers and 'diet experts' that losing weight is all about 'energy in and energy out', and if you do not burn more than you take in, you will not lose weight. Sometimes they even say that *"you can't change the laws of physics"*.

In a broad sense, this is true - you can't change the laws of physics and they do apply to us, even when we're trying to achieve and maintain our goal bodies! However, our bodies use different nutrients in different ways due to the physiological processes that our bodies use to digest and use nutrients. As you learned in the first section where we talked about metabolism, different calories are used by the body in different ways. There have been plenty of studies about the thermic effect of food, showing that protein calories take much more energy to absorb than other calories.

You've also seen evidence showing that proteins and dietary fats trigger peptides that make you feel full faster, while calories from sugars and high-GI carbohydrates make you want to eat more.

Sure, it is ultimately all just energy going in and out. But some kinds of energy make you want to eat more and can result in health issues such as heart disease and diabetes, while other kinds make you feel full faster, support lean muscle mass for metabolism, and are great for overall health.

This is where ACM guides you to ensure you get the right kind of energy in – clean, whole foods to keep you energised and lean.

2.4.2 Myth: Saturated fat is bad for you

This is one of the longest lasting myths, based on a study that only showed a possible correlation between saturated fat and heart disease. It is well known and accepted among scientific circles (and anyone with common sense) that **correlation does not imply causation**. For example, just because most people die lying in bed doesn't mean that beds are dangerous!

Since the original study by Dr. Ancel Keys in 1957 showed a correlation between heart disease and saturated fat[106], many more studies were conducted to further prove that idea. Study after study failed to come up with a concrete link between the two, even failing to find a possible mechanism for saturated fat to give you heart disease. It culminated in the Cochrane Group conducting an extensive meta-analysis of all studies conducted to date. A meta-analysis involves evaluating and standardising the results of all related studies, and compiling these to draw very accurate results.

The result was that saturated fat intake had no effect on death rate[52]. None at all. Straight away, this meta-analysis showed that the extensive body of research available contradicts the popular position that we must pursue low-fat diets and that saturated fat is a so-called 'bad fat'. **So let's be clear – both unsaturated and saturated fats are actually 'good fats'!**

Doesn't saturated fat increase LDL, the bad cholesterol, you ask? It actually does, but here's the part you probably don't know. There are two kinds of LDL – large fluffy particles and small dense particles. The large fluffy ones do not harm us and do not clog arteries, while the small dense particles are the ones that cause heart attacks. Saturated fat from animal products (the main form of intake) only increases large fluffy LDL particles, meaning that it does not do you any harm! On top of that, saturated fat also increases HDL, the so-called 'good cholesterol', which clears out LDL.

We've also seen studies that show swapping saturated fats with carbohydrates actually increase the risk of heart disease[107]. Another study, covering over 300,000 people, also came to the same conclusion – there is no link between saturated fat and heart disease[108]. Researchers have even looked specifically at red meat to see if it is related to heart attacks. Again, the study showed that there was no correlation[109].

Frustratingly, the health bodies that first accepted these trouble-causing studies are now so entrenched in their position that the overwhelming evidence proving the exact opposite has not yet been able to convince them to update their positions.

2.4.3 Myth: Eating cholesterol will increase your cholesterol

This is another one that seems logical, but is completely wrong. Your body needs cholesterol to function properly and it is definitely not the bad guy it has been made out to be! There is a common belief that cholesterol clogs your arteries and causes heart attacks, but that is just not the case!

One common area you'll see people worrying about this is when they avoid eating eggs due to the cholesterol in them. But in reality, studies have shown that where people introduced eggs (yolks and whites) into their normal diets, the results showed that their HDL (so-called 'good cholesterol') was the one that increased in their blood levels[110].

Of course, this doesn't mean your blood cholesterol levels doesn't matter – you still need to pay attention if your cholesterol levels are getting too high, but it won't be because you are eating saturated fat or eating cholesterol. It will more likely be due to too much grain or sugar in your diet. Those are the real risks for heart disease.

2.4.4 Myth: Lots of protein is bad for your kidneys

Even though we've mentioned this already, this is worth reiterating. This is one of those long standing myths that everyone seems to have heard of, but which is simply not true. There is no evidence to support this myth, and there has been plenty of research done to confirm that there is indeed no link between high protein diets and kidney damage.

Since high protein diets are frequently used for diabetes, there has been a lot of research on this subject. A study in 2013 from diabetes research showed that there is no link between high protein diets and kidney disease[111]. Another showed the same thing, finding that high protein does not affect the kidneys unless there is pre-existing kidney disease[112]. Similarly, another diet also showed exactly the same thing – no link between kidney damage and high protein diets[113]. Others have even postulated that too much protein will leach calcium out of bones, but this has also been shown to be false[114].

So rest assured – there is plenty of evidence that shows you are not going to damage your kidneys if you go on a high protein diet. At the same time, if you are really worried anyway or maybe have kidney damage already, then you can keep your protein portions smaller and eat more of the other food sources on the pyramid. It is that easy! You can always tailor and fit healthy eating to your lifestyle and choices. Just pick from the right foods, and ACM can still work for you!

2.4.5 Myth: Eating fat makes you fat

How could this not be true? It seems so obvious! First of all, as we've clearly set out in the Macronutrients section, there is a big difference between dietary fat and the body fat around our hips and waist. It's definitely confusing that we use the term 'fat' to refer to both of these, but they are very different!

Dietary fats are an important part of our diets. For instance, without fats, we cannot digest fat-soluble vitamins such as A, D, E and K. We also need fats as a source of energy, and since it takes longer to digest and absorb, it is a more constant form of energy as opposed to sugars which cause spikes, leaving us to ride an energy rollercoaster.

As we saw in the Dietary Fat section, they also make us feel full much faster than carbohydrates. This means that foods containing fats are less more-ish than sugary treats, meaning you'll eat less overall, helping you to lose weight! It is no wonder that the big push for fat-free foods coincided with the obesity epidemic, since suddenly foods that made us feel full were removed and replaced with foods that just made us want to eat more.

When our blood sugar spikes from sugary and high-GI foods, insulin is released to clear the excess sugar from the blood. Insulin first stores excess sugar as glycogen, and then when the glycogen stores are full, the excess sugar is stored as body fat. Unless you are doing a whole lot of exercise to keep using up the glycogen stores, your body will quickly start to store the excess sugar as fat. Fat taken on its own or with protein does not result in an insulin release, thus is does not promote fat storage nearly as much as sugars and high-GI foods.

2.4.6 Myth: Eating more frequently will speed up your metabolism

"Eat five to six times a day, and watch your metabolism go into overdrive!" We hear this all too often. So often, in fact, that it is preached by an astonishing number of diets out there. A lot of theories have popped up to support this idea, but the science shows us that it just doesn't work like that.

Study after study has failed to find any evidence that an increased number of meals leads to an increased metabolic rate and thus increased weight loss. Some of these studies included the use of Whole Room Calorimeters, where a person stays in the room while air supply and respiration is tightly monitored, along with all other waste and energy expended. Given that fat is metabolised mainly into carbon dioxide and water, these types of instruments can provide us with very accurate measurements on the metabolic rates of our bodies.

One result showed that eating one meal a day, while maintaining calorie intake, helps to reduce fat mass[115]. Another study measuring energy expenditure concluded that increasing meals from three to six per day may actually increase the desire to eat[116]. A further study concluded that increasing the frequency of meals does not help with additional weight loss[117]. Yet another showed that the resting metabolic rate largely depends on lean muscle mass, and is also very much determined by genetics[11]. One study simply concluded that changing meal frequency does not have any significant effect[118].

Through these studies, we can see that the frequency of meals does not help to increase metabolism[119], with one study even showing the opposite[115]. Still, some people swear by six meals, others love one meal a day (intermittent fasting), which is a testament to how adaptable our bodies are!

Eating more regularly can result in eating more calories overall. If your goal is to eat more, such as to build more muscle, then going for six meals a day is a good approach. To that extent, one study showed that people who eat at night time just before bed usually gained more weight and ate more calories in total than those who didn't[120]. This is a useful strategy to help gain muscle, or if you are struggling to lose weight and you are a night time eater, it might be time to change that habit!

If you really want to increase your metabolic rate, you'll need to increase your lean muscle mass, as more muscle needs more calories to function, even when you are resting[11]. As for how often you should eat, it is largely up to your personal preference. On ACM, you can eat often and you won't have to worry about putting on weight, so you can eat more regularly if you prefer. Otherwise, eating three or four times a day isn't going to damage your metabolism, so don't worry!

To keep that lean muscle mass, you will need to eat more protein, as this is what maintains muscle, which is where ACM will help you get results. By following the healthy eating plan, you can maintain muscle mass and thereby have a proportionally higher metabolism compared to low-protein diets. Use these proven techniques to your advantage!

2.4.7 Myth: We need to eat lots of fruit

We are often told how good fruit is for us and that we should eat lots of fruit each day. Just think of "An Apple a Day" and other slogans that advertisements have pushed on us. While fruits do provide some vitamins and minerals, they are also high in fructose which is a form of sugar that works against our weight loss goals.

The strange thing about fructose, which sets it apart from other forms of sugars, is that the body has to send it to the liver to be processed before it can be used. Other sugars raise blood sugar levels first, resulting in insulin trying to find a place where it can be used. When fructose is sent to the liver faster than the liver can process it, the liver starts to produce body fat cells and sends them off into the bloodstream, and you know where these get deposited!

One of the biggest problems with this myth is fruit juices. These sound like they would be healthy since they are made from fruit (the better quality types), but the truth is that they are pumped full of sugar, and often are high in fructose as well. This means we end up drinking lots of fruit juice, thinking that it is healthy, all the while we are gulping down a drink that contains more sugar than a sugary soda drink!

Where does this leave fruit? As we've worked through so far, fruits are not that great, since they contain fructose, but they are also not that bad, since they don't contain a great deal of fructose. That is why we leave it as a 'sometimes' food to be had in moderation. Eat no more than one a day, unless you want to get really low body fat (e.g. for competition prep), then you'd have to cut them out completely.

2.4.8 Myth: All foods are OK in moderation

There's an inherent problem here which is working out just how much is 'moderation'. Moderation differs for different types of food – a moderate amount of meat would be much greater than a moderate amount of sugar. So how do we know when we've reached 'moderate' and we need to stop?

The problem is that some foods actively work against us, such as sugars and high-GI carbohydrates which promote hormones and peptides that make us want to eat more. So to stick to moderation, we have to fight our natural impulses brought on by sweets and sweet foods. This makes it really difficult to eat those kinds of food in moderation, while other foods like meat and vegetables fill up us quickly so it is easy to stick to a moderate amount.

Stick to the foods in the Think Lean food pyramid and follow the guidelines on how much of each food group you should eat.

2.4.9 Myth: This or that food will give me cancer

How often do we hear that some new food has been proven to be a cancer-causing carcinogen? Luckily for us, most carcinogens found in food are so low in concentration that we are not at risk of developing cancer from them. Including broccoli.

The reality is that stressing about food is much worse for your health than the food itself. Yes it's true - all that stressing raises our cortisol levels. High cortisol levels have a huge range of negative effects on our health, especially if there is a constant amount of stress that is keeping our cortisol levels too high. It is more important to avoid stress than worry about foods.

So instead, relax. Enjoy eating the good foods on the Think Lean pyramid which will do much more for your health and the quality of your life than stressing about food!

> **What to remember:**
> - Focus on what has been scientifically proven, rather than taking anyone's word (including the media) on the latest fad
> - Stick to the Think Lean Method for healthy eating that is proven for weight loss and boosting health

The Second Key:

3 Boost Your Brain

*We often hear how important it is to look after our body and our mind, but what exactly do we mean by 'mind'? And how do we make sure it is healthy? The mind itself is very complex, so we need to take a broader view to understand how to make sure we have a healthy mind. To begin, let's look at the two parts that make up the mind - the **physical brain** and the **thinking and actions** that emerge from it.*

The brain plays a crucial role in our overall health and wellbeing, but it's easy to forget about it since it's always just there, doing its thing. You might even be wondering, "Why do we even need to learn anything about it? I'm just here to get a lean body!"

Good question – so ask yourself:

- *Do you often get **tired**, or experience consistent tiredness?*
- *Do you ever have **trouble sticking to a diet**?*
- *Do you get a kind of '**brain fog**' and have trouble focusing?*
- *Do you find you become **irritable for no reason**?*
- *Do you have periods of **low motivation** or apathy?*
- *Do you find it a **challenge to stay consistent**, day by day, meal to meal?*

Well guess what – all these issues originate from the brain! And do you know what the most commonly used strategy is to deal with these issues? *Live with it.* That's right – most of us don't ever resolve these issues and they just become part of everyday life. You may even notice your conversation starts to be about it too – "Around 3:00 in the afternoon I'm going to crash." "Tomorrow morning I'm going to be so tired." "Before I can start work I really need a coffee... or five."

But I'm here to tell you that it doesn't need to be like this! **Don't learn to live with it – instead let's find and fix the problem and get your brain working at its best!** A well-functioning brain will support you to feel happy, healthy and confident – that's what this section is all about!

Improving your thinking is an important part of helping you to stay consistent with healthy eating. After all, if your diet isn't keeping your brain healthy and it makes you feel tired and depressed, how can you ever manage to stay motivated every day to eat right? This is where the Think Lean Method is different – it focuses on what other diets leave out by teaching you how to identify what is going wrong in your brain, and how to fix it.

Let's take a look at how the brain fits in with supporting our thoughts, actions and feelings. Keeping this simple – we want to feel 100%. *Feeling 100% means we feel confident and ready to take on whatever tasks are ahead of us. We feel we can relax when we want to, that we can focus when we want to, and have an overall sense of being in control.*

So what does it take to feel 100%?

- The first 50% is the health of your brain. How well your brain is nourished, whether it has everything it needs to function well, or if there are deficiencies holding it back. Do all the neurotransmitters function well? Does the environment help the brain create new brain cells?
- The next 50% is about how healthy your thoughts are. If you are plagued with negative thoughts and self-criticism, have beliefs that are holding you back, and have a constant flow of emotions that are bringing you down, then there is no way you are going to feel 100%! We need to turn this thinking around into constructive, confident thoughts that support your goals and help you stay consistent

Some of the concepts we have talked through in the first section will apply here, and similarly, some of what we will work through here will apply to the Think Lean section. It is all connected, and all works together to help you live a life where you are healthy, lean and confident!

To get us that first 50%, we need to find out more about the brain, why it is important, and what can we do to boost it.

3.1 What is the brain?

Simply put, your brain is the single most important part of your body. Everything else, every organ, even your heart, comes a very distant second. Think about it – you can lose an arm or a leg, you can get skin grafts, you can get organ transplants, even your heart can be replaced, and you still stay *you*. Damage to the brain, on the other hand, can mean a total personality change, memory loss, paralysis, and more. It is only the brain that contains the essence of who you are. All your memories are stored in the brain. All your thoughts, actions and feelings come from the brain. So to speak, the brain is the *seat of the mind*.

Sure, some of us *wish* we could get a brain transplant, but lucky for us, the brain is an organ that we actually have a lot of control over. We can *change our brains*[121]. We can change it through what we eat, and also how we think! This was a big discovery when scientists learned we have the power to change our brains, as now we have a clear view of what we can do to improve not only our bodies, but also improve our minds to learn how to think constructively and feel great.

The brain itself is made up of brain cells called **neurons**. A *lot* of neurons – nearly 100 billion of them. These neurons are connected to each other, with some neurons having thousands of connections to other neurons. The connections between neurons create **neural networks**, within which signals are fired from neuron to neuron across the chain.

It is amazing to think that our whole experience of the world and everything we do is the result of signals firing across millions of connected neural networks. Even more amazing is knowing that we can change those neural networks to help us be more successful in achieving our goals, especially getting the body we want!

The ability to change our brains was a big discovery in **neuroscience**, the science of studying the brain. It was once thought that the brain didn't change over time, but a series of experiments in the 1970s showed that the brain can change and does change constantly through our lives[122]. This feature of the brain is called **neuroplasticity**[121]. It means that the neurons are 'plastic', in that they can make new connections.

New techniques in studying the brain have allowed neuroscience to make huge advances over the last few decades, which we can use to help us reach our goals.

> **Myth – we only use 10% of our brains**
>
> Let's quickly correct an old myth – the one that we only use 10% of our brains. The reality is that when we perceive something, there is a 'whole brain response'. There are no areas in our brains that are never used. In fact, all areas of our brains are used through our lives, though we only use parts of our brains for individual situations.
>
> Really, you do not want your whole brain to activate all at once. If your whole brain activated, your mind would be filled with a million incoherent thoughts, while every muscle in your body tries to both contract and relax at the same time, causing a massive seizure.
>
> It is more accurate to say that we only use 10% of our brains **at any moment**. Of course, it could be more or less, depending on how engaged we are. Through our thoughts, we can actually control which parts of our brain we want to use, since the different parts have different functions.

To get a basic idea of what is happening in your brain, let's have a quick look at some basic anatomy of the brain. Of course, since this is not a course in neuroanatomy (luckily!), we will focus only on the areas that play the most important role in helping you reach your goals.

- **Prefrontal Cortex** – As our brains evolved, this is the most recent part and is also where complex thought and consciousness takes place. It is what houses our personality, and what we use to solve complex problems

- **Amygdala** – Everything that we sense from the outside, such as sight, touch, sounds, is sent from another part of the brain called the thalamus to the amygdala to check if there is a potential threat to us. If the amygdala perceives a threat, it produces the 'fight or flight' response, and can also create powerful fear-based memories

- **Hippocampus** – This tiny part of our brain plays a very big role! It is crucial in forming short-term memories and assists with the formation of long-term memories. Damage to the hippocampus can result in memory loss, in particular of short-term memories. This becomes crucial when we start to build new clean eating habits. We need our hippocampus to be working optimally to help build our new healthy habits quickly!

To keep the discussions relevant to us, let's focus on how they influence what we eat and our weight, and also how we can influence them to achieve our goals for our bodies and minds. There are essentially two direct ways we can change and improve these parts of our brains so that we can reach our goals more easily:

1. Through healthy eating, sleep and exercise
2. Through how we think and our environment

To get a better idea of how exactly you can improve our brain, let's look at four key factors related to the brain, what we can do to influence them, and what happens if there is an imbalance. These components are:

- **Brain composition**
- **Neurotransmitters**
- **Hormones**
- **Brain-derived neurotrophic factor**

> A note on 'boosting your brain' – as we step through each element that make up the brain, we will be having a look at a few symptoms that you might be feeling if you have a deficiency or an imbalance. Take a moment to think through the symptoms and see if they apply to you. If they do, have a look at the solutions further down to resolve the deficiencies and imbalances and look for ways that you can bring it into your life. After we have worked through these four components, I will give you an action plan to 'boost your brain'. It might just make you feel like a whole new person!
>
> *Remember – The information here is not intended nor implied to be used as a substitute for professional medical advice. You should always consult a healthcare professional to determine the suitability of the information for your own situation or if you have any questions regarding a medical condition or treatment plan.*

3.1.1 Brain composition

To take good care of your brain, you need to know what it is made of so that you can understand what types of nutrients it needs. Imbalances in the basic composition of the brain can have a serious effect on our mental and physical health. The main ingredients are[123]:

- **Water** – The main component is water, no big surprise here! This includes water inside the cells themselves
- **Lipids (body fat)** – The second largest component is body fat! That's right, the brain mainly consists mainly of fatty tissue. This is one of the reasons why dietary fat is so important – our brains are made from the stuff!
- **Cholesterol** – This is also very surprising, given how negatively cholesterol is viewed. Our brains are around 15% cholesterol, making it one of the largest components! Of course, our bodies can manufacture cholesterol by itself, and if we eat more cholesterol, it means our bodies manufacture less
- **Choline** – Another interesting one, since we spoke about this mineral before in the minerals section. Around 8% of the brain is choline, which reminds us how important it is to get all our vitamins and minerals!

The Think Lean food pyramid has been constructed with the composition and needs of the brain taken into account. This gives you a clear guideline for healthy eating that not only keeps your body healthy, but your brain as well!

If your diet is very different to these guidelines, you could have imbalances in the basic makeup of your brain. Look through the symptoms below and see if any apply to you.

Symptom: Irritability, aggression and depression

Since the 1950s it has been known that high LDL cholesterol is a risk factor for heart attacks[124]. This view has resulted in a number of therapies and diets focused on reducing cholesterol levels. To some extent, they do work in lowering the risk of a heart attack, but it comes at a price – in more recent years, low cholesterol levels have been linked to higher rates of death from suicide, violence or accidents[125,126].

These studies often report that low cholesterol levels are linked with increased aggression and irritability. One study showed that this leads to an increase in death from causes other than heart attacks[126]. It showed that while treatment to reduce cholesterol resulted in 28 fewer heart attacks, there were 29 more deaths from accidents, suicide or violence per 100,000 people! So overall, lower cholesterol just made things worse!

The results vary and the actual mechanism has not yet been fully determined, but there seems to be a clear link between cholesterol and our moods. So much so that depression is often cited along with low cholesterol levels as leading to suicidal behaviour[127]. Along with what we've discovered before (that cholesterol is not the enemy it has been made out to be, and that saturated fats are actually ok), it would seem that the demonization of cholesterol can actually have very negative effects on our mental health.

Saturated fats (from meats, coconut oil) increases total cholesterol – that is both large LDL particles and HDL. These are both **not** dangerous to our health, and are exactly what we need to overcome depression and aggression caused by low cholesterol levels. On the other hand, small LDL cholesterol from sugars is dangerous and must be avoided!

Symptom: Poor memory, memory loss

Choline is required to manufacture a neurotransmitter important for memory and also plays a role in transporting cholesterol. Given the big role that cholesterol plays, it is clear that choline is something we need to get from our diets to keep our brains working well. If you are noticing that you have memory problems, then it could be a lack of choline in your diet!

Symptom: Psychiatric and neurodegenerative diseases

These include depression, schizophrenia and Alzheimer's disease, which are linked to low levels of omega-3. It has been shown that EPA (an omega-3 fatty acid) can help with treating and protecting against these neurodegenerative diseases[63]. In addition, low levels of omega-3 are also linked to major depressive disorder and bipolar disorder[128,129].

The studies have shown that supplementing with omega-3 in the short to medium term benefits the treatment of these diseases and disorders, but we have to be careful here. These are polyunsaturated oils, which easily become rancid. When they become rancid, they cause oxidative damage in the body. The problem is that a lot of oil supplements go rancid while on the shelves, and we just never notice when we take them in pill form. This is why eating fish is better than supplementation. At least it is fresh and you'll notice if it's not!

3.1.2 Neurotransmitters

Neurotransmitters are the chemicals that mainly send signals between neurons. There are many neurotransmitters in the brain, so we will focus only on some of the more important ones that have the largest effects on our mood and motivation. These chemicals can both increase and decrease activity in the brain. Below are the key neurotransmitters:

- **Serotonin**
- **Dopamine**
- **Epinephrine** (adrenaline)
- **Norepinephrine** (noradrenaline)
- **Gamma-aminobutyric acid** (GABA)

With all neurotransmitters, we don't want too much or too little of any one type. What we really want is for all of these to be balanced and functioning in a healthy state. If the body doesn't have the nutrients it needs to maintain and make new neurotransmitters, it can cause our moods to change and we'll have a hard time with motivation and staying focused!

For example, if our brains can't make enough GABA, then we can easily become overexcited, resulting in anxiety, stress and a feeling of fear. The same with each of the transmitters – their absence can result in responses to situations that are not helpful – like stressing about something that you know isn't important, or not enjoying something that you used to enjoy.

This is why it is very important to ensure we have what we need to keep our neurotransmitters functioning well, and why we take a particular interest in them. Later on we will also see how transmitters like dopamine help us form new habits, using our new understanding of how the brain works to change itself and help us reach our goals.

Symptom: Food cravings

Carbohydrate-rich foods like bread and sweets create an insulin response, as we've seen before. We've looked at how this insulin response causes us to gain weight, but we haven't yet looked at how this affects our brain. Beyond storing additional body fat, insulin also removes **large neutral amino acids** (LNAA) from the bloodstream. These compete with **tryptophan** for entry into the brain through the blood-brain barrier. When the LNAA's have been removed, it means more tryptophan goes into the brain[130]. Tryptophan boosts the amount of serotonin in the brain, increasing our mood and making us feel happier[131].

This is how eating carbohydrates make us feel good, and it would be fine if it didn't come with some nasty side effects:

- First of all, there's the obvious point that eating a lot of carbohydrates (especially breads and sugars) makes us gain weight. Constantly eating a lot of carbohydrates means we store a little bit of body fat each day, which adds up over time to a lot of numbers on the scales!

- Secondly, chronically increased serotonin results in resistance to serotonin[132]. This can cause depression and mood disorders, in addition to feeling like you need to eat more to get the same feeling of happiness, leading to binge eating

- Lastly, the anticipation of the serotonin release (and feeling good) causes a dopamine spike[133], which strengthens the neural network that drives you to crave carbohydrate-rich foods. This strengthening of the 'craving neural network' forms a habit where you crave carbohydrate-rich foods whenever you want to feel better, need a boost or want a 'pick-me-up'. This is because when we get a dopamine spike, we are motivated to repeat the action. This plays a major role in developing both good habits (good dopamine releases) and bad habits (unhelpful dopamine releases). Once these kick in, they become second nature!

The weight gain factor is particularly troubling, since this causes a complex set of conditions, including reduced self-esteem. Reduced self-esteem and 'feeling low' causes us to want to feel better, initiating a search in the brain to find ways to feel better. Of course, the brain knows one really good way to feel better – eat carbohydrate-rich foods!

This then causes a vicious cycle, where we eat more carbohydrates, gain more weight, feel even worse, and develop serotonin resistance, causing us to have to eat more to feel better, resulting in us gaining weight faster. And on it goes! These 'craving neural networks' can eventually become so strong that we experience uncontrollable eating. We just cannot stop.

Essentially, we are using carbohydrate-rich foods as an antidepressant. Why? Because most antidepressants (like Prozac, Zoloft, Lexapro) are Selective Serotonin Reuptake Inhibitors (SSRI's). Long story short, they increase the amount of serotonin available in the brain, making you feel better. Sounds familiar? Yes, it is the same way that carbohydrates make you feel better.

This means we are self-medicating with food in the same way a drug makes us feel better. And just like most drugs, we become desensitised over time and we need to increase our dosage to lift our mood. With drugs like speed (methamphetamine), an overdose can cause death. With carbohydrates, an overdose results in obesity, and can even result in diabetes and death. We can plot out this overall process by using our mood and time as two sides of a graph.

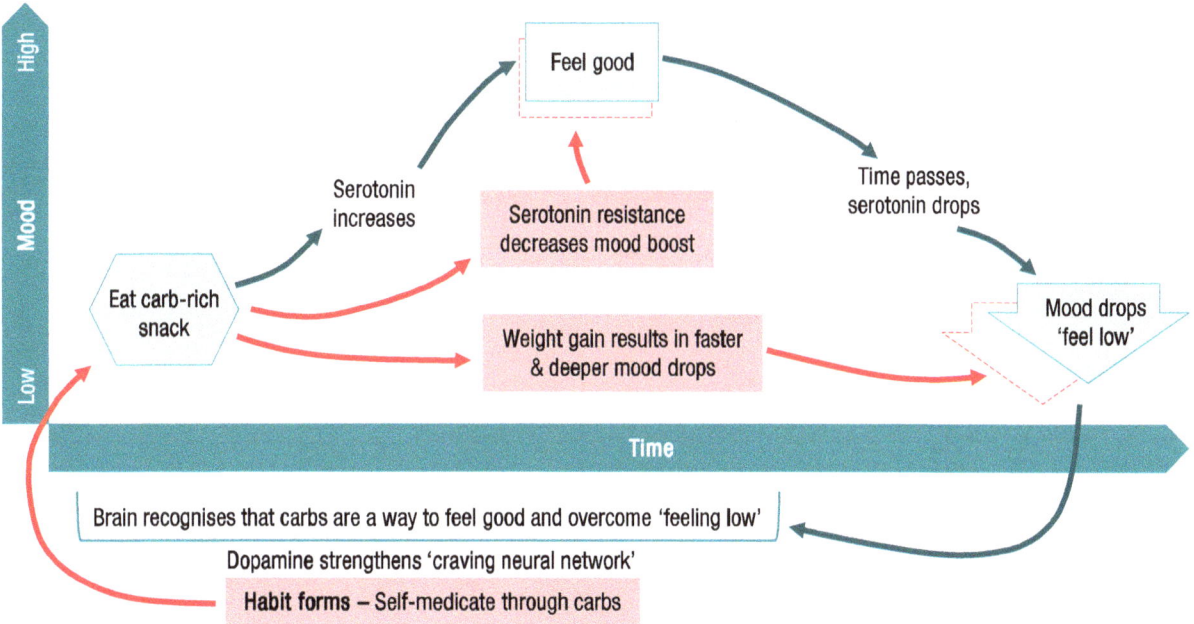

On the graph you can clearly see how our carbohydrate-rich snack increases mood, while at the same time increasing serotonin resistance and making us gain weight. The serotonin resistance means we don't feel as good as we did when eating this snack previously, so we increase our portion sizes. The weight gain makes our mood drop faster than in the past, meaning we need a lift sooner than we did in the past. All this increases the strength of our 'craving neural network', making us want to eat more carbohydrates more often to feel good.

Of course, the good news is that **you can break this cycle**!

The key is to break the 'craving neural network'. Through Hebb's work on how neurons connect, we know that *"neurons that fire together, wire together"*[34]. More recently the opposite finding was made, showing that *"neurons that fire apart, wire apart"*[35]. What this means is we have the power to **break neural networks**.

Having this overview of what happens to us during cravings makes it easier to see how our new healthy eating plan can help overcome cravings and break the cycle:

1. Cutting out carbohydrate-rich foods (grains and sugars) evens out our mood, meaning we are no longer on the rollercoaster, needing an up when we are down
2. When we lose weight and get closer to our goal, self-esteem and confidence increases, meaning our moods do not drop as low as before and we don't need to self-medicate with food
3. We start to overcome conditions like serotonin resistance, making normal life (when we are not high on carbohydrates) feel better
4. By not activating our 'craving neural network', we start to break the neural network through the principle of 'neurons that fire apart, wire apart'. Eventually the network dissolves and we are free from cravings!

To achieve this, we need to stay consistent with our new healthy eating plan. Otherwise occasional activation of our 'craving neural network' can keep it strong and it will still hold power over us.

Symptom: Tiredness and fatigue

This is often a result of drinking too much coffee or caffeinated drinks. To understand this, we have to take a look at a molecule called **adenosine**. In the brain, adenosine binds to adenosine receptors, which causes us to become drowsy while also having an inhibiting effect on cell activity. This means our brains slow down and we start to feel sleepy.

Caffeine is very similar in structure to adenosine, which allows it to bind with the adenosine receptors[136]. The difference is that caffeine doesn't decrease cell activity and the neurons speed up instead, preventing us from getting drowsy. The increased brain activity results in the release of adrenaline[137], possibly due to the brain perceiving the increased brain activity as a threat response.

The adrenaline boost activates our 'fight or flight' response, making our heart beat faster, increasing our breathing and blood pressure. The problem is that the 'fight or flight' response is a stressful state, and it wears out our bodies and our minds. After a stress response like this, our bodies need a break, which is when you feel the 'come down' and you feel tired and even irritable. At this point, you might go get another coffee to get you going again.

This really becomes a problem when we drink coffee later in the day. Caffeine can stay in our bodies much longer than the 'pick me up' effect that we feel. Because caffeine stays in our brains, it continues to interfere with the adenosine receptors, which are needed to make us feel drowsy and get a good sleep at night. A study has shown that even drinking coffee six hours before bed time can result in an hour's less sleep and reduce the quality of sleep overall[138].

In fact, it is well known that coffee is a cause of insomnia, as well as a number of other psychiatric disorders such as anxiety, eating disorders and schizophrenia[91]. Many don't realise they have a case of insomnia, which is mostly experienced as difficulty falling asleep, lower sleep quality and frequently waking up during the night. This leaves us feeling tired the next day, waking up groggy and needing another coffee to get us going, thus continuing the cycle.

We also need to be mindful of the impact of coffee and caffeine on the neural system – more about this when we discuss supplements and the brain. For now, this is just one aspect of how misuse of something like coffee can have a strong effect on our brains. What is really troubling is that coffee is supposed to reduce tiredness, and ends up causing it, meaning we need to take more!

As mentioned before, tiredness and fatigue can also be caused by a number of vitamin and mineral deficiencies, especially B vitamins. We've also talked about how sugar and high-GI foods cause spikes in blood sugar, giving an energy rush followed by a dip in energy, causing us to feel tired and needing another boost. In this way, tiredness can be a combination of many factors, so we need to provide our body and brain with the best conditions overall, such as healthy foods and just one coffee at the start of the day, so we can still get good, restful sleep at the end of the day.

> **How do antidepressants affect our health?**
>
> Serotonin is used in many body functions, including mood, attention, digestion, gut movement, blood clotting and more. This means that if we disrupt it through the use of antidepressants (SSRI's in particular), there can be all kinds of side effects. A recent study looked into these health effects and showed that there may be a large range of effects, including[139]:
>
> * **Attention** – increased risk of driving accidents
> * **Digestion** – diarrhoea, constipation, upset stomach, nausea, abdominal pain
> * **Blood clotting** – abdominal bleeding, increased risk of stroke
> * **Mood** – risk of depression relapse when medication stops
>
> These and other findings resulted in the researcher to call for SSRI's to be used only when the negative effects outweigh the risks. As in other cases we may be better off maintaining the body's natural balance and treating depression through talking therapies instead of resorting to medication.

3.1.3 Hormones

The body is regulated by a large number of hormones that play a major role in the brain. We previously talked about insulin, which plays an important role in our weight, but there are a great many more that are needed by our bodies to work well. Hormones also include the peptides that we have mentioned before, like the ones that influence whether or not we feel full after meals. We will not be looking at all of these here, but rather, we want to consider how hormones relate to the brain.

Hormones originate from many areas in the body and work through the endocrine system. The endocrine system connects with your whole body, and allows the body to communicate with neurons in the brain. Based on the signals that the brain receives, it tells the pituitary gland to increase or decrease certain hormones within the body.

Hormones can come from many areas such as the pancreas, thyroid, kidneys, heart - even body fat produces hormones. Some of the hormones and peptides we have learnt about so far are:

* **Insulin**
* **Glucagon**
* **Glucagon-like Peptide-1 (GLP-1)**

- **Peptide Tyrosine Tyrosine (PYY)**
- **Ghrelin**
- **Leptin**

These are all hormones that play a part in how hungry we feel, or in the storage of body fat and regulation of energy. If they are not functioning properly, they can easily cause us to eat too much or even result in eating disorders. In addition to these, there are a great many other hormones that play major roles in our bodies. These include hormones such as:

- **Oxytocin** – Increases the feeling of trust between people
- **Growth hormone** – Stimulates muscle growth and cell reproduction
- **Estrogen** – Gender characteristics and multiple other roles
- **Testosterone** – Libido, muscle growth and multiple other roles
- **Cortisol** – Stress hormone
- **Adrenocorticotropic hormone** – Stress hormone

The reason these are being listed is not to give you a lesson in biology, but simply to highlight the importance of looking after our brains. All of these hormones, and many more, are regulated in some way by the brain. Some imbalances can have serious and obvious negative effects like diabetes, while other effects can be vague and hard to put your finger on, like poor memory and concentration, or an overactive appetite.

Let's have a look at how an imbalance in hormones may manifest itself in some diet-related symptoms:

Symptom: Uncontrollable appetite

An uncontrollable appetite often results from the type of food we eat impacting our hormones. This is particularly the case when we consume large quantities of food that our ancestors did not have access to, such as high-GI carbohydrates and sugar. When we eat these foods, our brains react by releasing hormones to make us want to eat more of it so that we can store some of the energy as fat for times of famine.

Obviously, this survival technique now causes trouble when we consume high-GI and sugary foods, since our brains motivate us to keep on eating.

If you find that you just can't stop eating, look at the foods you are eating and check if they are high-GI. Or maybe you are missing protein from your meals and snacks. Over eating is a big reason why you need to include protein in every meal – it nourishes you and makes you feel full! Protein-rich foods are a preferred snack food, as they make you feel full faster, help build lean muscle mass and provide less calories than carbohydrates due to the thermic effect of food.

Symptom: Always having room for dessert

To properly explore this symptom, we need to head back into neurotransmitter territory and take another look at dopamine. As we learned before, dopamine helps to strengthen our neural networks, which is where our brain makes the connection between action and reward. In this instance, a carbohydrate-rich dessert provides a serotonin release, making us feel good (refer to the Food Craving graph). When the connection is made between action and reward, dopamine is released, strengthening the neural network and our desire for dessert.

If you have grown up eating dessert after meals, just imagine how ingrained and strong this neural network has become! Since dopamine releases *in anticipation of a reward*[133], the very thought of dessert activates that strong neural network and the brain says *"Never mind how full we are, this serotonin release is gonna be awesome!"*

Because we now understand how this works, we can make an informed decision about whether we want to give in to these cravings or not. We can plan ahead and prepare to say no to dessert. We can play tricks with our brains, by focusing on how good it will be to get the figure we want and focusing on how good it feels to tick off another successful day on our healthy eating plan, instead of focusing on how good dessert will be.

Symptom: Obesity

Obesity has many causes, but one is known as **leptin resistance**[140]. We've read before about leptin, and how it inhibits our appetite. Leptin is produced by body fat, so the more body fat we have, the more leptin we produce. Theoretically, this should mean that the more body fat we gain, the less hungry we become.

However, in reality, when there is too much body fat, the levels of leptin become so high that the brain assumes there must be something wrong with the leptin and builds up a tolerance which reduces its effectiveness. This results in the mechanism losing effectiveness, causing us to not know when to stop eating.

The good news is that you can reverse leptin resistance[141]. Studies show that a change of diet can bring back sensitivity to leptin, meaning we will naturally start to decrease our calorie intake. This return can take a number of weeks, however, which is important to recognise so that you are prepared to resist urges to eat while your sensitivity is returning.

3.1.4   Brain-derived neurotrophic factor (BDNF)

Brain-derived neurotrophic factor, or BDNF for short, is a crucial protein needed by your brain to allow it to continue to grow and learn.

We talked before about neuroplasticity, which is your brain's ability to continue to change and learn over time. Part of what enables this process is when your brain produces new brain cells through a process called **neurogenesis**[142]. It used to be thought that the brain does not produce new brain cells after birth, but the discovery of neurogenesis gave us a new view of how the brain grows. This discovery showed that throughout our lives, neurogenesis continues through a constant production of new brain cells.

The amount of new neurons that the brain produces depends on the amount of BDNF available. If we have more BDNF, the brain produces more neurons which make it easier for us to learn and adapt to new situations. When we have less BDNF, our thinking can become rigid, resulting in us doing the same things over and over, even if we are not having success. BDNF also has a role in ensuring that existing neurons survive. Without it, or with lower levels of BDNF, existing neurons can die, resulting in looser or broken connections in our neural networks.

Here we start to see that if we are not feeding our brains the right foods and treating it the right way to produce enough BDNF, it can actually start to affect your behaviour and your success in reaching your goals. This is a very important concept – *if you do not treat your brain well (resulting in low BDNF levels), it can have a serious negative effect on your emotional wellbeing in the long term.*

3.1.4.1 BDNF and the hippocampus

We briefly looked at the hippocampus before as a small cluster in the brain that plays a big role. The hippocampus stores short-term memories temporarily, allowing us to quickly refer back to something we just heard or saw. If the event is determined by the brain as important to survival, the memory has a greater chance of being stored as a long-term memory. If it is seen as not important to survival, it is discarded. It is now well understood that without the hippocampus, *we cannot form any new memories*[143].

This means the hippocampus is something we definitely need to look after! As it happens, the hippocampus is a major source of BDNF. This makes the hippocampus crucially important – it helps us to adapt to new situations by retaining important memories, while facilitating changes in neural networks through BDNF and the generation of new neurons.

The hippocampus is active all the time, including while we sleep when it works on integrating and storing memories. This means sleep is very important for the hippocampus and for our memories to work properly. You'll notice during periods where you haven't been sleeping well, the hippocampus does not get enough time to integrate memories, leaving you with increasing feelings of confusion as it overloads and waits for you to finally get some decent sleep!

This is not even all there is to the hippocampus and BDNF – they have also been shown to play a role in depression[144], with BDNF being a key to maintain plasticity during recovery from depression. This plays a crucial role in assisting us to adapt and form healthy and productive mindsets.

Symptom: Depression, poor memory, difficulty dealing with change
Each of these symptoms can happen individually, or together, and may all be related to issues with BDNF and the hippocampus. For example, we've already talked about how these impact memory formation – the hippocampus along with BDNF are crucial for memory formation. It has been found that depression can lead to a smaller hippocampus and lower BDNF levels[144], meaning that while we are depressed, we have a harder time adapting, learning and forming memories.

Within the hippocampus, BDNF also acts in opposition to cortisol, the stress hormone. This means that when cortisol increases, BDNF decreases[145]. So when we are under stress with high levels of cortisol, we become more rigid in our thinking and have less ability to learn and adapt effectively to changing circumstances. This may all sound like very long-term stuff, and certainly can be hard to notice day to day, but it is very important to our long-term health and happiness.

Otherwise, we end up in those situations where we wonder *"How did I get here? How did things get so bad?"* You may even find yourself trying the same old approach, even though the environment has changed and you are not getting good results anymore.

The good news, of course, is that we can fix this! There are a few key ways we can increase our BDNF levels and boost our hippocampus:

- **Exercise** – Research shows that exercise causes a very strong boost to BDNF. This even works later in life, helping us to increase learning and overall mental performance[146]. Exercise also helps to reduce cortisol, which in turn increases the levels of BDNF

- **Healthy eating** – A diet high in refined sugars and dietary fat has been shown to decrease BDNF[147]. As we've learned before, sugars and other high-GI carbohydrates are the real enemies due to their effect on insulin, while dietary fats are OK to eat. This means if we cut our sugars and high-GI food (as we know we must) we can boost our BDNF and our learning abilities

- **Quality sleep** – The hippocampus needs good, restful sleep to store and consolidate memories. Sleep is also crucial for BDNF, which helps change our neural structures[148]. If we improve the quality of our sleep, we can improve our brains!

- **Enriched environments** – Studies have found that 'enhanced environments' (those that you find stimulating and rewarding) increases BDNF and promotes learning[149,150]

The above provide a good overall summary of what we need to do to boost our brains and we will look at them in more detail later on to see how they fit into the big picture and some easy steps to help us implement them.

What to remember:
- The brain is where all our thoughts, feelings and actions come from. We must keep it healthy!
- The brain components include neural networks, neurotransmitters, hormones and BDNF. We can control and improve these
- Look after your brain health by focusing on healthy eating, exercise, quality sleep and maintaining a positive environment

3.2 What affects your brain?

The previous section gave us a good overview of some of the key components that make our brains work, the symptoms we may experience if something is wrong, and some ideas of what we can do to resolve individual problems.

Our next step is to combine the lessons from these and take a different perspective, by focusing on different factors that affect our brains and what we should do about each. This will set us up for the next section, where we develop a plan to *boost our brains*.

3.2.1 Diet

Even though our bodies have an amazing ability to adapt to what we eat, it often takes a long time to really start to feel the effects of an unhealthy diet. This is why we can easily make it through our early years eating everything in sight and our bodies just seem to cope. We feel great, we feel invincible, like we don't need to eat healthy. Soon after problems start to creep in – weight doesn't seem to come off, joint pains, headaches, tiredness and more. This is where we need to realise that we should fix our diets and eat healthy instead.

The reality is that many things (like oxidative damage and omega-6 overload) accumulate over time. An unhealthy diet now might take many years before you realise the damage it's doing to your body. On the other hand, if we start to eat healthy sooner, we can reap the benefits of longer lasting health and vitality. Think of it as investing in a lean body now and in an improved quality of life in later years. You are not only investing in your body, but also in your brain and your mental health.

3.2.1.1 Macros for the brain

In terms of brain health, we really need to build our healthy eating habits around the following concepts from a macronutrient perspective:

- **Plenty of protein** – Proteins are needed by every single cell in the body, including the brain. While neurons themselves are mostly made of lipids, they communicate with each other through neurotransmitters which are manufactured from proteins. Quality, complete proteins are needed for a healthy brain, just as it is needed for a healthy body

- **Include dietary fats** – Dietary fats are essential in our diets, including unsaturated and saturated fats. They provide fuel (ketones) for our brains which is a healthy way to feed your brain. In fact, ketogenic diets (very low in carbohydrates) are actually used to treat some neurologic disorders like epilepsy[151]. Omega-3 in particular helps to boost our brains and fight inflammation. Inflammation not only affects our bodies, but can also cause headaches and migraines

- **Stick to low-GI carbohydrates** – Carbohydrates are the only non-essential macronutrient, but there are still a lot of good sources of carbohydrates that we can include for health and variety, such as vegetables, legumes and nuts. We've seen the evidence of how grains and refined sugars negatively affect our bodies and brains. Keep these out and keep the good carbohydrates in to start healing your brain!

 Getting the right macronutrient balance for your brain is simple – eat according to the Think Lean food pyramid!

3.2.1.2 Vitamins and minerals for the brain

Vitamins and minerals play a major role in our brain health. Our neurons and the components that make them work require a variety of different chemicals that we get through our daily meals. We've already looked through these in the first section, so let's do a quick recap on what is important for the brain:

- **Vitamins** – From a neurological perspective, B vitamins are the most important vitamins for your brain. Not getting enough B vitamins can result in depression, poor concentration, tiredness, delirium, irritability, and many forms neural damage. This damage adds up over time and can result in neurological disorders such as Alzheimer's

- **Minerals** – Minerals are more basic substances, which help to serve as the building blocks for many parts of your brain. These play a role throughout your body, but you can especially notice them when they affect your brain, since an imbalance can result in you experiencing effects such as headaches, insomnia, tiredness, feelings of apathy, confusion and irritability. All of these are feelings produced by the brain when it is not getting what it needs!

If you have had a very unbalanced diet, you might have some deficiencies that we will need to address as you go on the diet. Addressing those will help to get you to feel 100% again!

Use the Think Lean Method for long-term micronutrient balance, but address any deficiencies you have through the action plan at the end of this section.

3.2.1.3 Caffeine

We already know how caffeine affects our brains through its action on the adenosine receptors. The way it interacts with our brains produces dopamine through our reward system which makes coffee an addictive substance. Caffeine is actually ranked as the most used drug, used by around 85% of people[152]. Coffee and energy drinks are really just delivery vehicles for caffeine, so we really need to think of these together to get a realistic view of how much caffeine we are taking in. Even chocolate contains a bit of caffeine!

Coffee makes us feel energised, but it also comes with side effects like insomnia and anxiety. This can result in us increasing our coffee intake over time when we start to rely on it to get us up and going, while it also reduces our sleep quality, resulting in us needing more coffee the next day to keep us going.

Most of these negative effects happen when we consume too much caffeine. 'Too much' is estimated to be more than 400mg of caffeine per day[152], which is equal to about three cups of coffee a day, or two to seven energy drinks, depending on their caffeine content. Some energy drinks have 400mg of caffeine in a single can, so check the label when you pick one! Going above the recommended levels can result in these side effects[91]:

- Anxiety and mood disorders – mood swings, depression
- Sleep disorders – insomnia, leading to tiredness, irritability
- Eating disorders – anorexia, bulimia
- Schizophrenia – making psychosis worse
- Withdrawal symptoms when trying to reduce caffeine intake

That's not to say that coffee is bad for us overall. In fact, there have been studies that show a moderate intake of coffee can be beneficial for us. For example:

- **Short-term benefits** (a few hours)[153]:
    - Lift in mood
    - Improvement in reaction time
    - Increased cognitive performance
    - Better performance during exercise
    - Endurance increased
    - Increased metabolism[90]
- **Long-term benefits**:
    - Lowers risk of diabetes[154]
    - Lowers risk of Alzheimer's disease[155]
    - Reduces risk of Parkinson's disease[156]
    - Somewhat reduced risk of death from all causes[157]

The key to getting the benefits of caffeine without the side effects is balance and moderation. As we saw previously from the sleep disorder study, it turns out that the mornings are the best time for us to have a coffee or energy drink, as by the time we get to bed, caffeine has done its work and we can have a night of quality sleep[138].

If you like caffeinated drinks, limit yourself to one at the start of the day.

3.2.1.4 Alcohol

Alcohol is often used as a 'social lubricant', it makes us loosen up and feel good for a while. But it can also tear apart relationships, families and communities. Alcohol abuse can strip your body of vital vitamins and minerals, resulting in deficiencies. Taking a look at what alcohol does to your brain is very eye opening. Excess alcohol consumption does the following:

- It makes your memory worse[158]
- Can result in irreversible brain shrinkage[158]
- Impairment of neurotransmitter function, needed for normal brain function and feeling good[158]
- Inhibition of the frontal cortex which reduces complex decision-making ability[158]
- Reduces hippocampal function, needed for short and long-term memory consolidation, as well as BDNF needed for learning and adaptation[158]
- Strongly related to depression and suicide[159]
- And much, much more...

Still, there are at some good effects you can get from a moderate consumption of red wine. It may not be good from a weight loss perspective, but it is the best choice if you really do want to have a drink, because:

- It contains **resveratrol** which one study has shown to fight cancer[160]. White wines also have some resveratrol, but not as much as red wines. However, this is contentious as more recent studies indicate that resveratrol may not have any benefits to longevity[161]
- It contains **polyphenols** which are powerful antioxidants[162]

Of course, you also get resveratrol from grapes, mulberries or peanuts, and polyphenol from broccoli, blueberries, onions, grapes, and other sources which are much better for you than red wine[161,163]. So, if you absolutely want to drink, keep your intake moderate – one or two glasses once or twice a week. It all comes down to your goals:

- If you want to lose weight as fast as possible, cut out alcohol
- If you still want to enjoy alcohol along the way and are not in much of a rush to lose weight, then you can still have drinks now and then

Stay away from alcohol if you can, otherwise keep it to one or two glasses of red wine once or twice a week.

3.2.1.5 Supplements

There are an impressive amount of health supplements available in the market today. For that reason, we're just going to focus on the few that are proven to have some health benefits. The key word here is 'proven'. The majority of supplements on the market have either no evidence that they are beneficial, or have taken scientific studies out of context so they can pretend to be beneficial.

This may sound surprising, but it is standard practice in the supplement industry. The usual course of action is something like this:

1. Some chemical compound is proven to be helpful to people with a particular disease
2. The study is picked up in the media which then exaggerates its effects
3. Supplement companies notice the increased public interest in the compound (or creates interest themselves)
4. A new product is created, selling the compound in doses much smaller than used in the original study to people without the particular disease
5. The product is marketed with bold health claims, generating millions of dollars of revenue on something that was *never proven to be beneficial for healthy people*

We need supplements that are proven to benefit healthy people. Most supplements only work when you have a certain disease or deficiency, while very few actually do anything if there is nothing wrong with you. If you are interested in particular supplements, see if you can find any studies that prove they actually do something for healthy individuals. If you can't find any studies, it likely means it is not proven.

Below we will look at a few supplements that have proven benefits.

Vitamins

As mentioned before, if you don't have any vitamin deficiencies, then taking vitamin supplements is not going to have any effects. However, if you have been maintaining an unbalanced diet, particularly one with lots of fast foods, drinking lots of alcohol, and so on, then you are likely to have a deficiency or some sort.

We know vitamin supplements work due to the research we covered before and their frequent use in hospitals and medical centres to treat deficiencies. The important thing for us is that we preferably want to get our vitamins and minerals from whole foods, rather than pills. The Think Lean Method will help with that, but to get you feeling 100%, we first need to sort out any deficiencies you might have right now with supplements so that healthy eating can take over afterwards.

It can take a long time and lots of tests to find out if you have any particular deficiencies, so below we will find a way to do this efficiently so that you can quickly resolve any deficiencies, getting our neurons, neurotransmitters and hormones working well, so we can feel 100% sooner!

Take vitamin supplements if you notice any particular symptoms that are related to vitamin and mineral deficiencies.

Fish oil\flax oil

We've seen that fish oil and flax oil are good sources of omega-3, and that omega-3 is great for brain and body health. It would seem logical that fish oil would be a great supplement, but unfortunately we have a problem here. Thing is, these are polyunsaturated fats that become rancid very easily. When these become rancid, they become dangerous to our health, as they cause oxidative damage to our bodies.

In fact, very few of the studies done that shows an improvement in fish oil supplementation has been longer than one year. Oxidative damage can take much longer to manifest, meaning one year may be too short to determine if there are any long-term risks.

One long-term study that followed up with participants between three and nine years actually highlighted these risks. What did if find? It showed that supplementation with fish oil capsules actually increased the risk of death from heart attacks[164].

That's a bit scary, especially given how much fish oil is pushed as a great supplement for overall health! Thinking about it more, it doesn't seem that unlikely as fish oil is very unstable as a polyunsaturated fat, and generally sits on store shelves for a long time before being bought and consumed. In addition to that, we usually take it in pill form, meaning we can't even smell if it has gone rancid.

The same applies to flax oil, which is another often used supplement for omega-3. We need to take much more flax oil than fish oil to get the same amount of omega-3, which means it is usually taken in exposed, liquid form. This at least makes it more likely that you would smell if it has gone rancid. They are also usually stored in refrigerators in stores, making them a little safer. Still, they are usually transported without refrigeration, so there is still the possibility for them to go rancid on the way to the store.

At the end of the day, we are much safer if we stick with our ACM rule – **Whole foods only**. Get your omega-3s from eating fresh fish like salmon! That way you can avoid oxidative damage and you still get your omega-3s to boost you brain health.

Don't use oil supplements. Instead get your omega-3 directly from eating fish.

Choline

We know that choline is needed for a good memory, where if you have too little, you can even suffer from memory loss. Choline is needed to produce a neurotransmitter called **acetylcholine**, which is crucial for memory function. Getting enough choline will help you maintain a good memory, but it has been found that supplementing with choline can help improve you memory even more[165]!

This is significant, as we mentioned before, there are very few supplements on the market today that have actually been proven to work. The majority of supplements you see on the shelves either are not proven to work at all, or are taking research findings out of context. This means that they usually only help people with a specific disease or condition, and do nothing for normal, healthy people (the majority of consumers).

So having some actual evidence that backs up the claim that choline supplementation helps to improve memories, it gives us a good incentive to include it in our diets and boost our brains! One way to get additional choline is through taking pills, but we can actually do it naturally as well. Sometimes we have to take medication where we really can't get something from whole foods, but wherever we can get nutrients from real food, we should do that!

Choline has also been shown to:

- **Improve hippocampal function**, helping with **neurogenesis** needed for memory, learning and adaptation[166]

- During pregnancy, choline supplementation **improves child hippocampus function**, BDNF and memory, and helps to **protect against neurodegenerative diseases**[167]

A great source of choline is eggs. In fact, eating three to four eggs a day already gives you a high enough dosage of choline that has been proven to boost your memory! This is great news for us, as eggs are on the menu for both Core and Complete ACM. Eggs are also great for protein and other nutrients, and keep the yolk in since cholesterol isn't bad for you!

> I get about 800mg of choline through four eggs, meat and vegetable sources every day. Since starting with healthy eating, I have noticed that my **prospective memory** has improved a lot.
>
> Prospective memory is your ability to remember to do something that you intend to do later. Such as *"I need to remember to call that person"*, *"I need to remember to buy more eggs"*
>
> My prospective memory used to be terrible, resulting in me writing lots of notes and forgetting things all the time, but now I can decide to remember something, and then actually remember it later!

The research showed that the most important aspect is that you need to have a *consistent intake* of choline, meaning you need to eat it every day. This luckily is easy, since we can have eggs for breakfast and then have vegetables and meats through the day for our normal healthy eating, giving us a natural boost to our memory.

Eat three eggs for breakfast a day with their yolks to get a boost in memory.

Theanine

Not to be confused with thiamine which is also known as vitamin B1, **theanine** is a different amino acid with a very different effect. Theanine is totally natural substance mainly found in green tea and there have been a number of studies in the last few years showing some remarkable effects that it has on our minds.

Taken on its own, theanine supplementation has been proven to produce a calming effect[168] - it lowers our heart rates and also reduces the stress hormone cortisol[169]. This reduction in cortisol is a great benefit to our hippocampus and BDNF, which helps us learn and adapt to change. On top of that, theanine has also been shown to fight cancer and microbes, and also reduce the symptoms of cold and flu[170].

Theanine blocks **glutamate** from binding to glutamate receptors[171]. Glutamate is one of the main neurotransmitters, and plays an 'exitatory' role, meaning it stimulates nerve cells to function faster. Sometimes we get too much glutamate binding to the glutamate receptors, causing us to feel stressed and anxious, and can even lead to 'exitotoxicity', which is where nerve cells are damaged or killed by too much stimulation from glutamate. Theanine blocks this process by preventing glutamate from stimulating the nerve cells, producing that calming effect.

This already makes theanine a useful supplement, especially if you feel stressed or anxious. What is unique about theanine is that it produces a calming effect *without making you drowsy*. If you are looking for something to help calm you down through the day without reducing performance, a cup of strong green tea will do great. Note it has to be strong green tea, otherwise the dose will be too low to have an effect.

There is also another side to theanine which has been getting much more attention – *its effect alongside caffeine*. A number of studies have come out showing a synergistic relationship between caffeine and theanine. These studies showed that if caffeine and theanine is taken together:

- It increases our **speed** and **accuracy** with mental tasks[172,173]
- It helps to increase **concentration** and **stay focused** on a task[174]
- It increases **reaction time**, faster **working memory**[175]
- It **reduces headaches** and **reduces tiredness**, while making us feel more **alert**[175]

That is a very impressive list of benefits that we can get from taking these two together. Of course, if you are generally relaxed and don't have the kind of job or hobbies that require those attributes, then you don't need it!

A lot of people are currently taking coffee together with a theanine supplement (which can easily be bought online), to get the kick from caffeine without the added feeling of stress and anxiety. *The result is a calm and relaxed boost in mental function.*

Incorporate theanine depending on your needs.

- *If you want something to help calm you down during the day and improve immune function, take a theanine supplement on its own*
- *If you enjoy a strong cup of coffee (or energy drink) but would like to have a calmer and more relaxed boost, take it along with a theanine supplement that you can buy online*
- *If you want a more natural, lower dose boost of relaxed energy, drink a strong cup of green tea*

3.2.2 Exercise

Apart from the benefits of exercise to your weight and body composition, a great reason to do exercise is how it improves the health of your brain. This is where exercise plays a major role. Here are some of the health benefits of exercise for the brain:

- In the short term[176]:
    - **Increases cerebral blood flow.** Our brains heavily depend on blood flow to be able to function, so more blood flow helps our brains work better!
    - **Improves neuroplasticity** by boosting hippocampal function
    - **Releases endorphins** and can help with treatment and prevention of stress, depression and anxiety[177]

- In the long term:
    - **Enhances brain plasticity** and **increases BDNF**. This helps to stimulate the process of neurogenesis which is the production of new neurons to help our brains grow. This helps us **improve learning** abilities and overall **mental performance**[146]
    - **Protects against cognitive decline** as well as declines in complex decision making skills and memory[176]
    - **Helps our brains grow** and contributes to a larger brain size[178]

> I have been consistently exercising for between four to six days a week for about eight years now doing various types of exercises. During this period I have made major improvements in my thinking patterns, building healthy habits and made great improvements to my own personal resilience.
>
> Was exercise responsible for that? Not entirely, but the benefits it provided to my brain definitely helped me to achieve what I have over the last eight years!

That's right – exercise literally gives us *bigger brains*.

The main form of exercise that has been shown to boost our brains is aerobic exercise. This is the kind of exercise that gets your heart rate up, although recent evidence has shown that weight training also provides a boost to your brain[179].

The conclusion here is simple – if you care about your brain (and you should) then exercise! The positive benefits to your brain can be achieved by exercising just three times a week. How long you train is important, as you should not overtrain either[180]. Working out for long sessions (more than 1.5 hours) for upwards of six days a week can result in raised cortisol levels, fatigue and tiredness.

On the whole, incorporating a basic exercise routine in your schedule will have some serious positive effects on your brain and overall feeling of wellbeing. Do it!

 Boost your brain along with your body by adding at least three sessions a week.

3.2.3 Sleep

Quality seep is essential to health, and especially to your brain – just ask anyone who is not getting enough sleep! We need sleep to help the body and brain recover, but the brain in particular needs sleep. Not getting enough sleep quickly becomes apparent. You might notice[181]:

- Lack of concentration, reduced attention span
- Loss of coordination
- Increasing pressure to fall asleep
- Negative impacts on perception – we are less able to see and hear correctly, resulting in more mistakes
- Inconsistent emotional states and mood swings
- Loss of inhibition and control
- Increased cortisol levels that makes it harder to cope with stress[182]
- Reduced BDNF levels and hippocampal function due to increases in cortisol[145]

These are examples of the powerful effect that poor sleep has on our brains and in fact play a part on why poor sleep is closely linked to weight gain.

A recent study showed that when we are sleep deprived, blood flow to our prefrontal cortex goes down (meaning we become worse at higher-order thinking) and the amygdala is drastically more active than normal (meaning it starts to run the show with impulsive decisions)[183]. When people are given a choice between a healthy meal and junk food during this state, the results are startling – while the amygdala is running the show, a sleep deprived person's brain lights up when they see junk food, making them want to eat it far more than non-sleep deprived people.

This study shows us that if we get quality sleep, we are much better at resisting unhealthy food. Get poor sleep, and you may find it incredibly hard to resist because your amygdala is trying to help you survive by picking the most calorie-dense foods it can find!

What can cause poor sleep?

It is one thing to know that lack of sleep or poor sleep is bad for us, but another thing entirely to know what causes it, and more importantly, how we overcome it. Let's look at some causes and what we can do about them:

- **Alcohol** – many people use alcohol as a way to get to sleep each night. While alcohol might help you fall asleep, your overall sleep quality is reduced, even if the drink was six hours before going to bed[184]. If you regularly drink alcohol before bed, it can add up to sleep deprivation over time, even if you still manage to get a full eight hours of sleep each night.
  Action - skip alcohol to get better sleep!

- **Too much light** – is there any light making its way into your room at night? Such as street lights coming through thin curtains, cracks in the curtains letting light through, glow from an alarm clock or other electronics? Even if the light source is small, it can seriously reduce the quality of your sleep, and has even been linked to obesity, increased risk of breast cancer and mood disorders[185]! Have a look at your room tonight and see how dark it is and whether you can see any light. If so, eliminate all the light sources! Put in blackout curtains, remove night lights, put phones upside down, or get a decent sleeping mask. You'll be surprised how quickly you notice the difference!
  Action – eliminate all sources of light that makes it into your bedroom at night

- **Caffeine** – we went through caffeine before and the effect it has on your sleep, even if taken six hours before going to bed. While it is still possible to go to sleep, the quality of sleep is reduced (very similar effect to alcohol, just different mechanism). If you are drinking a lot of caffeinated drinks and struggling with getting good sleep, it might be time for a change.
  Action – stick to one caffeinated drink per day at the start of the day

- **Stress and a racing mind** – you might be going to bed each night at a good time, but lying awake for hours trying to fall asleep without any luck. You get stuck thinking about this and that, stressing about what happened today, what is going to happen tomorrow, trying to remember this, worrying about that... It is extremely frustrating. I know because this absolutely used to be me. I would lie in bed for about two hours each night trying to fall asleep, ending up with chronic sleep deprivation. This *was* me, until I went through the transformation that we will talk through in the Think Lean section. Now I fall asleep within a few minutes after getting into bed – every night!
  Action – read the next section!

- **Too much to do!** – you might just have a lot of trouble actually going to bed on time in the first place, or staying in bed. Newborn baby? Goodbye sleep! That is a tough situation, but there are always ways to improve the situation. For example, becoming more efficient at doing tasks, better division of tasks in the house, preparing meals in bulk to get some time back in your day. If you can start to see that lack of sleep is affecting you, negotiate with your partner or others in the house so you can get more sleep. If you tend to watch TV each night, cut back a bit and prioritise sleep instead. It will make you more relaxed than TV does anyway!
  Action – fight for your sleep!

- **Noise** – too much noise can make it hard to fall asleep and can constantly wake you up during the night, interrupting deep sleep cycles. Find ways to cut down on any noise in the house, like closing the door and shutting down appliances and computers that might be making noise. If all else fails, some earplugs can also do the trick!
  Action – eliminate sources of noise, or get some earplugs

- **Sleep medication** – as much as they help you fall asleep, they are not very good for quality sleep. Drugs like benzodiazepines (Valium, Xanax and many others) have been shown to increase sleep duration, but lower sleep quality[186]. They also interfere with hippocampal function, which can prevent new memories from forming[187]. It might be easy just to take one to fall asleep faster, but it's better for your health to find the real issue and fix it instead!
  Action – avoid medication and fix the real problem!

Fighting for your sleep is important. By 'fighting', I mean to make it a priority and ensure that others understand that it is a priority to you. If you need to negotiate this with your partner or others, try to find solutions that can benefit others around you as well, but make sure that sleep is a priority and you will be amazed at the difference it can make.

How much sleep?

Research shows between seven and eight hours of sleep each night is ideal for adults[188]. Dipping below seven hours each night for a few nights in a row can cause significant declines in brain function and cognitive abilities.

On top of all the benefits that good sleep has for your brain, sleep is also necessary for muscle repair and healing. This is especially important if you are exercising, as your body needs time to repair itself and build muscle. Many people don't realise it, but your muscles do not grow while you are in the gym – they grow during sleep when your body increases growth hormone and sends protein to the damaged muscles to make them stronger. If you don't have enough protein, the muscles can't improve, and if you don't get enough sleep, the body doesn't have enough time to repair them. As you would remember from before, more muscle helps to increase your metabolism, which means you can eat more and still stay lean! Good, quality sleep is crucial for overall health, so make it a priority!

Get at least seven hours of sleep each night. If you are struggling with sleep, identify why you are struggling and fix it. Fight for your sleep!

What to remember:
• Healthy eating is crucial for your brain - The Think Lean Method is designed to give you brain what it needs for long-term brain health
• Exercise is important, not just to look good, but to increase BDNF and enhance you brain's ability to adapt and change
• Aim for around seven hours of sleep each night. If you struggle with going to bed, look for what is wrong and fix it!

3.3 Take action to boost your brain

We've learned a lot by now of how we can boost our brain. Some of it is through healthy eating, through better sleep, exercise and even having a healthy environment around us. What we need now is an action plan to put all this in action and boost our brain! Our plan includes eight components:

- Healthy eating (Think Lean food pyramid)
- Vitamin and mineral supplements
- Include theanine or green tea
- Quality sleep
- Exercise
- Less caffeine (one hit at the start of the day)
- Less alcohol
- Supplement with choline

3.3.1 Fast action plan

If you want a big brain boost right away, the best course of action is to start with all of these as soon as possible! Our action plan has a few temporary actions as well as lifestyle actions.

- **Temporary actions** include taking supplements. Over the long term we want to get our vitamins and minerals from our diets, so we only want to use supplements to overcome deficiencies now and then let the Think Lean food pyramid carry us in the long term
- **Lifestyle actions** include permanent changes like quality sleep, the Think Lean food pyramid, less caffeine, etc. These are actions that add to our overall health in both the short and long term, so we need to include this into our lifestyle!

Here is the action plan:

Action type	Do this	Month 1	Month 2	Month 3	Ongoing
Temporary actions	Vitamin and mineral supplement - Multivitamin	✓			
	Vitamin and mineral supplement - Magn. Vit. D, Calcium	✓	✓		
	Include theanine or green tea	✓	✓	✓	
Lifestyle actions	Healthy Eating Plan (Think Lean food pyramid)	✓	✓	✓	✓
	Quality sleep	✓	✓	✓	✓
	Exercise	✓	✓	✓	✓
	Less caffeine (one hit at the start of the day)	✓	✓	✓	✓
	Less alcohol (one or two glasses of red wine)	✓	✓	✓	✓
	Supplement with choline (three eggs a day)	✓	✓	✓	✓

Note that the vitamin supplement is split out into a multivitamin and also a magnesium supplement. The ideal magnesium supplement is one that comes with calcium and vitamin D as well to help with absorption. The split between a multivitamin and magnesium supplement is because a lot of people especially have a deficiency in magnesium, so including that one for a month longer will help to properly resolve any deficiencies that may be present.

The theanine supplement is something you can actually include as a lifestyle choice, though I would recommend not relying in the long term on a supplement to reduce stress. If you want to include it for its neuroprotective properties, then you absolutely can.

You'll notice that a lot of the actions are lifestyle actions. Where it says 'Ongoing', it means you continue with them as a permanent lifestyle choice! That is because they are generally good for brain health as well as healing your brain. If you make all of these a permanent part of your lifestyle, you will enjoy a healthy brain and stay mentally sharp until old age!

3.3.2 Staged action plan

If introducing it all at once feels like too big a step for you, then you can take a staged approach. This option allows you to bring in all aspects at a more controlled pace, but you need to keep track and stick to the plan! You can use this option as presented in the table below:

Action type	Do this	Month 1	Month 2	Month 3	Ongoing
Temporary actions	Vitamin and mineral supplement - Multivitamin	✓			
	Vitamin and mineral supplement - Magn. Vit. D, Calcium	✓	✓		
	Include theanine or green tea	✓	✓	✓	
Lifestyle actions	Healthy Eating Plan (Think Lean food pyramid)	✓	✓	✓	✓
	Quality sleep	✓	✓	✓	✓
	Exercise		✓	✓	✓
	Less caffeine (one hit at the start of the day)			✓	✓
	Less alcohol (one or two glasses of red wine)				✓
	Supplement with choline (three eggs a day)				✓

Remember that if you exclude items from the plan, you will not be able to boost your brain as much as possible! The lifestyle actions in particular are key to building long-term brain health. You have the power to apply this to your life and make it fit!

> Follow one of the simple action plans above and feel how quickly your brain responds. You may notice increased energy, better concentration, better memory, less fatigue and less cravings. This will set you up for the next section where we learn how to **Think Lean**, giving us what we need to feel 100% on a consistent basis!

What to remember:
- Do temporary actions only for the timeframe indicated and make lifestyle actions a permanent part of your life!
- Use one of the templates to put in place an action plan to boost your brain and help you feel 100%

The Final Key:

4 Think Lean

*What is the single most important factor for getting real results with a diet? Is it the food, the exercise, or some trick to boost your metabolism? No. There is just one thing that is absolutely crucial for you to succeed – **Consistency**.*

Consistently eating healthy means deciding every day to eat the right foods. It means choosing the right foods when you're eating out, when there's a party going on, when things are stressful or when you are bored. No diet can give you real and lasting results if it is not consistently followed. The truth is that eating one low calorie meal is not going to make you thin, just as eating one high calorie meal is not going to make you fat. You have to consistently eat right to get results.

Despite our best intentions, life just seems to get in the way of us trying to be consistent. Some emergency comes up and messes up our day, the lunch place is out of salad, the pressure and stress is piling on, time runs out and the fast food place seems like the only chance to get something to eat... The list goes on and on.

Still, through all of this, some people just seem to be able to cope with everything and they maintain consistency in their diets and achieve great bodies. So how do they do it? The very fact that there are people out there who manage to stay consistent is proof that it is possible. And you know what? You can learn how to do it too! It is not some special trait that some people are born with – instead, it is a **skill** that you too can learn.

Learning this skill is what can give you your goal body along with serious, long-term success. *This can be a total transformation of your life.* This is where **Think Lean** comes in:

> **Think Lean** *is a method that gives you the skills to develop the ideal mental state of* **relaxed determination** *and* **effortless discipline** *– a state of mind where you find yourself* **consistently eating right***, not because you have to, but because* **you truly want to***.*

That would be fantastic, wouldn't it? This is what you can achieve through the Think Lean Method. While we will focus specifically on how it applies to healthy eating, you can apply the Think Lean Method to all areas in your life.

Think Lean consists of three basic concepts that will guide you towards developing this ideal state of mind:

1. *Personal resilience* – Improving resilience means that you develop the ability to bounce back from difficult situations and stay focused on what is most important
2. *Quality beliefs* – When you improve your beliefs, you can improve all aspects of your life since all your emotions, thoughts and actions flow from your beliefs
3. *Clear goals* – By understanding what is important to you, your motivations and learning how to translate your desires into specific goals, you can gain a level of clarity that makes anything from the smallest to the largest decision simple and rewarding

Think Lean is about teaching you to become a resilient person with clear goals supported by quality beliefs. In this section we will explore each of these concepts and learn how to make the Think Lean Method real in our own lives. To get there, we need to know what stands in our way and how we overcome it. We need to know **what threatens our ability to stay consistent and, well, why do diets never seem to last?**

Why do diets fail?

Some diets can make you lose weight faster than others. Some are healthier than others. Some are better researched than others. So why don't we get consistent results from all these diets? The answer is that we are terrible at sticking to them[189]!

Still, we know that some people can manage to do it which is proof that it is absolutely possible to achieve consistency. As I developed and adopted the Think Lean Method, I found that I had developed the ability to stick to healthy eating habits for years and years on end. Not only that, but I found that the Think Lean Method helped other aspects of my life improve too. This was because the same three concepts that helped me stick to clean eating also helped me to look clearly at other parts of my life that weren't working either.

So, just what are the main obstacles that get in the way of us sticking to our dietary goals?

- **Stress** – Chronic stress from work, relationships, health issues, even sudden high pressure moments. Stress can sap our energy and raises cortisol (the stress hormone). Too much cortisol can damage the hippocampus[190,191] and create traumatic memories
- **Challenging events** – Relationship troubles, accidents, natural disasters, health issues, retrenchments at work. These are the crises that life keeps throwing at us and which can easily throw us off track with our diets if we are not prepared
- **Social pressure** – Hanging out with friends and work colleagues often results in pressure to eat and drink with the rest of the group. This is one of the most common situations that prevent consistency with healthy eating

- **Toxic environments** – Sometimes we are in an environment where we face bullying, verbal or even physical abuse. We need to deal with these if we are to achieve success – and not just with body goals

- **Information overload - mental whiplash!** – We live in an information age where there is a constant inflow of new diets and new research. All this information can result in 'mental whiplash', leaving us feeling like it is just too hard to eat right!

- **Too impatient for results** – Let's face it, we want results fast and when they don't come fast enough, we are prone to giving up and trying something else instead. This results in us spending months or years looking for a quick fix that never comes

- **All-or-nothing thinking** – Ever had a day where you found yourself eating something that is not on your diet so you decide that the diet is ruined for the day and you just keep eating more and more? You are not alone, this all-or-nothing thinking happens to many people!

- **Dieting as a temporary fix** – We often take on diets to lose weight quickly. We may try to do too much too soon, resulting in a big change that is not sustainable long term, which makes us think *"It didn't suit my lifestyle"*, *"It was too restrictive"*, *"It just didn't work"*

- **Unclear or bad goals** – Not having clear goals means not having a clear path to achieving the right results. This means we waste time getting results we didn't want, causing us to feel frustrated and to give up. Clear goals are essential – not only for our diets, but for our lives overall!

As you can see, there are loads of reasons that can cause our diets to 'fail'. No wonder so many diets end up not giving us the results we want! As we have all experienced, dieting it not as simple as just knowing what to eat. We need to have the mental strength, discipline and willpower to make these choices every day so we can get results. We need to set ourselves up for success, which means having the right goals in place and the motivation to succeed.

This is where many diets fail - they tell you what to eat and when, but then don't prepare you mentally to turn the diet into a complete lifestyle change.

We need to overcome the mental blocks that prevent us from achieving results and find practical ways to overcome them to set ourselves up for success. Considering the reasons why diets fail, we can overcome these through the Think Lean Method as follows:

Issues	Fix it with:
Stress Challenging events Social pressure Toxic environments	4.1 Personal resilience
Information overload - mental whiplash Too impatient for results All-or-nothing thinking	4.2 Quality beliefs
Dieting as a temporary fix Unclear or bad goals	4.3 Developing goals

Think Lean

You can see in the diagram above that each of the factors that stop diets from succeeding is addressed through one of the concepts of the Think Lean Method. This combines with the section on how to Boost Your Brain to provide an environment that is ready for the Think Lean Method to get you feeling 100%.

> Our first stop is Personal Resilience. How can we be more like those people who just seem to bounce back from anything in life and not let everyday stresses affect them?

4.1 Personal resilience

Personal resilience is defined as the ability to **positively respond to difficult situations**[192]. There's a key word here that is important to point out – it is not just our ability to respond to a difficult situation, but our ability to **positively** respond to a difficult situation that is important. The addition of the word 'positive' highlights that there is more to resilience than our normal ability to make it through adversity.

It is important to realise that resilience isn't something you either have or you don't – in fact, you can be more, or less, resilient, and it is a skill that you can learn. We all have some amount of innate personal resilience – otherwise we wouldn't have made it this far through life! Yet some people seem to manage stress and crises better than others, and some come out the other side with less scars than others. So why is this?

The difference is in how **positively** we respond to these moments in our lives. Think of a scenario – let's say you are on your way to work and your car breaks down. Do you:

1. *Start to panic, get angry at the car and the situation because this stuff just shouldn't happen, finally get into work late, have a terrible day, eat some sweets to feel better, go for some drinks after work to relax and eat whatever you can find. Oh, and diet? What diet?*

2. *Or do you recognise that these things happen, that yes, it is frustrating, but you can call someone to come and sort it out. You call you manager to let them know you'll be a bit late and do everything else as you normally would on any other day. You keep your smile and you eat healthy like any other day*

There are so many situations which are like this and, quite simply, the difference between panicking and taking it in all your stride comes down to your level of resilience and being able to **positively** respond to the situation. And being able to positively respond to situations is something I want to help you achieve.

4.1.1 What is personal resilience

Personal Resilience consists of five components that are driven by clear goals that we set to help us achieve our own goals. This is especially important for reaching body goals. Let's take a quick look at each of the components that make up Personal Resilience:

- **Realistic optimism** – A grounded and realistic sense of hope for your future and your ability to reach your goals

- **Involve others** – Your relationships with family, friends and work colleagues are crucial. Don't do it alone!

- **Look after yourself** – Proper sleep, exercise and nutrition keeps you physically ready for anything. Boost your brain and go on the Think Lean Method

- **Embrace change** – Each change is a challenge and a chance for you to improve yourself and move closer to your goals

- **Self-assurance** – Develop confidence and be centred within yourself. You are the only one that needs to approve of yourself and your actions

These components are all connected and support our ability to positively respond to anything – even the most difficult situations. We will work through each of these components in turn, though here is a challenge for you – don't just read! Instead, take your time with this section and compare these ideas with your own beliefs. You will feel when something is different from what you believe and how you behave. If you feel or notice that difference, don't skip over it – really think about it and consider if your current beliefs are giving you the results you want, and if not, open yourself to the idea that there might be a better way.

This section may be confronting, and really, it *should* be confronting. If you don't feel challenged by some of these ideas, then you probably haven't opened yourself enough to be able to seriously consider the possibility of a personal transformation. The key is not to run away - if you feel challenged or uneasy, go towards that feeling and take comfort that it is exactly how you should feel, and that it is the beginning of your own transformation. It all starts with having clear goals.

4.1.2 Clear goals

Clarity. Clarity is something we all should aspire to have in our lives. Clarity of what our goals are, clarity of what we want to achieve. How often do you find yourself having trouble making a difficult decision? How often do you feel like you keep making the same mistakes? Or that you just have no direction? Are you doing a bit of this and a bit of that, anything that makes you feel good for a while? Or maybe you feel as if you are being pulled in too many directions, by too many goals and too many people?

This is what happens when we don't set clear goals. Setting *clear goals and also understanding how to use those goals to make decisions gives us an incredible amount of clarity in what the right and wrong decisions are.*

First we need to understand our own goals. We need to set real, achievable and meaningful goals, and we need to identify what motivates us to achieve our goals, even if it seems trivial. As the driving force behind our Personal Resilience, our goals need to be clear to us to provide clarity to the rest of our lives.

After all, actually pursuing your goals is not a complex process. Once you know what you need to do, you only really have to do two things to make it a reality:

1. **Decide to do it**
2. **Do it**

It's that simple. From a dietary perspective, if you want to make it a lifestyle, there is a third step:

3. **Keep doing it**

What more is there than that? It is really simple once you consider it like that. On the other side, not having clarity around goals makes it difficult to decide what to do in the first place, meaning you can't get to step two. Or you may constantly decide to take on different goals - constantly doing different things, meaning you get no consistency and don't actually manage to

> **Goal-directed thinking**
>
> Think of learning to play a musical instrument – if one month you try the piano, the next month the flute, then the drums, then a guitar, and so on, after a year you still won't play any instrument and you will feel like you just wasted a year. Instead, if you pick one and stick with it, then you'll actually have a real skill by the end of the year.
>
> By picking one instrument and focusing on it as a high priority goal, you will start to naturally spend more time on learning it. Anything else would not be part of the goal, so you eventually start to subconsciously move other things aside to make time for what is really important.
>
> *That* is effortless discipline. *That* is goal-directed thinking.

achieve anything worthwhile. This is why we need to look more closely at our goals. Overall, having clear goals allows us to:

- Make decisions that enable us to keep our actions focused on our goals. It gives us something to consistent strive for. If we don't have something specific we are working towards, we can't be consistent, and consistency is what we need to be able to achieve results with our bodies
- Maintain our perspective in difficult circumstances. Even during a crisis, focus on what is really important
- Be proactive, rather than reactive. You get into the driver's seat of your own life. You make your own opportunities and actively take your life in the direction you want

Even if you take on board nothing else in this book, the simple act of developing clear goals in your life is already enough to cause a personal transformation. You will find you will start to see through the noise of everyday life, put events and decisions into perspective and actively work towards where you want to be.

If you are familiar with the corporate world you may have heard of setting SMART goals, an acronym for Specific, Measurable, Attainable, Relevant, Timeframe. Using this method can help you to set realistic goals that you can actually achieve. However, this doesn't help you with the main issue – which goals should you set in the first place? Setting bad goals can be just as damaging as not having any goals at all. To be able to develop and set clear goals, we need to have a deeper understanding of ourselves, our needs and our motivation.

Goal development involves:

- **Understanding what is really important – understanding our needs.** If we neglect our needs when we set goals, we will find it hard to consistently work towards our goals
- **Developing a vision of yourself.** This can be extremely difficult, but I will show you an easy way to create a powerful and motivating vision
- **Setting clear goals.** Determining goals and learning how to set meaningful body goals
- **Prioritising goals.** This one is often forgotten, but clear prioritisation will improve your ability to make decisions and stay consistent with your goals

For now, we will leave the goal setting until after we have worked through the rest of the Personal Resilience section and the section on Quality Beliefs. The reason for this is simple – while you need to understand the importance of setting goals now, the goals that you end up setting might change after having read through the next sections.

4.1.3 Realistic optimism

We are often told to *"Be positive"*, *"Look on the bright side"*, or my personal favourite, *"Just be happy"*. Book after book, article after article tells us about the virtue of being optimistic, but there is a line between being optimistic and being overly optimistic. Sometimes when we are not optimistic ourselves, we look at people who are overly optimistic and feel that they are just totally deluded.

The difference here is **realism**. Optimism needs to be grounded in reality for it to be useful to us – otherwise we will have unrealistic expectations of how we should feel or what should be happening. It is important to clarify that the choice is not just between 'optimism' and 'pessimism'. In fact, it is a sliding scale stretching from being deeply pessimistic at the one end to overly optimistic at the other end. In the middle is realist. In this context, being a 'realist' is essentially someone who is neither particularly negative nor positive.

| Deeply Pessimistic | Pessimist | Realist | **Realistic Optimist** | Overly Optimistic |

Personally, I used to be a 'realist' by that definition, but have since shifted towards being a 'realistic optimist' as I have clarified my goals and vision for myself, and gained a better understanding of how to get there. Also keep in mind that we can be optimistic about some things and pessimistic about others at the same time. We don't need to be one or the other about everything. What is important is that we have *a realistic sense of optimism about what is most important to us*.

We need to find that balance between being realistic and being overly optimistic. This balance ensures that we have realistic expectations about how easy it will be to achieve our goals and get results with our diets. In fact, this is where many people and many diets fail as have been proven by recent studies.

- One study showed that women who expected to succeed lost a lot more weight than those who didn't[193]. Interestingly, having a positive image of what you want to achieve on its own doesn't help you realise your goal. You need to have the confidence that you will succeed!
- Another study revealed that when thoughts of a positive fantasy (like having the confidence to succeed) were contrasted to the negative reality (like being overweight right now), people started to feel that they could turn their fantasy into a reality, and thus achieve their goals[194]. Suddenly they were motivated into action!

Fantasies on their own result in us being overly optimistic. We form the expectation that reaching our goals will be easy and quit the moment it becomes hard. Overly positive fantasies have even been shown to drain our energy[195], as we feel that the fantasy should already be a reality.

To be motivated into action, we need to have realistic fantasies, but we need to be confident and positive in our expectations that we will succeed. Confidence in part comes from knowing **how** we will achieve it. If we know the steps we need to take and we know these steps will work, then we gain confidence in how to get there.

What should our internal dialogue look like? Essentially, it could be something like this:

- *"I want a lean body and want to weight X"*
- *"Currently, my weight is Y and it is not where I want to be."*
- *"I know what I need to do and I am confident in the steps I need to take."*
- *"It will be challenging along the way, but I am confident that I will stay consistent and I expect to succeed."*

> **Try it!**
> Give yourself a quick test by using the internal dialogue to the left on yourself. Talk to yourself about your own goals, and say each of the lines to yourself.
>
> What does it feel like? Do you believe yourself, or do you feel like it is untrue? If you don't believe yourself just yet, don't worry – we will go through the steps in more detail as we go so that you get the confidence you need to follow through with healthy eating and get the success you want!

This simple dialogue shows what we've been talking about so far – know where you are, know where you are going, have confidence in the method to get there and have confidence that you will do what you have to in order to be successful.

This creates that realistic optimism that motivates us into action and increases our chance of success.

Visualisation

I'll share with you a mental trick that has dramatically improved my own personal resilience over the years. This is one of those techniques that really sets resilience apart from our everyday capacity to manage personal crises – this is not just about managing crises when they do come up, but instead is about preventing crises, and limiting the impact on yourself when something does happen. This is where we get 'ahead of the curve' – in the same way as regularly servicing a car reduces the chance of it breaking down, or regularly visiting the dentist prevents cavities.

So what is 'Visualisation'? It was originally developed by the Stoic philosophers in ancient Greece. They called it 'negative visualisation' which in short is when you imagine personal crises as if they are happening now.

But why on earth should we want to do this?

The Stoics used this technique to reduce the mental impact of negative events and maintain a 'level head' when something bad happened. This makes us less reactionary (less emotional) when something happens, allowing us to better manage difficult situations. This technique is very useful for us on our healthy eating journey, especially considering common events such as people pressuring us to eat cake, or when we get cravings for sugary foods!

I have successfully used this technique for a long time for a few specific purposes:

- **Maintain perspective during adversity** – This is one of the original purposes of the technique. It starts to become clear that every crisis can be managed – there is always something that can be done, and certainly no reason to panic. In fact, once it becomes clear that emotional reactions during crises are not useful, it becomes easier to stay rational, allowing you to focus on solving the problem

- **Appreciate what you have** – This technique reminds you that nothing lasts forever, but rather than detach from it, you should enjoy everything as much as you can while you can. Visualisation reminds you to make the most of your life, including pursuing your goals with passion and to fight for what you want!

- **Prevent crises** – As you consider events and feel your emotional response to it, you also start to identify which events would impact you too much and which you need to do something to prevent. If a goal or project is very important to you, focus on what you can do to keep it on track. Consider what can go wrong and do whatever you can to prevent something from going wrong. Get advice from others – learn from their experience to help you stay on track and avoid the common pitfalls – especially with dieting!

- **Motivate yourself to take action** - Visualisation is essentially the same as negative fantasies. From what we read about in the study earlier, negative fantasies are actually better at making us feel energetic than positive fantasies[195]. This is because negative fantasies motivate us into action to prevent that vision from becoming a reality. Combine that with an expectation that you will succeed and you find a powerful motivational tool that builds personal resilience

Putting this ancient technique into context with the modern world, a similar technique called 'exposure' therapy is also used as a modern psychology treatment for anxiety[196]. This involves gradually exposing someone to something that they deeply fear, resulting in a gradual 'depowering' of the emotional reaction. Gradually the patient becomes more rational in response to the trigger. In the same way, visualisation is powerful in building your personal resilience.

So how can you do it too?

Early on in using this technique, it can be quite confronting to imagine negative events – all kinds of emotions come up, it is painful and you might want to stop thinking about it. The easy way to begin practicing is to start thinking about smaller events. This gives your brain practice with thinking in that particular way. Then you can build up to bigger events. Keep pushing through and contrast one event with worse events for perspective. You can start with questions like these – what would happen if:

- You lose your phone or wallet?
- You lose your keys?
- You lose your computer/laptop/tablet?
- Someone gives you a chocolate while on the diet?
- There's a party and people pressure you to have cake?
- You don't lose weight as fast as you like?
- You don't lose weight at all?

> **A note on anxiety**
>
> We start small so we can gradually build up our ability to think through scenarios. It takes time to build this ability, so be patient!
>
> However, if thinking through a simple scenario like losing your phone starts to give you feelings of anxiety already and you can't continue, stop and discuss it with a therapist or psychologist before attempting again.

Each of these lines of questioning can motivate you into action. You can make backups of all the information on your phone and computer. You can have spare keys with a friend or partner. You can get insurance for loss of income. Same goes for eating healthy – you can prepare for any situation so that when they do come up, you'll be ready and you can stick to your diet!

This adds to our sense of realistic optimism as something that is not just overly optimistic thinking, but as something that motivates us into action to achieve our goals. When we contrast our hopeful vision of our future selves with the reality of the present and we have a realistic understanding of what we need to do to get there, then the steps we need to take become clear and we become motivated to act.

Practicing visualisation causes physical changes in our brain that help us solve complex problems. Having a strong ability to solve problems means we can better manage whatever situation comes up since we can come up with useful and practical solutions. Let's take a quick look at our brain and neural networks to get a better understanding of how problem solving works.

The prefrontal cortex houses our ability to perform complex thought and think abstractly. This is where we come up with creative and useful solutions to complex problems. When we are not mentally prepared for adverse situations, the process in our brain is as follows:

1. The perception of the event enters through our eyes, ears, etc. and the signal is transported to the **thalamus**
2. The thalamus sends the signal to the **amygdala** for threat assessment
3. The amygdala does a quick check with the **cortex** to find out if it should stay calm (downregulate)
4. If the cortex doesn't tell the amygdala to calm down because it is not a real crisis, then the amygdala activates the **'fight or flight'** response. This reduces blood flow to the cortex, disabling complex problem solving and we start to behave impulsively and emotionally

In the moment itself it is hard to control this response if you are not prepared for it. The easiest way to overcome this response is to change step 3. This is where we have control as we can prime our cortex to respond to the amygdala and tell it to calm down. An easy and reliable way to prime our cortex is, of course, through visualisation.

As we start to practice visualisation, we simulate the signals that we would get from an actual crisis. Imagining a negative event passes through the thalamus and into the amygdala as it normally would. The amygdala does its check with the cortex to see if this is bad or not. If the cortex is silent on the imagined event, the amygdala activates 'fight or flight', just as it normally would, and you start to feel panicked. So, even though you are just imagining it, the amygdala can have a hard time telling apart real signals from imagined signals, providing very similar feelings as you would in a real event.

> **Practice visualisation**
>
> To change your brain and benefit from visualisation, you need to practice. The brain is plastic and changeable, but you need to practice for change to happen on a neural level.
>
>
>
> *Your task:* Once a day, think of a scenario. Visualise what it would be like, how you would react, and see what feelings come up. Start small (like losing your wallet).
>
> Start small to make it easier to think through the scenario in a calm way. If it starts to make you feel anxious, look back at the purposes of why we do this. You can even talk a scenario through with someone else and get their perspective. This can be an easier way to start. As you become more comfortable with working through scenarios, take on bigger ideas and challenge yourself more!

This is why we need to start small. Don't think of too heavy subjects right away, as it will just cause you more harm than good. What we want to achieve through visualisation is to change the response that the cortex gives to the amygdala when a crisis happens. We do this by building our beliefs around our ability to manage crises so that the cortex will tell the amygdala to stay calm.

As we do this, the structure of our brain begins to change and we start to become able to use our whole brain during a crisis. Without this, our responses are limited to our primitive impulsive brain, which is not able to do complex problem solving. A **whole brain response** gives us the ability to think clearly, even when terrible things happen, allowing us to respond in a useful way.

To illustrate this, here are some basic beliefs that we can use to shield our amygdala from overreacting (note – from here on we will mention beliefs quite often. Beliefs will be highlighted with a light coloured stripe behind them, like the bullet points below, so you can easily identify them):

- *"Every crisis can be managed."* (and I do mean *every* crisis)
- *"Before I react, I need to understand the situation. What exactly is the problem?"*
- *"I might have misinterpreted what I heard/saw. I need to clarify so I react in the right way."*
- *"This is not the end of the world. I will survive this."*

Imagine these beliefs as a nice, comforting blanket that the cortex throws over the amygdala when there is a crisis.

"There, there, amygdala. It's not so bad. Everything will be ok."

The key here is to prevent a hasty and impulsive response and give ourselves the time to come up with a useful response. For example, when you are unexpectedly presented with a slice of cake, the thinking shouldn't be *"OMG I didn't expect this it looks so good I can't resist this oh I'm never going to lose weight so might as well eat it!"*

No, we'd rather be prepared for that situation so that we can think something like this *"Oh, I have prepared for this. I'll just say I'm being healthy"*, or *"Like I've decided before, I'll take the slice of cake, eat a few bites and throw the rest away when no one is watching"*, or *"I'm very consistent with healthy eating, so I can eat a slice of cake now and then without having to worry about getting fat. So I'll eat it and enjoy it!"*

Whatever your strategy, if you are prepared, your cortex can keep the amygdala calm and you can come up with a useful response without getting stressed. As we slowly introduce visualisation exercises, our cortex builds neural networks that are better at down-regulating the amygdala, helping us to stay calm and focused. Building these neural networks take time, so don't expect to suddenly change overnight.

A physical brain change takes a while, but the more you practice it, the stronger it becomes. This is like a workout for your brain and your reward is calm focus, even in the toughest situations. Practicing this also means there is less adrenaline and cortisol released when you experience a traumatic event. This action and the calming effect that the cortex has on the amygdala means that the hippocampus will be less prone to form traumatic memories. Without those, it is easier to move past the event and get on with your life. Brain derived neurotrophic factor (BDNF) is increased and you learn from the event rather than getting stuck on the past!

> **The meaning of dreams**
>
> A leading theory of the meaning of dreams is that it is a way for the brain to test different scenarios and find out which responses would help to reduce anxiety, stress and frustration[197]. The strategies that best do this are kept and integrated into the brain, while others are discarded.
>
> The brain runs these scenarios based on what is available in your brain and what you are focused on, which is why certain people and situation might come up often in your dreams. As the brain tests scenarios, we can find ourselves having very confronting dreams. We wonder why we dreamt it, but really the brain is trying to test which responses would be best for difficult situations in a dream state in an effort to help us cope better in real life.
>
> If we change our brains through visualisation and build realistic optimism, our dreams will become more constructive and less disruptive. I experienced this myself, as I used to have nightmares and disturbing dreams, but now my dreams are interesting and enjoyable. Sometimes they still feature challenging scenarios, but my response in them is always useful.
>
> If you have trouble with dreams, this can help you a lot!

This is also why it is important for us to do visualisation in the context of realistic optimism – we need to maintain a realistic sense of hope of the future to be able to maintain the belief that we can manage and get through any crisis, no matter how small or large.

4.1.4 Involve others

Being independent is fantastic. Having the ability to do things on our own is a great skill to have. But that doesn't mean you need to do everything on your own! In fact, a recent study has shown that when it comes to weight loss, it is best to do it with someone else[198].

Research shows that weight loss spreads across social groups. Basically, this means that if you connect with other people who are losing weight, then you are more likely to succeed in losing weight yourself. So if you have friends and acquaintances who share your plan to lose weight, you are also more likely to lose weight[199].

The mechanism for this is simple – when you have friends who are also looking to lose weight, you can keep each other on track and focused on losing weight. You can also help each other through the tough times and stay consistent.

There are even more reasons to involve others – when you tell other people about your decision to reach a body goal (or any goal for that matter), then those people can help to make it easier for you to reach your goal. Believe it or not, most people are actually decent and will try to help you towards your goals when you share your goals with them. After all, if they do not know that you are trying to lose weight, then how will they know not to constantly put doughnuts under your nose?

Sharing goals with other people allows them to provide two types of support:

- **Emotional support** – Helping you to stay focused and helping you through tough times. Being interested, offering concern and being compassionate with your efforts to lose weight
- **Physical support** – These are the practical things, like choosing restaurants that supports you in eating healthy, helping you avoid tempting situations, bringing healthy snacks to office parties, and so on

When you let people in, they can be powerful in helping you stay motivated and consistent. Of course, not everyone will care that much, but I can tell you that around 95% of people will be supportive of your goal in one way or another. That 5% of people who don't support us, we just ignore. There's no need to worry about them and their opinions – you don't owe them anything, so stay focused on your goal!

For the rest of the people, you can even ask them to help you stay consistent and stay focused on your goal. As you have probably found, one of the toughest times to stay consistent is during social gatherings where the pressure comes on to 'let loose' and enjoy yourself with everyone else. Naturally, 'enjoying yourself' usually equates to drinking alcohol and eating carbohydrate-rich foods. Not helpful. But let others in on your goals, they can help you avoid and navigate these situations. Even better is if you have a friend there with the same goal. It is much easier to say "No" to some cake when there is someone else also saying "No".

> *Important note!* *If you ask someone to help you stay consistent with healthy eating, and they come around and offer you a chocolate, it does not mean they are working against you. It does not mean they are out to get you. It does not mean they are your enemy!*
>
> *Remember that everyone is fighting their own battles, and sometimes they forget about what you asked for. It does not make them bad. It does not make them your enemy. They simply forgot, just as we are all prone to forget things. Plus, if they are offering chocolates to everyone else, they probably feel it would be ruder not to offer it to you as well, than it would be to skip you because you are eating healthy.*
>
> *Similarly if you asked someone to help you and during a social gathering they tell someone not to offer you cake because you are eating healthy, don't get angry at them for 'making choices for you' or something like that. After all, you asked for their help, and even if they are saying this semi-sarcastically, what they are saying is in line with your goal, so be glad they said it. Again, no reason to get angry at all. It works towards your goal and that is what's important.*
>
> *Remember that everyone is trying to do the best they can. Stay focused on your goal and be patient with people.*

Perceived support

If you are in the corporate world, you might have heard the often repeated phrase that *"perception is reality"*. To many, this doesn't seem to make sense, as, reality is reality, right? Not so, unfortunately. You see, we are limited by our senses and our brain. We can only see and hear so much, and from the amount of information that our senses do take in, we can only focus on a small amount of it. From the small amount that we do focus on, we can only integrate a small portion of that into our thoughts and memories!

Think of watching a movie – during the movie we see and hear everything, but right after you have probably forgotten the names of the characters already. A day later we only remember bits of the dialogue, parts of the sounds, and we can only recall specific scenes when someone reminds us of the scene. A while later, most of the movie is forgotten other than the general plot and maybe some specific scenes that really stood out.

We can only experience the world through our perceptions. Sure, we can imagine things, but even our imaginations are based on perceptions of the world. Since our perceptions of the world are what we act on, it starts to become clear that, indeed, our perception *is* our reality. Even if we perceive the world incorrectly, we would act on our incorrect perception rather on the reality, as we are not aware that our perceptions are wrong.

This is why research has consistently shown that it is not actual **received support** that is important to us, but rather **perceived support**[200]. Received support is when someone actually does something for us, but perceived support is your belief that someone will help you when you need them. Interesting, isn't it? It is more important for our mental health to *believe* that we will get help when we need it, than to actually get it.

The reason for this has to do with our *biases*.

Back to the movie example, what stood out for me would be different than from what stood out for someone else. We all have different interests, different senses of humour, and more. These differences cause us to focus on different parts of the dialogue and events. These are our biases. We all have biases through which we look at the world. If we did not have biases, we would not be able to cope with the flood of information constantly coming in. Biases help us to put information into a context that makes sense to our way of thinking.

It is important to know that people all have different biases. This explains why four people can leave a meeting and every person has a different take on what was said. And as much as it would be nice, it is not possible to just force everyone to abandon their biases and think your way. Our biases are integral parts of us, and every person needs them to function.

Our belief in whether or not someone will help us during a time of need is also a bias. If we have a bias that people will help us during difficult times, then it affects our actions as we become more confident in taking risks, as we know that people will be there to help us if we stumble. Even if this is not entirely true, our belief in it being true gives us the peace of mind we need to fight for our goals.

If you are worried that you might not have the support you think you have, or if you already believe that you don't have much support, just go and talk to some people you know and ask if they would help with eating healthy. The vast majority of people would be happy to help you. More than that, most of our friends and family would help us if we have a major life crisis. It is ok to believe that you will get support when you need it! For your own mental health, you need to have the perception that you will get support. If you really feel you don't have that perception, there are many you can talk to:

- Friends
- Family
- Your partner
- Colleagues
- Pets (yes, even dogs and cats can be great sources of support!)
- Therapists and psychologists
- Meetups and support groups in your city
- Online forums and support groups

♦ Social welfare for really difficult situations

There absolutely is support out there!

Of course, the best situation is to have both the perception of support and also real support provided by the people in your support network. Stay in touch with your friends and family. Let people in on your goals, and support others as well with what they want to achieve. Be a friend, and maintain your friendships.

4.1.5 Look after yourself

Taking care of your body and mind is a crucial part of personal resilience. Health issues, both chronic and sudden can be a source of constant disruptions in our lives. Disruptions like these can make it extremely difficult to stay consistent with healthy eating. Health issues sap our energy and take up the little time we have available. It adds stress to our lives and we fall behind on work and personal tasks.

Simply put, *a resilient body supports a resilient mind.*

Good nutrition, sleep and exercise

Looking after yourself involves many components that we have already discussed in the previous sections as this mainly involves maintaining good nutrition, getting enough sleep and including exercise in your routine.

- **Good nutrition** – This is what the Think Lean Method is all about – healthy eating that is proven to be beneficial to the health of your body and mind. It not only helps you lose weight in a healthy way, but also helps to provide your brain with the right nutrition to help you feel energised and ready to take on the world!

- **Sleep** – We saw before that when we are sleep deprived, there is less blood flow to our prefrontal cortex and more to our amygdala. This results in more impulsive behaviour and makes us more likely to crave and eat unhealthy and fattening foods. This reduction of blood flow to the prefrontal cortex also lowers our ability to solve complex problems and we feel like we can't 'think straight'. When we are constantly not getting enough sleep, it can be hard to properly process information as it comes in, like properly putting in context what people say and events we experience. This can leave us feeling like 'everything is just too much' and we feel as if we don't have any control of our lives. These days, I fight for my sleep as I know I need at least seven hours to be able to function properly the next day. Fight for your sleep!

- **Exercise** – In the Boost Your Brain section we also found out that exercising enhances brain plasticity and stimulates the creation of new neurons to improve learning ability and mental performance. It releases endorphins and improved blood flow to the brain, and even protects against cognitive decline. Of course, this doesn't even bring into account the most basic benefit of exercise – feeling strong and looking good! Even if you don't feel all the other effects of exercise, the confidence boost of having a body you are proud of in itself can be a massive benefit to your ability to handle the day to day stress of life (any time you feel stressed, you can at least look in a mirror and think *"Well, at least I'm making progress!"*)

All of these factors contribute to having a healthy hippocampus that produces plenty of BDNF, which in turn helps your brain to continually grow and adapt to your environment as it changes. This allows you to have that 'whole brain response' that gives you the ability to creatively solve complex problems and make good decisions in difficult times.

In the Boost Your Brain section we touched on enriched environments. Let's take a deeper look into that, and also its opposite – toxic environments.

Enriched environments and cognitive reserve

Our brains have the capacity to withstand a certain amount of damage, making the brain in itself 'resilient'. This capacity of the brain to withstand damage is called **cognitive reserve**. Studies have shown that the more cognitive reserve we have, the more resistant our brains are to damage and disease, such as Alzheimer's and other degenerative diseases[201,202].

Studies have also shown that we can *increase our cognitive reserve*, especially in our earlier years[203]. The best way to do this is by engaging in activities that are mentally stimulating - like studying topics that interest you and doing additional courses and certifications for work or for hobbies. We are also much more likely to do this if we are in an environment that is healthy for our brains.

What does an environment like that look like[204]?

- We feel supported by others and, where we have constructive relationships
- We have a sense of control over our environment and that things make sense
- We find positive experiences that support our goals and limit negative experiences
- We can enhance our self-esteem and constantly improve how we feel about ourselves

These factors make up a high quality, or **enriched environment** where we feel at our best. Think about what it is like at home or at work – do you feel that these factors are present in these environments? Do you get the chance to be your best, or are there some factors missing? If so, why are they missing?

There is a great deal we can do to create an enriched environment for ourselves. Our own actions, thoughts and decisions are what we have control over. By taking accountability of our own state of mind, we can change how we relate to others, how we respond to situations and how we interpret events. Through these changes, we can transform an environment that we previously thought of as negative into a positive environment.

Toxic environments

While we should take responsibility for the environments we find ourselves in, it doesn't mean it is necessarily all our doing, or that we need to put up with it. The main example of this is when we find ourselves in situations where we experience abuse. This can take many forms, for example:

- Living with a verbally and/or physically abusive person (partner, parents, roommate, even children)
- Living with someone who has an addiction (drugs, alcohol, gambling, etc.), possibly refusing treatment
- Working in a place where there is bullying, verbal or physical abuse
- A work environment that constantly puts unrealistic expectations on staff and reprimands them for not meeting these unrealistic expectations (evidence for this would be people regularly getting fired for performance issues.)
- Friends who belittle you, subvert your efforts, and constantly drag you down. Beware of 'friends' that suck energy out of you without ever adding to your life

As you can see, when talking about toxic environments, we are not talking about living next to an asbestos factory, but rather about psychological environments we may live in where our basic needs are regularly violated. We want control, but it is taken from us. We want safety and positive experiences, but we are attacked and harmed. We want positive connections with people, but they betray us and belittle us. We want to feel good about ourselves, but we are made to feel worthless.

These are toxic environments, and if it sounds familiar to something you are experiencing right now, then you need to know something – *you are going to struggle with sticking to healthy eating until the situation is resolved.*

> **Talk to someone**
>
> If you feel you are in a toxic environment, talk to a therapist or psychologist. Remember that part of personal resilience is to involve others. It is a hallmark of personal resilience to recognise when you need help and asking for it. Don't do it alone – ask for help!
>
> Keep in mind that when you find yourself in a toxic environment, the people closest to you may not be the best to help you out of it. In these situations, having someone from outside (like a psychologist) may be better to give you a realistic and objective view of the situation and how to get out of it.

Toxic environments add huge amounts of stress to our lives through constant disruptions and upsets. Sometimes it feels like there isn't even one single day where things are ok and we can get on with things. This makes it incredibly difficult to stay consistent, which is what we need to get results and reach our body goals.

Often, toxic environments are out of our control. We can't just stop someone from being addicted to alcohol. We can't cause a sudden personality change in a bullying manager. We can't suddenly stop a partner from being abusive. If you are subjected to abuse, *it is not your fault*. It is the fault of the abusive person. When we can't change the situation, sometimes the only real solution is to get out. **This is drastic action, so talk to a therapist or psychologist if you feel you are in a toxic environment.**

Remember, *it is a hallmark of personal resilience to involve others*. There is absolutely no shame in asking for help – in fact, it is a sign of strength and resilience to recognise when you need help and ask for it. You deserve to be in a positive environment. You don't need to subject yourself to abusive treatment. You may be ready to soar, but you can't do it if someone is constantly breaking your wings. You may feel that you need to put up with the situation because you need the money, or for the kids, but remember – you can't look after others if you don't look after yourself first. There is always hope, so remember – talk to someone and involve others!

4.1.6 Embrace change

Change is often something we fear. It represents a disruption to our normal routines and patterns, and when we detect that these routines are being forcefully changed, our amygdala can easily start firing and make us feel like panicking. When we are not prepared for change, it can feel like a loss of control – a violation of one of our basic needs.

But let's face it – change is everywhere and it is constant. It is the one thing we can count on in life. There will always be change in our lives. Just think of these examples of change:

- A change/loss of job
- Changes within your job or projects you are working on
- A new relationship, or breakup of a current one
- Moving house/countries

- People changing
- Conversations that change your perception of people
- A new coffee machine or microwave (you mean I have to learn this device all over again??)
- Not being able to eat certain foods anymore
- Eating out less and making more food ourselves

Most of us are here to make some positive changes to eat healthy and get great bodies, but it can be challenging to make the mental shift. So what holds us back?

Why change is so hard

When we do not have clear goals, we tend to spend our time settling into our environment (work, home, relationships, diet) until we feel nice and comfortable – not too stressed, we know what to do, have our routines, and we want things to remain as they are. Even if we are not getting the best results, the environments become routine, so we want to protect that and fear any change. Here our brains become sensitive to any perceptions that there might be a change (threat) to our environment, leaving the amygdala to fire up as soon as we sense a change. This quickly leads to feelings such as anger, fear, stress, frustration, or depression.

We can feel as if we have wasted all the time and effort we have put into a task, a job, a relationship. Now that it is changing, it was all worthless, and we just hate to think that our efforts didn't mean anything! Of course, this is absolutely not the case. Even though a change has happened, our efforts contributed to us building new skills, having new experiences, making new contacts, making new friends. Yet we have a hard time remembering all these benefits in the middle of a change.

The reason we tend to overlook all the benefits we received before change is due to our amygdala firing, causing us to experience 'tunnel vision'. The blood flow to our prefrontal cortex is minimised, meaning we can't think straight and have a hard time solving complex problems that change often brings. We are in 'fight or flight' mode, and this really does not help us to deal with the situation!

Still, we know that there must be a better way. To get there, we need to think differently about change.

Improving how we think about change

One major change that you will feel over time when you start doing **visualisation** is that you become far better at calming down your amygdala and you become much more clearheaded during periods of change.

As we practice visualisation, we also start to think through possible changes to our environment, so that when something does happen, we will have already considered the possibility and consequences of it. This makes us prepared and ready to handle any change and disruption.

> **It's all connected!**
>
> The components of personal resilience flow into each other and support each other. This is why it is important to work on all these aspects. Skipping one can compromise your overall resilience!
>
> You can work on them one by one, but remember to work on all of them eventually to build true and lasting personal resilience that helps you stay consistent with healthy eating in all situations!

Combine that with having **clear goals** and suddenly change becomes an opportunity. When we have clear goals we are working towards, we can assess change through the lens of our goals and identify opportunities to move closer to our goals. When we know what we want to achieve, we can even become *instigators of change*. This is when we proactively start to create our own opportunities to move closer to our goals.

For example, if we want to build a specific skill at work, we can push to join certain projects, join a different team, or swap tasks with someone else in the team. We can build persuasive arguments for why we or the team needs to do something different and change how the team operates. Sometimes simply being honest with your manager about what you would like to achieve can help bring about a positive change and give you the opportunity you want.

So often we feel as if our job is rigid and we can't change anything, even if we want to. But the reality is that everything is negotiable. In a single team, there are likely some people who have a far better deal than others, simply because they negotiated it. Remember - you have to fight for your goals to achieve them!

This also applies to our diets – we may feel like control is being taken from us because we can't eat this or that anymore. We love our food and when our brain detects that some of our favourites might be taken away, our amygdala starts firing and we become resistant to the change. Even though it wouldn't be hard to change our diets, the amygdala decreases blood flow to our prefrontal cortex, limiting our complex problem solving skills. This makes it harder for us to think of ways to incorporate healthy eating into our lives, and we get feelings like *"This is just too hard"*, *"It's just not going to work"*, while ignoring evidence that it absolutely is working for others, so it can work for us too!

If we apply clear goals to the idea of healthy eating, then we can improve how we think about doing it. No longer is healthy eating a threat to our favourite snacks that we are comfortable with, instead healthy eating becomes a fantastic opportunity to get healthy and create the body we've always wanted!

Improving our beliefs about change

Our beliefs about change shape the emotions and thoughts we have when we experience change. For example, if we have a general dislike of change, then a change in our job environment will likely cause us to get angry and stressed. On the other hand, if we are actively pursuing change as opportunities to reach our goals, then a change can be a time of excitement.

A simple way to start changing our beliefs about change is to consider a few good beliefs about change. Read over each of these and pay attention to your emotions as you do so:

- *"There will always be change. Change is a natural part of relationships, business and life in general."*
- *"I can manage any change, because I can manage any situation."*
- *"Change brings opportunities to move closer to my goals."*
- *"When change happens, I will look for hidden opportunities."*
- *"I will proactively manage change towards what is most important to me."*

A note on the last belief listed above about proactively managing change. This one goes a bit further in than simply controlling our reactions to change by proactively staying on top of what change might be coming. If we keep sight of possible changes on the horizon, we can better prepare for the change, or we can even fight the change where we are able to prevent the change from happening. Fight change? Yes, we need not always blindly accept change. Sometimes people want to change situations when they are better left alone.

So, do the sentences above grate against your beliefs? Do you feel like you disagree? What comes up instead in your mind? If you feel as if you don't like any of these or don't believe them, ask yourself why you disagree. What is holding you back? The simplest way to challenge your own beliefs is to simply ask yourself: *"Why do I believe this?"*

That leads to more questions:

"What is my evidence?", "Where did I hear that?", "Does my evidence actually make sense?"

Once you start digging a bit, you'd be amazed at how many of our beliefs come from distant childhood experiences that we misconstrued, but never challenged, so they've always been around colouring our lives. Remember, you are only talking to yourself – there is no shame in admitting that you have been wrong. The only shame is continuing to be wrong once you've realised there is a better way! Being able to update your beliefs is a crucial aspect of personal resilience and quality beliefs (the next section). Challenge yourself and don't back down if it feels a bit confronting!

Knowing when to fight change and when to accept it is an art form, and a lifelong learning experience. We can get better at making this distinction by improving our understanding of our environment, the people in it, and that we have the power within ourselves to make change happen. One of the scariest realisations is that we have far more power than we think we do.

Of course, some change will still bring pain when it involves loss of something important to us. But this is about building personal resilience – your ability to bounce back from that change. Visualisation helps you be prepared for that situation and improves your ability to deal with it by increasing blood flow to your prefrontal cortex. Clear goals help you filter the event and see opportunities to move closer to what you want to achieve. Even if the change involves major disruptions to your life, it can still end up being a positive event.

Now you can see the power of embracing change - *our emotions change and our attitudes change because we know change is an opportunity.*

4.1.7 Self-assurance

Now for the final component of personal resilience – being centred within yourself. Having confidence in yourself. You are the only person that needs to approve of your goals and the pursuits you choose to follow!

Take a moment and think about how you feel when others show their disapproval, particularly when someone disapproves of what you are doing. Let's say someone comes up to you and tells you your diet will never work:

1. Do you immediately start to question yourself and start to worry that maybe you are not doing the right thing?

2. Or can you easily handle their comment because you know you've done your research and you are confident in your decision?

When someone challenges a position you've taken, challenges an idea or belief of yours, or says something you don't agree with – do you find yourself getting angry, upset, flustered, offended, or hurt? Again, these feelings come up when our amygdala senses that we are vulnerable and it engages its 'fight or flight' mode.

In this instance, the amygdala does a quick check with the cortex to see if it can handle the idea or belief being challenged. If the cortex is silent on the challenge, the amygdala takes over, reduces blood flow to the cortex and floods our system with adrenaline so we can protect ourselves. Of course, this response really doesn't help when our ideas are being challenged, as this is a time when we especially need our prefrontal cortex. At these times, outsiders find us to be 'hard headed' and 'stubborn', because we keep repeating familiar and safe ideas and refuse to listen to their ideas.

On the other hand, when our brain contains beliefs that we have already extensively challenged within ourselves, then no challenge from the outside comes as a surprise. In this case, when the amygdala checks with the cortex when the challenge comes in, the cortex will reply that *"Yes, we have considered this and it is not a threat."* Then the amygdala calms down and you think with your prefrontal cortex, allowing you to think clearly about the challenge and respond without feeling threatened.

To be able to manage these situations effectively, we need a resilient sense of confidence, which consist of the following:

- Be committed in our actions
- Build firm values, principles and beliefs
- Be decisive and trust our own judgement
- Believe in our own self-worth
- Bounce back from mistakes

These build strong neural pathways to the prefrontal cortex with good cortical blood flow, which in turn helps to downregulate the amygdala during these situations. This translates into a stronger feeling of confidence in these situations, since we can stay calm and collected. Let's take a look at each of these.

4.1.7.1 Be committed in your actions

When we take action on anything in life, we prefer to know what we are doing and have some assurance that our action will result in success. Often when we take action, we are very unsure about it, and we are filled with self-doubt as soon as we run into adversity. Just think of buying a used car – it can be a nerve-racking experience because we just don't know the history of it, or if it will break down right after we buy it! The same goes for diets – will it work, are you going to be able to stick to it?

If we are not sure of our actions, then the first sign of trouble can make us give up. Luckily, we can secure our actions in a few ways:

- **Do research** – This is why the Think Lean Method has so much research behind it – it gives you the confidence that this diet is proven and has the evidence to support it. Therefore, you know it works, and if someone else challenges you on it, you can point them to the research! You can also look up research on your own, investigate what other people did, and gather evidence

- **Think through alternatives** – Consider different ways in which you can accomplish the same task and what the potential results would be. Having thought through alternatives means you won't be surprised when someone else comes up with a different way and causes you to question your methods. Talk to others about your ideas to get alternatives before you start. Read the next section on Certainty for more about this

* **Don't worry about perfection** – It is more important to be consistent than to be perfect. You can never do anything perfectly, it is simply impossible, so don't even try. In particular with diets, aim for consistency rather than perfection. If you are consistent, you will get results!

4.1.7.2 Build firm values, principles and beliefs

If there are certain things you definitely do not want to be part of, or do not want to do, then take a stand and do not give in. For example, if you do not want to do drugs, or don't want to drink alcohol anymore, make the decision and stick to it. Often when we make these decisions and do not stick to it, it can diminish our sense of self-worth as we feel like we can't even follow through on simple decisions.

> **My experience with drinking**
>
> Sure, I used to have a few drinks. Then one day I decided I've had enough of drinking, so I stopped. Given the drinking culture in Australia, not drinking involves constantly declining drinks, but using these techniques, I have stayed consistent with not drinking and I have not had a single alcoholic drink in ages.
>
> The same goes for my eating habits. Once I decide to eat a certain way, I stick to it using these same techniques. It can take a while to develop this kind of discipline, but it is absolutely achievable, and the Think Lean Method gives you the tools to achieve it as well.

Being able to stick to it involves preparation. You can use visualisation for this as well, where you picture yourself in a situation where you get pressured to drink alcohol (let's say you have decided not to). You probably know how it will go – people keep pushing you to drink, different people put the pressure on. Someone just hands you a drink, and you feel it's rude to refuse now that they have already paid for it, so what do you do?

As you visualise the situation, rehearse what you will do. For example, if someone just hands you a drink, take the glass, say thank you and that you are not drinking. Then put the glass down and carry on with conversation. You can offer it to someone else, and if no one wants it, it can just sit there. You are under no obligation to drink just because someone bought it for you. Even if your friend bought you the drink, if you have previously expressly said that you are not drinking, and they still buy you a drink, *then they are not your friend in that moment*. They might still be your friend overall, *just not in that moment*. If they were really your friend in that moment, they would respect your wishes.

In this example, it is only your choice if you end up drinking or not, but it is important for your own self-worth to be able to make decisions and stick to it. Same goes for drugs, gossiping, illegal stuff, and more. If you do not want to do something, make a decision, rehearse how you would resist it, and stick to it. Even if it is stuff you used to do before, you can make a decision today to be different. Involve others and tell them you are not doing something anymore, and ask their help to stick to it.

As you practice saying no and sticking to your decisions, you will become better at it and it will take less effort! If you do find yourself giving in, do not view this as a failure. Instead tell yourself you need more practice. Also, just because you start something, doesn't mean you need to finish. For example if you catch yourself with a bite of cake in your mouth, it doesn't mean you now have to finish the rest. You can have that one bite, and put down the rest. There is no universal law stating *"If thou taketh one bite, thou shalt finish the rest!"* No. You can take one sip, take one bite, and put down the rest. Simple.

These same principles especially apply to eating healthy:

- **Decide** that you will eat healthy and follow the guidelines in this book
- **Visualise** yourself in situations that might challenge you and rehearse how you will manage it (such as parties, going out drinking, office functions, etc.)
- If you know some event is coming up, **be prepared** and take along healthy meals and snacks
- **Involve others** and ask them to help you stay consistent
- **Stick to your principles**, values and beliefs. Do not give in – you owe it to yourself!

At the core of all this are our beliefs. Having firm beliefs help us to feel centred and secured.

4.1.7.3   Be decisive and trust your own judgement

When you make a decision, especially a big decision, do you find yourself calm and collected, knowing that you did the right thing, or do you become riddled with doubt? A big part of confidence is being able to trust yourself and that you know what is the right thing to do. You need the ability to trust yourself to collect the right information, make the right decision, and take the right action.

Do you see other people who are confident and decisive, and wish you were like that? I'll let you in on a big secret – they are just as uncertain as you are! That's right – everyone has doubts. Everyone struggles with indecision. So how do most people deal with it? Mostly by the *fake it till you make it* approach, or sometimes even the *fake it till you can fake it better* approach, along with not questioning themselves after they have made a decision.

Faking confidence and faking being decisive can actually help to build confidence. Try acting confident at work tomorrow and you might just notice something surprising – that you actually start to feel confident! This is not just some illusion, either. Studies have shown that standing in powerful poses (where your body takes up more space and limbs are open and away from your body) actually increases the circulation of testosterone and lower cortisol, causing you to feel more confident and powerful[205].

Low-power poses (where you take up minimal space and your limbs are closer to your body) does the opposite by increasing cortisol and decreasing testosterone. This is why slouching make you feel less confident. Studies show that you can adopt a powerful pose for just one minute and you will feel a difference. In fact, try it right now! **Try one of the following poses for one minute:**

- Put your feet up on the table, sit back and put your hands behind your head (like you are an executive sitting at their desk thinking about buying a bigger boat)
- Stand up with your feet about shoulder width apart, hands on your hips and chest up (the Superman pose!)

As you hold the pose, testosterone starts to increase, making you feel more decisive and confident, while cortisol decreases which reduces feelings of stress. Feeling more confident yet? Just think of managers and leaders who adopt these poses all the time in meetings and presentations. Think of the confident people you know who do this in social situations.

Now we start to notice something – faking it is not even faking at all. **It is practice**. Confidence is actually something you practice! By faking it, you might simply be allowing yourself to trust your own judgement, an ability that has been there all along! A large part of actually being confident, *is acting confident*. By acting confidently, you practice *being* confident and build habits like keeping

good posture that physically increases testosterone and feelings of confidence.

Of course, confidence must still be supported by quality beliefs, clear goals and personal resilience. So take this on as a task – act confident in your daily life, keep a good posture, and remember that you need to practice being confident to actually be confident!

4.1.7.4   Believe in your own self-worth

Can you look in the mirror and give yourself a genuine smile? We need to be able to trust that we are worthwhile, and that those close to us value us, just as we value them. We are so good at finding fault, especially with ourselves, that we often have a hard time just looking in the mirror and being able to smile at ourselves regardless of all the faults we see.

Finding faults in ourselves is actually ok, as long as we do it in a *constructive* way. This is called **constructive self-criticism**, and is a way for us to look within ourselves at what is and isn't working, and take action to help us move towards our goals. When we get better with constructive self-criticism, we also become better at handling criticism from others. If your criticisms of yourself leave you feeling sad and depressed, then you need to change to constructive self-criticism. You will know you are doing it right when you feel energised afterwards and want to take action.

Follow these guidelines to change to constructive self-criticism:

- **Don't judge yourself** – Don't make broad negative personal judgements like *"I am useless" "I'm so stupid"*. Universal judgements like these serve no purpose other than making you feel even worse about yourself. If you are going to make broad judgements like these, make them positive, like *"I'm great at [something]", "I'm actually ok",* or even *"I'm awesome"*. If you feel you can't do that just yet, then continue to the next point

- **Be specific** – If something didn't go as well as planned, then focus on what specifically went wrong. There is no need to judge yourself for what happened – focus on the specifics of what went wrong, whether you can fix it, and how you can prevent it from happening again. If a report was wrong because it didn't contain some information, then it doesn't mean you are useless. It just means that next time you should double check that area to make sure it has what it needs. By focusing on the specifics, mistakes become a learning experience that help you improve!

- **Discard the words 'always' and 'never'** – *"I always mess that up", "I never get that right"*. These two words sneak in so easily and they wear down our sense of self-worth. After all, if you always mess up something, then you are making a prediction that you will mess up again next time even though you might actually succeed! In fact, you are more likely to succeed if you believe you can succeed. These two words are far too absolute and we are all better off without them. And while you are at it, don't use them in reference to other people either!

- **Recognise when external sources share the blame** – None of us are immune to the effects of our environment and the people around us. Usually, we are not the only ones to blame for something going wrong. Recognise when others are also involved in what happened and hold them accountable as well. Talk to them about what went wrong and try to find a constructive way to prevent it from happening again. There is no need to dwell on the past, but there is value in analysing it to prevent it from reoccurring

Be constructive with yourself. Be specific when looking at things that went wrong, and absolutely avoid making negative judgements about yourself. They are just not useful. Taking these steps will help you have more respect for yourself, and once you have more respect for yourself, you will notice that others will start to respect you more as well!

4.1.7.5 Bouncing back from mistakes

It is easy to get stuck on old mistakes and we often exaggerate and dwell on them for far too long. Be constructive about mistakes and challenge yourself with the beliefs below about mistakes.

- *"Everyone makes mistakes. I too will make mistakes."*
- *"I am not my mistakes. Mistakes do not define me."*
- *"When I make a mistake, I take responsibility for it and I fix it."*
- *"I am not afraid of making mistakes. I can overcome any mistake."*
- *"I will think constructively about my mistakes and how I will prevent them from happening again in the future."*

Depending on your job or situation, you might throw in another belief:

- *"If I am not making mistakes, then I am not working fast enough."*

Obviously that last one applies less when you are an air traffic controller or surgeon. But for most of us, we have colleagues and managers around us who can catch mistakes, and we can be vastly more productive if we allow ourselves some mistakes and trust the people who support us to catch occasional slip-ups. Internalising these beliefs changes your mindset, and you become appreciative when someone catches a mistake, rather than feeling threatened by it.

Bouncing back from mistakes also includes letting go of old mistakes and incorrect beliefs and letting go of feelings of guilt and shame.

These are the components of personal resilience. These concepts can be quite a lot to take in, especially if much of this is different to your current beliefs. Don't worry about internalising it all at once – you can focus on small parts to begin with and work your way through it in time.

This way you can work your way through each part of personal resilience, gradually building it up in yourself and making it a reality. It will take time and effort, but all good things do! So be patient with yourself and stay the course. The benefits are incredible!

> **What to remember:**
> - Personal resilience is the ability to positively respond to difficult situations
> - Resilience is driven from clear goals which give clarity and guide your decisions and actions
> - Boost your resilience through realistic optimism, involving others, looking after yourself, embracing change and being self-assured

4.2 Quality beliefs

The personal resilience section already called out a few good beliefs, but let's take a step back to consider what beliefs are and why they are important. Beliefs are thoughts and ideas about the world that we hold to be true. Beliefs are important as they set our expectations about the world, and guide our thoughts, actions and emotions. We act on our beliefs. We form ideas from our beliefs. In fact, beliefs are at the very foundation of who we are.

Most of our beliefs are set as we grow up and experience the world. Of course, we often misinterpret events when we are young as we have a limited concept of the world we live in at that age. This means that many of our beliefs are not as accurate as they could be. This leads us to the first of three important *beliefs about beliefs*:

1. *"Not all beliefs are equal"*

As the saying goes *"Everyone is entitled to their opinion."* In the same way *"Everyone is entitled to their beliefs."* While sure, anyone can believe whatever they want, there is a practical reason to want better beliefs, because:

2. *"Better beliefs help me to be more successful in life"*

Think about this from a dietary perspective – Person A believes that eating lots of cake will make them leaner. Person B believes that eating protein and vegetables will make them leaner. Both go out and act on their beliefs. Who do you suspect will get to their goal of being leaner? Hint - it's not cake. The reason that some beliefs are better than others is because in the real world, physics and cause and effect come into play. The better we understand what really works and is proven to work, the better we can align our beliefs and act on those beliefs to get real benefits!

This is really why we should strive for quality beliefs. If you find that you keep doing the same thing, but it is not working, or you find that you are just not achieving the goals you want, despite your best efforts, then there might be old beliefs holding you back. Since beliefs shape our very experience of life, the better our beliefs are, the better our success in achieving our goals! But what if we don't have good beliefs already? Well luckily:

3. *"I can change any belief"*

We can challenge any belief we have and change it to something more useful and practical to help us be more successful. Changing a belief is actually very easy – you simply have to challenge a belief with new information and possibilities. The hard part is being open to change it in the first place!

Think of having an argument with someone, and somewhere during the argument, you realise you were wrong. How often do we announce *"Oh, I just realised that I'm wrong and you are right."* Yep, pretty much never! We absolutely hate to be wrong. 'Saving face' is crucial to us.

This tendency to resist being wrong is the main obstacle that gets in our way when we try to change our beliefs. Remember that part of personal resilience is having the ability to bounce back from mistakes, and this includes letting go of beliefs that turned out to be wrong. Updating beliefs can be really easy. For example, we may believe that Transylvania is only a fictitious place where Dracula comes from. But it only takes a quick search to find out that Transylvania is actually a real place in Romania. Just like that, we have updated our belief about Transylvania!

Essentially, every time we learn something, we form new beliefs and update old beliefs. In this way, our beliefs are the things we 'know' to be true at a certain point in time. To change a belief, we need to challenge it, which means we need to do a bit of introspection and challenge our own ideas.

Once again, our amygdala often comes barging in when we attempt to change beliefs. If we are not prepared to be wrong, then as soon as we sense that we might actually be wrong about something, the amygdala fires up in an attempt to defend us against the threat of being wrong. Our adrenaline starts to spike and we lose higher reasoning skills so our arguments deteriorate and our thinking becomes rigid. Definitely not helpful when we are trying to improve our beliefs!

As we get better with challenging ourselves, our cortex gets better at calming down the amygdala as we start to understand that being wrong is not a threat to us. Being resilient means we can handle being wrong, and we actually appreciate learning when we are wrong because it means we have the opportunity to improve our thinking and use that improvement to be more successful!

> **Beliefs don't change overnight**
>
> When we first realise that a belief is wrong, the updated belief is held in the brain as a memory. This memorised updated belief stands in conflict with the old belief that exists as a strong neural network. The updated belief now has to slowly break down the old neural network and form a new one that is more resilient than the old one.
>
> While this happens, the memorised updated belief and old belief can cause some conflict and we might feel confused when we need to act on it or think about it. But rest assured! The plasticity of your brain allows the old belief to be dissolved and replaced with the updated belief. This takes a bit of time, but stick to it. I promise you it is absolutely worth it!

To give ourselves a better chance at overcoming the initial reaction from the amygdala, we can prime our cortex with this thought:

- *"I think I could be wrong about (belief in question)"*

Starting with this thought about particular beliefs immediately opens us up to considering alternatives. Once we are open, we can engage our whole brain to consider new ideas and new possibilities. This means when we integrate the new belief, it is linked through wider neural networks. Wider networks mean we can think broadly and more creatively, using our whole brain to solve problems and come up with useful solutions to issues we face. As we do this, our brains become our friend and we start to trust ourselves more as we know we can come up with useful ideas to overcome problems and reach our goals!

Types of beliefs

When I say you can change any belief, I do mean *any* belief. Now, you can convince yourself that you are a pony made of rainbows, but that would not be a very useful in reaching goals in general. What we need are beliefs that are grounded in the real world - beliefs that we can rely on to make accurate predictions about the world and guide our decisions.

We can broadly set apart two types of beliefs:

- **Core beliefs** – These are broad beliefs that we base a lot of other beliefs on. These are beliefs like what is 'good' and 'bad', what is 'right' and 'wrong', if the world is fair, whether people are good, etc. These tend to be harder to change and are formed earlier in our lives. They exist as heavily ingrained neural networks that have been strengthened over many years, making them resistant to change

- **Outer beliefs** – These beliefs surround our core beliefs, and are more specific in nature. They include things like what we know about our job, our general knowledge, specific beliefs about specific people. These tend to be a bit more changeable, depending on our mindset as the neural networks that contain them are not so strong yet

Usually, we don't spend much time strengthening our core beliefs, so in an effort to protect these core beliefs, the brain surrounds them with more rigid outer beliefs. The outer beliefs need to be more rigid, because if they change, they can affect the core belief, which would threaten our sense of self!

For example, Jane is overweight and has a core belief that "Dieting just doesn't work". This belief comes from growing up in a family that has always been overweight and compounded by not having had any success with dieting herself. This core belief conflicts with reality, as obviously there are many people around the world who are maintaining lean bodies through healthy eating. Naturally, she is often confronted by these lean people, so to protect her core belief from reality, she constructs rigid outer beliefs around it.

To protect the core belief, she has, amongst others, an outer belief that "All thin people are starving themselves and have eating disorders". This gives her a way to explain what she sees and is a way to dismiss the lean people she runs into and challenges her view. Some lean people try to tell her that they are not starving, and that they do not have eating disorders. She can even see them eating lots of (healthy) food, but despite the evidence, she sticks to her outer belief. If she allowed evidence to get past the outer belief, then she might have to face the fact that "Dieting does work". Since that would challenge her core belief which underpins many other beliefs, it would make her wrong about a lot that has been ingrained in her since childhood! And we all just hate being wrong.

This is why her outer beliefs need to be rigid and unyielding even to strong evidence – to protect the vulnerable core beliefs she holds inside.

The bouncy ball of beliefs

To illustrate the example above, you can imagine these beliefs as layers of a bouncing ball. This ball bounces through life and hits all kinds of obstacles (difficult situations) along the way. Following on the example above, the very outer layer of the ball is made up of beliefs we don't worry about too much and are willing up change if we get new information. This thin layer gives a bit of flexibility as the ball bounces along.

'Soft' centre consisting of unchallenged beliefs

Next is a thick layer of rigid beliefs which do not yield even to strong evidence. They are rigid, because they protect the vulnerable core beliefs in the centre. The centre is 'soft' because they have not been examined and a challenge might mean that we need to admit (to ourselves at least) we were wrong, which would affect many other outer beliefs.

Large set of rigid beliefs that are resistant to change, even if new evidence is presented. Tries to protect the 'soft' centre

Few flexible beliefs to buffer against challenges and change

So you can imagine a ball like this with a thin flexible layer on the outside, a thick rigid layer, and a soft centre. As it bounces through life, most of the little bumps along the way are absorbed by the thin flexible layer. However, when we hit some larger bumps that make it through the outer layer and hit the rigid layer, the ride starts to get rough - like driving in a car without shock absorbers. These larger bumps shake us to our core, bringing up all kinds of feelings such as anger, confusion, and frustration.

This rigid bouncy ball shows us the opposite of personal resilience, because it does not have that ability to bounce back from big blows in life. It does not have the flexibility we need. And importantly from a dietary perspective, it can cause many events in our life to ruin our consistency because every now and then we have to recover from another big shock! To overcome this, we need a more flexible model.

A resilient bouncy ball

This time, imagine a bouncy ball with a big outer layer of flexible beliefs, open to change given new evidence. At the core is a solid centre, made up of quality beliefs that have been examined and challenged. These core beliefs are solid, but not rigid. There is always the understanding that they might be wrong, and we can change them, but we need strong evidence to change these.

- 'Solid' centre consisting of quality beliefs
- Events interpreted through clear goals give direction and further stabilises the core
- Protected by flexible beliefs and understanding of the world that is open to change and new evidence

In the middle, we have a new layer that is made up of our clear goals. This layer also has a bit of flexibility, and further stabilises the core by allowing us to make better use any jolts or bumps from the outside. In fact, this layer allows us to bounce back even higher when we hit a big bump in the road. This layer provides us with true resilience!

When we are like this, we have a nice thick layer to absorb even the biggest blows in life. With our solid core we feel centred, in control and relaxed. Even if a bump gets all the way through the thick flexible layer, we can consider it and rebound to become even stronger than before. The middle layer of our goals helps us to keep our direction and bounce back higher.

This brings us back to our original definition of resilience – **to positively respond to adverse situations**. We don't want to just bounce back, we want to bounce even higher and do even better after a tough situation. This way, we get stronger and stronger through adversity in life, and nothing in life can beat us down!

Changing core beliefs

Sounds good? It is! But the road to get there can be challenging and we need to prepare ourselves for it. I'll be honest - changing core beliefs can be a frightening experience. When we truly hit that point where we feel we are about to challenge and change a core belief, it feels like our whole world is in jeopardy. It feels like, if we were wrong about this belief, how many other things may we have been wrong about?

In that moment, the most frightening thing is not knowing what kind of person we may become if we change the belief. That uncertainty of how it might affect us at a deep level and how it might affect our perception of life is huge, so we need to prepare our brains to be ready for a change. So ask yourself a couple of tough questions:

1. *"Are my current beliefs actively helping me reach my goals?"*

2. *"Is my current way of thinking giving me a positive and useful experience of life?"*

3. *"If I do not change, I will keep feeling like I do now – is it maybe better to be open to a new way of thinking and change?"*

In fact, that last one is a guarantee – **if you keep your beliefs as they are, nothing will change**. Once you can honestly say to yourself *"Yes, I'm ready for things to be better"*, then you become willing to update your beliefs. You can look more honestly at your beliefs and recognise where a belief is not helping you be successful and have a positive experience of life.

Just take this core belief as an example:

- *"People are terrible."*

That is a massively broad belief that surprisingly many people have. Except for a very few people very close to us, we can believe that everyone else is just bad, so we close ourselves down to new people, we judge their actions as 'mean' and we easily get angry at people for being the way they are. But we can replace this with a more realistic quality belief:

- *"Everyone is doing the best they can with the information they have."*

Suddenly, we realise that everyone is just like us – trying to make the best decisions and take the best actions given the information they have available. Realising this, it makes it hard to get angry at people as we know they are fighting their own battles, just as we are, and they are fallible and make mistakes, just like us. This belief builds compassion and opens us up to others.

If you are challenging your beliefs in this way, it could be a bit scary. So what should you think if you feel frightened when you are challenging a core belief? You should think *"This is fantastic! I'm scared and that is great!"* That is because if you feel that way, you are making progress! Don't turn back - push through. At that point, you know you are about to make a real change in your life. *This is the point to have courage and go all the way.*

What is important now is to look at a few common pitfalls we need to avoid when choosing and internalising beliefs:

1. **All-or-nothing thinking** – This sets traps for us and makes us give up far too easily in the face of adversity. What is a better way to think to help us stay consistent?

2. **Certainty** – We want to be certain about something before we take action, but is this the best way, especially when going on a diet?

3. **Rationalisations** – What are these and how do they stand in the way of us staying consistent with our diet?

> **Hanlon's razor**
>
> One of my core beliefs is a paraphrase of Hanlon's Razor:
>
> *"Never attribute to malice that which is adequately explained by ignorance or misunderstanding."*
>
> This essentially means that it is extremely rare that anyone does something because they are 'bad' or because they are 'evil', or because they are specifically out to do something 'bad'. Instead, usually it is just because people don't realise what they are doing, or were mistaken about something and it happened to affect us in a negative way.
>
> For example, imagine getting cut off in traffic. Did he do it on purpose? No, it is more likely he didn't see you, or is in a rush for some emergency. The result? No need to get angry – just deal with the situation and move on!

As we go through these, we will turn our focus specifically on eating healthy and staying consistent. That is the ultimate aim here after all!

4.2.1 All-or-nothing thinking

A trap we frequently fall into is thinking that we need to totally commit to something and do it 100% correctly 100% of the time. How often do we find ourselves having a chocolate in the morning and deciding that the diet is now ruined so we might as well pig out for the rest of the day? Then after a day like that, we figure that the diet is now ruined for the week, so we'll get back to on diet next week!

This kind of all-or-nothing thinking means that any little failure causes us to postpone our efforts to eat healthy. You probably picked up that this kind of thinking is definitely not resilient, and it is a threat to our ability to stay consistent with healthy eating. We need to be able to look beyond this at the reality of the situation.

What is the reality? The reality is that **the healthier we eat, the more we benefit**. We don't have to eat healthy either 100% or 0%. If we eat healthy for 90% of the time, we get nearly all the benefits. At 80% we still get most of the health and some weight loss benefits. Even if we only follow it 50%, it can still help us to live healthier.

Trying to follow it 100% might just be too restrictive and unrealistic for many people – but that does not mean it is hopeless and not worth it! Just think of it this way – if you are following ACM 95% of the time, it means you get one free meal a week. Not bad, right? You could even split that free meal into three snacks through the week and you'd still be around 95% clean eating!

The people I know who are most successful at maintaining their weight in the long term realise that they can treat themselves every now and then, enjoy it guilt-free, and get back to healthy eating right after. Having a chocolate or a piece of cake for them doesn't mean their healthy eating is now ruined for the week and you might just as well give up. For them it is a treat that they can comfortably have now and then, and they can get right back to eating healthy straight after and they know that one treat is not going to make them overweight.

That is important to realise – it takes consistent overeating to put on weight and maintain an overweight body. One meal doesn't make you fat, just like one healthy meal isn't going to make you lean. You need to eat consistently to go either way!

Another area where we tend to apply all-or-nothing thinking is when we look at our results – we eat healthy for a while, then we look at our bodies and our weight and decide that this just isn't working fast enough, so we decide it is not worth the effort and totally give up. The reality is that good results take time, and they come gradually. Think of this common scenario:

> *Chloe wants to lose 10kg quickly. She looks around and finds a diet that promises that she can lose 10kg in two weeks. She goes on the diet and after two weeks, she notices that she's only lost 2kg. Disappointed that she didn't lose all 10kg, she drops the diet and looks for something else. While looking, the 2kg comes back on with an additional 1kg for good measure. Now she wants to lose 11kg, and spends a few weeks looking for a better diet. She finds another one, and the same thing happens. Six months go by and she ends up weighing 5kg heavier than when she started! This all builds a belief in her that "Dieting is totally useless!"*
>
> *Instead, if she realised that all-or-nothing thinking is counterproductive, then she would recognise that losing 2kg after two weeks is a great start. Not as good as it could have been, but still she's making progress to her goal. That way, if she just stuck with the first diet and stayed consistent with it, she could have lost all 10kg in less than three months!*

Our drive to want it all and want it now blinds us to what we can have if we just stayed consistent and waited a bit longer. What belief can be distilled from this?

- *"Consistent healthy eating pays off far more than a burst of dieting."*

Perfectionism

Are you a perfectionist? If so, it is important to realise that 'perfect' does not exist. **To seek perfection is to guarantee failure** because it is not possible to achieve perfection. Ask a number of people what their perfect meal is – they will all answer differently. Ask people what their perfect man or woman is – again all different.

And so it is with trying to stick to a diet perfectly – it takes a lot of dedication to perfectly follow any diet. If you try to do anything perfectly, you will nearly always be disappointed as perfection is an illusion. Besides, everyone's idea of perfection is different!

Nothing can ever be perfect, but hey, that's OK! We don't need perfection! Instead of aiming for perfection, **aim to be better than you were before**.

This is what is really important – instead of aiming for perfect healthy eating, aim to be better at healthy eating than before, then aim to do it better day after day, week after week. Now you start to use yourself as something real and tangible you can measure your success against. Don't measure against other people! Instead measure against yourself, and each time try to do a little bit better than you did last time.

You can write that report a little better than last time, deliver that presentation a little bit better. Improve your relationships, bit by bit. Learn from last time and improve. *Perfection never tells you what you did wrong, it only tells you that you've failed yet again.* This is an important distinction, as the one is constructive, and the other destructive. Measuring against yourself shows you what you can improve and where you can do better. Aiming for perfection just results in failure without constructive feedback on where you can improve. So forget about perfection and aim for improvement instead!

> **Don't wait for perfect conditions!**
> How often do we say *"Oh it's not the right time for a diet"*? Far too often! The timing may never be perfect, but the best time to start is still right now! Don't wait for the perfect conditions, as they may never come. Instead, start right now!

Holidays and healthy eating gaps

If you are going on holiday, eating out for a special day, or so on, then go and enjoy it! When you come back, get back to healthy eating and pick up where you left off. Sure you might be a kilogram or so heavier, but these moments are so important to life and you should never feel guilty about enjoying them. If these moments happen all the time and your goals start to suffer, then you can look for strategies to limit the effect. For example:

- If there is a cake every day at work because somehow every day is someone's birthday, then you can eat just a few bites of the cake and throw out the rest
- If there are a lot of office functions, stick to the healthier food and stay away from the rest
- Take along your own healthy snacks and stick to those

Strategies like these can help you stay consistent even through difficult circumstances. Otherwise, if you generally follow the ACM 95% of the time and you are going on holiday, then go and enjoy yourself – try the local foods, make the most of it, and get back on ACM the day you get back. No problem! Forget about the weight and just get back to eating healthy. No guilt, no shame.

So let's turn this into two quality beliefs:

- *"I do not have to eat perfectly healthy all the time."*
- *"The healthier I eat, the more I benefit and the closer I get to my goal."*

Here's what you should get out of it – if you are aiming to stick to ACM 95% of the time, then enjoy that 5% totally guilt free! Sticking to ACM 95% of the time is a fantastic achievement all on its own, so enjoy that free meal like no tomorrow! And then get back on ACM right after. If someone asks you *"What happened to your diet??"* Then I recommend sticking your tongue out to them.

4.2.2 Certainty

Closely related to all-or-nothing thinking is the idea of 'certainty'. We like to be certain that we are doing the right thing. People often ask us *"Are you certain?"*, *"Are you certain healthy eating will work?"*, *"Are you certain this is the best way to lose weight?"*

The answer? No. We are not certain about anything and we can never even be certain about anything. In fact, we can't even be certain that we can never be certain about anything! This is a bit of a philosophical point, but it has important implications for us when we are eating healthy.

Many people think we only make a choice when we are certain about what we need to do. This is nearly the opposite of how the brain actually works. The brain does not work on certainty, but instead it is 'fuzzy' and works on **probability**. Probability essentially means the brain picks the choice that it thinks has the highest chance of success.

When faced with a choice, the brain throws the different choices at its own model of the world to try and make a prediction of what will be more successful. The model comes back with a few different potential outcomes, and the brain translates these into which choice is preferred. You know this when you say *"I think I need to do this and not that."*

> **More successful predictions**
> Our model of the world in our brains is essentially our knowledge and understanding of the world and how it works. The better our model, the more accurate our predictions and the more successful choices we can make. This is actually a very important point, and is a reminder of why we should always try to increase our education and general knowledge.

We spoke a bit earlier about perception and here is another important point about it. Our senses (vision, hearing, touch, etc.) are not perfect. For example, our eyes can only see objects when there is light on them or around them. This means when we see something, we are not actually seeing the object, just the light bouncing off the object. Since there are many different types of light, some outside our visual range, we only get a very limited perception of the object. In fact, if we saw it in different types of light, we would have an entirely different perception of the object.

> *Imagine a table. If the light was coming from behind us, we only see that it is a table made of wood, and we think it has a rough, wooden texture. If the light it moved to the other side of us, we see that there is a glare on the table, which tells us that the table is actually smooth. When we touch it, we notice that it is not smooth, but is actually a bit sticky because someone did a bad varnish job on it.*

So, each time we learn a bit more about the table and our perception of it changes. Each time we make a bunch of assumptions based on what we see. We might even be 'certain' that we know the table is smooth, until we learn it is actually sticky and then we are 'certain' that.

Bottom line is that we our senses give us very limited information, and it is never enough to be certain about anything. In fact, we can't even be certain that we are reading right now, because we might be asleep and dreaming all of this in a very vivid dream. At any time our 'certainty' about something can be dissolved when we learn more. So it is best to realise first and foremost that we can't be certain about anything. This gives us a new core belief:

- *"I can never be certain about anything."*

Though this belief can cause a lot of distress since how are we going to be able to do anything if we can never be certain about anything? That is why we must consider this one with another belief:

- *"It is not **necessary** to be certain about anything."*

Given that we have never been certain about anything, instead we have only ever had the illusion of certainty, it follows that we have never actually needed to be certain of anything because we have been making choices just fine for our whole lives. So why are we talking so much philosophy in this book? Well, this is what it means when we realise we can't have any certainty:

- **We understand the importance of evidence** – We now see that the more we know, the better decisions we can make, and the more evidence is behind our healthy eating plan, the more confidence we can have that healthy eating is right for us

- **It adds to our personal resilience** – Knowing that we do not always have a perfect perception of situations means we don't jump to conclusions too quickly. Instead, we look for more evidence and confirm our understanding before we react. Especially with some new diet fad or something someone else said

- **We understand that our choices do not need to be perfect** – Most important of all, we know that sometimes we make mistakes with our diets, but consistency is far more important than perfection! If something turns out to be wrong, we fix it and we move on and stay consistent

4.2.3 Rationalisations and excuses

To really be able to overcome the habits and behaviours that hold us back, we have to be open and honest with ourselves about what these habits and behaviours actually are. This can be surprisingly difficult, as often we have spent so many years rationalising and making excuses, even to ourselves, that it becomes very daunting to look past what we have accepted all these years. Just think of the excuses we use so often:

- *"I'm not feeling well, I just want something sweet"*
- *"I'm so stressed, I need some ice cream"*
- *"Oh one cookie wouldn't hurt"*
- *"I'm just too busy today to eat healthy"*
- *"It's been a rough day, I deserve it"*
- *"Just one more bite"*
- *"I'll start tomorrow"*
- *"At least it's not like I'm eating a whole cake"*
- *"Today is an off day"*

You know what, some of these are not bad in themselves, but the problem is that we use these every day! How often do you wake up thinking to yourself *"I'm feeling great! I'm going to eat healthy today!"* Or *"I'm so relaxed today, who needs chocolate!"* Pretty much never, right? Instead there is always something happening or something wrong that gives us another opportunity to use our excuses and keeps us from getting the body we want. So we end up using the same excuse over and over, feeding our bad habits. In psychology this is known as **rationalisation**.

Rationalisations are explanations we use to provide a more socially or personally acceptable reason for our behaviour, *while avoiding the real reason*. Rationalisations can be powerful and last for a whole lifetime if we let them. Just think about how often we use the trusty old rationalisation: *"I'm just too busy"*. When are we ever not busy? Yet we seem to make plenty of time to watch our favourite TV shows, go out drinking, go to restaurants, and more.

We use these as a way to rid ourselves of responsibility and present our actions in the most favourable light. This makes it sound like our actions are not that bad, all the while concealing the real reason for our action. The real reasons tend to be something more rudimental, like we made a mistake, we were scared, or commonly, we're just lazy.

> *For example, I am lazy. I really am. Sure, usually I would present this more politely as "I value efficiency", but the reality is that I am lazy. And you know what – I totally accept that about myself. But more than enjoying laziness, I like results, so when it comes to healthy eating, I take into account my own laziness and I make very simple meals that are easy to cook. I cook in bulk so that I have less prep to do during the week. I eat consistent meals, so I don't have to bother making decisions during the week about what I want to eat. Having meals prepared means I don't have to walk to restaurants or shops to get food. It's all in the fridge ready to go!*

So, the real reasons behind our rationalisations need not be something we have to be afraid of. In fact, you can take anything and turn it into a strength, just as I have turned my own laziness into a strength that helps me be more productive and achieve my goals.

Sometimes, we really are that busy, but often this is because we cram our lives full of stuff that doesn't really matter. I have seen time and time again people unnecessarily overcomplicate tasks, making them feel as if they are overloaded with work, but in reality they have overloaded themselves by making mountains out of every molehill they come across. Instead of taking responsibility for their own choices, they blame others for having unrealistic expectations!

Looking past rationalisations can be confronting and difficult, but **the reward is that we take control of our own lives**. Rather than letting people and circumstances dictate our lives, we take charge and start making choices for ourselves, while knowing and accepting ourselves. This is a far more powerful position to be in and also much more fulfilling!

Your task – Investigate your rationalisations

At the end of the day, do we want rationalisations and excuses to stop us from getting results? No! So here is some homework for you:

1. *Look through the rationalisations and excuses listed above. Do you see any you use? Think about any other excuses that you use. Sometimes you might not even be aware of frequent excuses anymore, so ask a good friend what kind of excuses you use to keep yourself from healthy eating*

2. *As you find out about these, **write them down**. Once you have a few written down, look past the obvious and try to identify the real reason why you are using the rationalisations and excuses*

3. *When you feel you are getting closer to the real reason, work on turning it into a strength. Accept who you are, and take responsibility for your own actions and decisions. Work with yourself, rather than against yourself*

Stop making excuses – figure out what is wrong and fix it. Take control of your own life!

Resolving our rationalisations can take time, so don't expect to be able to suddenly overcome all the old excuses overnight! Taking it one step at a time is a more reliable way to make lasting long-term changes. We also need to make these changes with something to guide us along the way so that we can always check if we are heading in the right direction. This guide is our goals. Next, let's find out just how to set real, meaningful and motivational goals!

What to remember:
- Quality beliefs are rational and based on strong evidence
- Overcome all-or-nothing thinking, certainty and rationalisations
- Challenge your own beliefs and change them where they are not giving you good results or a positive experience of life

4.3 Developing clear goals

Before we can jump in and start writing down our greatest aspirations, we need to learn how to develop goals that take advantage of how the brain works and what it needs to thrive. New research in the growing field of neuropsychotherapy (psychology enhanced through neuroscience[206]) has revealed the **four basic human needs** for healthy brains. These basic needs drive our behaviour and also are what we need to consider when we set our goals so that we maximise our success and maintain a healthy brain[204]:

- **Attachment**
- **Control and orientation**
- **Pleasure and avoidance of pain**
- **Self-esteem enhancement**

Klaus Grawe wrote about the four basic needs and summed it up fantastically well, saying that we are in our most positive state (happiness and fulfilment) when *"...current perceptions and goals are completely congruent with one another, and the transpiring mental activity is not disturbed by any competing intentions"*[207].

What does this mean? It means that we feel our best when:

- We have clear goals
- We are working towards those goals
- We are seeing results in line with our goals
- The goals and actions do not clash with other goals

Thus, setting clear goals gives your brain a way to determine when it should reward you with dopamine releases and when it shouldn't. When we get this right, we get more motivated to do things like eat healthy and exercise, or study for an exam rather than watching some TV instead. In the last example, we'll be motivated to study because the brain will know that it is part of an important goal, and even though TV would provide short-term pleasure, it does not compare with the pain of failing the exam!

As you read through the four basic needs below, consider if you recognise them as needs that are important to you

Attachment

We have evolved as social beings and we draw an amazing amount of energy from being with others and feeling connected. These connections may be to a few special people, a large group of friends, clubs, work, and more. This is why Think Lean places such an emphasis on *Involving Others* because it is crucial for our own personal resilience! It can be hard making the shift to eating healthy when you are doing it by yourself. When tough moments come along, it can be easy to give up if you feel like *"No one cares anyway"*. When you set your goals, remember to get someone else involved, even if it is just one other person you are close with like a friend, parent or sibling. Doing this will support the fundamental wiring of your brain, making the journey to your goals more fulfilling and building a healthy brain in the process!

Control and orientation

We all have a huge desire to have a sense of control and feel that the world makes sense to us. To do this, we create a model of the world through which we interpret events and use that model to try and gain perceptions that satisfy or align with our goals.

Having **control** also means that our basic physiological needs are met, such as having enough food to eat, having a place to live, being physically safe, and having the security that these things will not be taken away. Sometimes we have a lot of anxiety about our jobs because of the subconscious realisation that if we lost our jobs, we would not be able to afford food and a home. As you can see, these are very basic things, but they are also very important! If we lost these, everything else in our life would go on hold while we focus on this need.

We feel we have more control when we have more options available to us. This is why it is important to understand the rules and guidelines of healthy eating, allowing you to be in control of your eating habits and knowing what you can change and tweak along the way.

Orientation refers to being able to understand events and situations. This helps us to recognise options which help us feel in control. If we don't know enough about a diet and we are faced with a difficult situation, we can feel out of control, become anxious and give up because it is all too hard.

When it comes to eating healthy, we can improve our sense of control and orientation by building *Quality Beliefs*. This gives us a more accurate model of reality, which we can use to make more accurate predictions about our actions and options. When we do that, our brains get positive feedback when the consequences of our actions meet with predictions and our goals become real. This is when we have a real sense of control, and we get the body we want!

Pleasure and avoidance of pain

The reward system in our brain releases dopamine (the feel-good neurotransmitter) when we have pleasant experiences. This wires the brain towards having more of those experiences. In the same way, the amygdala can quickly form memories to help us remember what bad experiences to avoid.

These are very well developed processes in our brain that motivate us throughout our lives to do more of the things that give us pleasure and less of the things that result in pain. The problem, of course, is that our brains need a bit of higher thinking to guide them towards what *should* really give us pleasure and what *shouldn't*.

Take **pleasure-eating**, for example. Pleasure-eating is when we are eating solely for the serotonin and dopamine releases given by tasty foods[208]. As we saw before, sugar and high-GI carbohydrates particularly have this effect, resulting in a cascade of peptides and neurotransmitters that make us just want to eat more and more! Just the mere sight of a piece of cake can trigger a dopamine release in anticipation[133].

This is in contrast with **hunger-eating**, which is focused on replenishing nutrients which we need to live. Pleasure-eating can thus be a powerful habit that causes obesity, and unless we do something about it, will continue to get stronger and stronger! This is a good example of why we need to put some higher thinking in place to guide our reward systems and where our goals play a huge role.

In all, while we are powerfully motivated towards doing things that give us pleasure, we need to be careful and not simply go towards short-term pleasures. Instead, we need to set meaningful and clear goals that guide our motivation so that we are rewarded when we achieve our goals. This provides long-term fulfilment and a greater sense of joy in life.

Self-esteem enhancement

Increasing and protecting our self-esteem is critically important for brain health. This includes our sense of self-worth, self-respect and how we feel about ourselves overall, and allows us to feel confident about ourselves, our actions and our goals. This gives us the mental freedom to explore our own creativity, effectively solve complex problems, and confidently engage in higher brain thinking.

> **Talk to someone**
>
> If you feel that you have a significant problem with any of these four areas and it is causing you distress, anxiety or depression, talk to a therapist or psychologist.
>
> Especially if you feel that things are not getting better and your own efforts aren't working. Recognising when we need help is crucial for our own resilience, so reach out and involve others!

Our pursuit of self-esteem enhancement can sometimes be held back by the other basic needs, as our need for safety, health, attachment, control and pleasure can take precedence if they are not currently being met. They can also get in the way where we might be considering a self-esteem enhancement goal that might interfere with another basic need.

Overcoming this means breaking down some old habits and having our brains firmly set on clear goals to guide our motivation! Much of the concept of *Personal Resilience* is focused on increasing our self-esteem, as well as helping to increase perceptions that our basic needs are being met. Again, we talk about perceptions, which is not always the same as reality. We often do not realise that our needs are being met in reality, and therefore we do not have the perception that our needs are being met.

> *For example, we might have a lot of friends and family ready to support us during tough times, but we don't believe it, so we feel alone. The reality is there, but the perception is not, therefore we feel a gap in our basic needs.*

If you feel that a basic need is not being met, challenge yourself and consider what evidence you have that it is not being met. Look beyond negative evidence and you might find a lot of positive evidence that you missed before.

Setting clear goals is crucial to self-esteem enhancement, as it is a way to constantly improve and advance ourselves. Working towards goals and achieving them help us feel more confident and increase feelings of self-worth.

4.3.1.1 Basic human needs and healthy eating

When we consider the basic human needs, it is not hard to see why going on a diet can seem so daunting. The diagram below shows the four basic needs and how it often feels when we are going on a diet. Our need for attachment can feel threatened because we often enjoy foods with other people at parties, restaurants and more. Food is very closely tied to social activities after all. Our need for control can feel threatened as we have less food to choose from. Similarly, sugary foods can be a big source of pleasure, so cutting those out threatens our need for pleasure.

Lastly, our self-esteem stands to gain from this, but when we have so many of our other basic needs being threatened the potential self-esteem enhancement can feel like just not enough to justify a

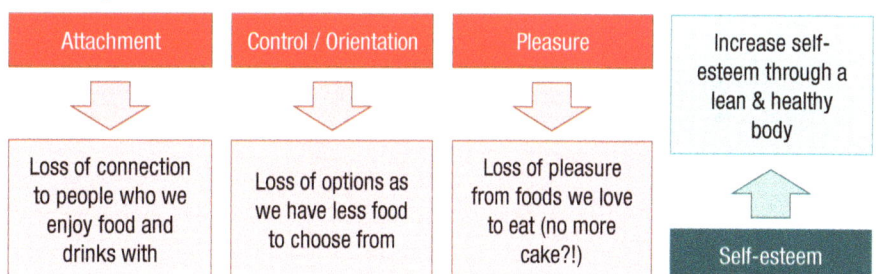

diet. This shows us why it is important to think differently and also be prepared for the challenges if we hope to succeed.

That is how we often feel about going on a diet, and the above is clearly **the wrong way to think** about healthy eating if we want to succeed! This can actively keep us from sustaining healthy eating, as we just can't see a way how we can permanently live like this if so many of our basic needs are reduced. Here we have basic needs in conflict with one another, so even if we manage to get some success in one, the reductions in others make us feel unhappy. Our actions constantly feel contradictory and the whole experience just makes us miserable. This is simply not sustainable, and is a big reason why many people fail with making healthy eating a long-term lifestyle choice.

Naturally, starting to eat healthy doesn't have to mean a reduction of so many of our basic needs. Instead, we can actually increase all areas of our basic needs through healthy eating. We just have to think about it in the right way! The diagram to the right shows a far more constructive state of mind when it comes to healthy eating.

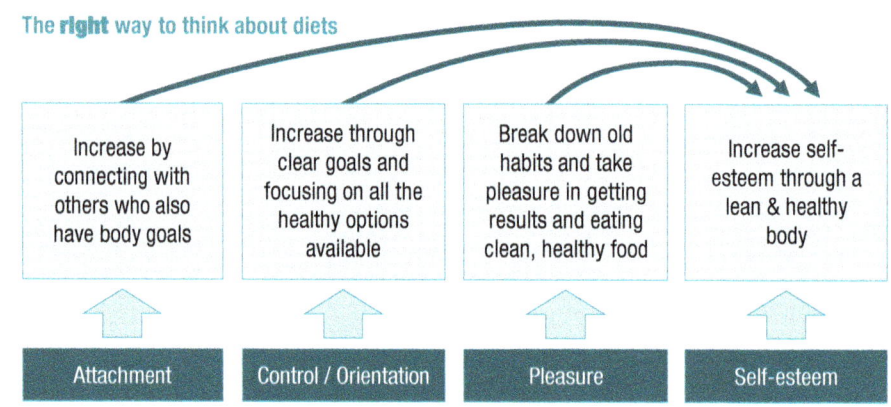

Let's look at each of our basic human needs and what is a more constructive state of mind:

- **Attachment** – By involving others, we can connect with others who also have similar goals and grow closer to our friends as they share in your goal and you share successes along the way. You can always still go out to restaurants, go to parties, and even eat some cake and snacks along the way. You don't need to follow ACM 100% of the time! Even 90% will still get you great results. So relax and enjoy being with friends!

- **Control and orientation** – Having clear goals around our bodies gives us a better sense of orientation, and focusing on all the healthy options available can give us a better sense of control as well. We are only giving up unhealthy foods that don't support our goals, so learn more about good, healthy foods and keep experimenting and learning about new options

- **Pleasure and avoidance of pain** – As we change our beliefs and focus on our goals, we start to get more pleasure from getting success in our goals instead. We break down the old habits of eating for pleasure and instead gain pleasure from pursuing our goals and seeing our progress towards getting the body we want. Over time the neural networks in our brain will change, and our success in sticking to our diets become more and more satisfying

- **Self-esteem enhancement** – As we change our beliefs, pursue our goals and progress to our new body, our self-esteem improves. We start to feel better about our ability to follow through on our goals, gain more confidence in ourselves and more!

What is crucial here is that all the other needs support our self-esteem enhancement. Enhanced self-esteem also makes it easier for us to keep doing the right things, and in turn supports our other basic needs. This means our body goal and our needs are now congruent with each other as they all support one another. This is the ideal situation and is **sustainable in the long term as a permanent lifestyle**.

This congruence prevents conflict in our actions and intentions. Remember that Grawe said we feel most fulfilled when our *"...current perceptions and goals are completely congruent with one another, and the transpiring mental activity is not disturbed by any competing intentions"*.

That can be a difficult sentence to really get your head around. It took me a few tries to really get it, but it is a powerful statement and worth spending a bit of time on as it helps you understand what your brain is striving for. Congruence with our goals and perceptions, and prevention of conflict is what we are aiming for here and what we can achieve. Achieving that sets us up for long-term success!

4.3.1.2 Goals and happiness

Now that we better know our basic needs and a bit about where the Think Lean Method fits in with those basic needs, it's worth talking a bit more about the idea of 'happiness'. Many people would say happiness is their main goal in life, but is this a good goal to have?

Taking a step back at the basic needs, we have seen that our happiness is highest when our actions and perceptions are aligned with our goals and there are no conflicts with other goals. What does this mean for happiness? Importantly, this means that **happiness is a side effect of pursuing and achieving our goals**. If happiness is really only a side effect, it means that happiness in itself can't be the end goal.

That's worth taking a pause over. So am I saying happiness can't be our goal? That's exactly right. Happiness shouldn't be, and precisely can't be our end goal – not if we want meaningful and fulfilling lives. Taking a look again at what happiness is at a neurological level, we find that it is essentially releases of neurotransmitters such as dopamine that gives us that feeling of joy and fulfilment. If happiness were really the end goal, then we would do what most effectively delivers those feelings, such as illicit drugs.

We have an innate desire to do things in an efficient way. We just hate to do things in one way if we think there is an easier way to do it. Why get up and change the channel if there is a remote? Why wash the dishes with our hands if there is a dishwasher? Understanding this basic drive for efficiency highlights why it is actually dangerous to have happiness as our goal, as it predisposes us to seek quick fixes, to seek instant gratification, even to use drugs as after all, it brings us happiness, right?

This is why having a goal of *"I just want to be happy"* is actually dangerous.

It is an aimless path that can prevent us from having meaningful and fulfilling lives. And it can go directly against developing a habit of healthy eating. After all, if chocolates and cake bring us happiness, then it serves our goal of being happy, right? So why not eat more! That is how your brain reasons, unless you program your brain with better goals.

Recognising that our happiness is a side effect of pursuing and achieving our goals opens us up to choose a new path that leads to more meaning and fulfilment in our lives. If you desire having a lean body and living a healthy lifestyle, then you need to align that goal with others. A goal of *"I want a lean body"* and a goal of *"I want to be happy"* can be conflicting goals, since there are many dopamine and serotonin releases to be gained from sweet foods that conflict with getting a lean body! And as we know by now, when there is conflict in our goals, we are less happy, which defeats our goal of being happy, so we need to eat more sweet food. Now *that* is a vicious circle that leads to obesity and overall unhappiness.

Think Lean - **Developing clear goals**

> **Important!** This does not mean I don't want you to be happy! On the contrary, what I want to help you achieve is real, lasting happiness that flows from a healthy lifestyle and the achievement of your goals. This kind of happiness comes from living a meaningful and fulfilling life. It is congruent with your goals, it is sustainable, and it can last a lifetime!

Some people intuitively understand that they need to pursue their goals to achieve happiness, and readily accept the struggles of pursuing goals as part of the process. This intuitive understanding can serve us well for a long time, but if we do not understand clearly that our happiness come from pursuing goals, then we can end up in trouble.

Imagine a person whose goal is to be happy and loves playing the piano as it makes him happy. Intuitively he understands that being an accomplished piano player makes him happy, though he does not realise this on a conscious level. After an injury, he struggles getting back into playing and the frustration is making it less enjoyable. He ends up stopping completely because playing no longer makes him happy, as his goal, after all, is to be happy.

He starts looking for anything else that can make him happy, and tries one thing after another with no success. He constantly tries new things, while at the same time getting more frustrated and depressed because he feels he is wasting time as he can't find something to make him happy. Because of this, he doesn't spend enough time on anything to get any real success out of it, so he never gets the same feeling as before!

This is where we sometimes see people 'lose their way'. People who used to be so clear in their path, but something happens and their lives just seem to spiral out of control. That is how a goal of *"I just want to be happy"* ends up leading to less happiness. We end up chasing one thing after another, and give up quickly on things because *"It's just not making me happy"*. And of course, we get *so* much sympathy from other people as well:

"Oh if it is not making you happy, then don't do it!"

Nod, nod "Yes, you're right. I mean I just want to be happy."

Why are we going into so much detail on this? One reason – if you currently have a life goal of "I just want to be happy", or some other variant, blow it away right now! Renounce it as a goal. **Write it down, and draw a line through it!**

Instead of that, we will establish new, clear goals that will do much more for your own personal happiness than that one goal ever did, because true happiness and fulfilment come from active pursuit of our aligned and congruent goals.

4.3.2 Develop a vision of yourself

Now that we have thrown out of happiness as a goal, we can move on to working on who we want to be and what kind of body and health goals we want for ourselves. The best way to do this is by developing a **vision of yourself**. Don't fear – we will keep this simple and practical! But first of all, why not just *"be ourselves"* as we are? After all, how often do we hear the good old advice:

"Be yourself"

The truth is that this is an absolutely worthless platitude. Just think of someone receiving this advice on their way to a job interview – what this advice really means is to stop stressing and be calm, confident and likeable!

This does not mean that how you are now is necessarily *"bad"*! In fact, you might be great right now, but there are ways we can all be better, and if you are reading this book to find out how to improve your body and mind, you are definitely on the right path.

A vision defines the kind of person you want to be

This is the starting point of helping us identify our goals. This starts to give us clarity, as we can clearly say what kind of people we want to become. So how do we do it? First of all, *remember that this does not need to be perfect*. Just put something together now, then as you come back to it over time, you can revise it and change as you improve your knowledge about yourself.

I'll show you a simple and practical way to develop a vision of yourself. All you have to do is write down a few words and sentences that describe what you want to be like – forget how you are right now – think about yourself five or ten years from now. What do you want to be like then? What values and traits do you want to work on? What do you want to enhance, and what do you want to develop in yourself? You only need about five or so bullet points of the most important aspects of this future vision of yourself.

Here are a few examples of characteristics that you might put in:

- *"I am confident at work and socially"*
- *"I am successful in my job"*
- *"I am reliable and true to my word"*
- *"I am a resilient person"*
- *"I follow through on my goals"*
- *"I am influential in my community"*
- *"I am compassionate and kind to everyone in my life"*
- *"I am persistent in all my goals"*
- *"I am reliable first to myself, then to others"*
- *"I actively help the people close to me and add to their lives"*
- *"I am adventurous in my social life"*
- *"I am precise and insightful in my work"*

> **More examples?**
> Having examples always makes it easier to choose! To find more ideas, go online and search for *"Personality traits"*.
> There are plenty of sources with long lists to get you thinking, and more importantly, visualising your future self!

These characteristics can relate to your work, your social life, you family, your body, your hobbies, etc. It's all about what you feel most strongly is what you want for your future self!

I'd recommend not writing down something too specific about having a particular job, being in a particular place, being with a particular person or anything like that. Really specific personal vision statements can be less resilient, as it makes success unduly difficult and may even demotivate you. Instead, statements like the examples above are more **broad positive characteristics** that we want to have, and there are multiple ways in which we strive towards them.

This also applies to your vision for your body. Keep it general here, as we'll get more specific when we set goals to achieve these. Here are some examples of body vision statements:

- *"I have an athletic body"*
- *"I have a body I'm proud of"*
- *"I live a healthy lifestyle"*
- *"I look after my body and mind"*
- *"I have a body that looks and feels strong"*
- *"I have a lean and elegant body"*

There are a huge amount of these that you can choose from. Go with what you best connect with. Don't pick a vision for yourself that you think other people want from you – pick characteristics that you want for yourself! If you want to be adventurous but other people want you to be dependable, then go with adventurous! You are the one who is important here, so focus on yourself and what is important to you. Put yourself first. After all, you can't effectively help others if you do not help yourself first.

Note – when you write down these, avoid words like 'good' or 'great'. For example, "I am a good person", or "I am a good mother". Both of those don't actually mean anything because there is no definition of a 'good' person or a 'good' mother. Is a good mother one that spends every moment with her child? Or one that displays independence by staying on with her career? Everyone's idea is different, so be particular in what you want to be like.

Need help?

There is much to be said about personal visions and what is good, better and best. Focus on what feels right to you. If you feel like you need help with defining this, talk to a psychologist, therapist or trained life coach. They are not just there for when something is wrong – they can also help you go from good to great!

If you already have some positive characteristic, then you don't need to include it. Include the things you want to have that you do not have currently. So if you are already confident, then don't write that down, unless you want even more confidence, then write that and be specific about what is different from now. For example, *"I want to be confident when talking to large audiences"*.

This way you are constantly building and improving yourself. Each of the positive characteristics you work on becomes part of you and your personality, which means that you are always becoming better and better. This is how you '**become yourself**', as you are always working towards that evolving future vision of you!

Your task – Write down your personal vision!

Your personal vision should consist of around five personal **broad positive characteristics** that you want to work on (like the examples above). These represent your future self, the person you will become.

Include as one of these your vision of your body. Remember to keep this one general as the examples above show. Write down a vision for your body that inspires you. It can be about health, about eating clean, or about getting lean. I'd recommend including "Be a resilient person" as well. Write it all down, and write it as if you have it now!

4.3.3 Setting clear goals

Now it is time to get specific and set your goals! Your vision shows you the general direction, but your goals are what get you there. For a goal to be 'clear', it needs to meet a few specific criteria:

- They are **specific and measurable**
- They are **attainable** and realistic
- They are **relevant** and congruent with other goals and needs
- They have a **timeframe**

Many of you will recognise this as the SMART criteria for goals often used by businesses. Well, as useful as it is for business, so is it useful for us when setting personal goals. However, one part that often is not used well enough is *"relevant"*. Here we strengthen the concept with our new understanding of the basic human needs, and use that understanding to define goals that are meaningful, support our own personal development and make us feel fulfilled along the way as we pursue them. This makes **clear goals** much more powerful and motivating. Let's look at each of these criteria and what it means for our body goals:

Specific and measurable

Let's get away from vague goals that we can't measure along the way, like *"My goal is to lose weight"*. If that is the goal, how would you know if you have achieved it? Is 1kg enough to lose? Or more? We need to be specific with our body goals so that we can track it as we go and adjust our efforts along the way to ensure we reach it. For example, more specific goals would be:

- *"Lose 10kg"*
- *"Exercise 30 minutes four times a week"*
- *"Follow the Think Lean Method 90% of the time"*
- *"Lose two dress sizes"*
- *"Cut out all grains"*

The last one might seem not very specific or measurable, but it actually is as we can count the number of times we ate grains vs a target of zero. As for how closely we follow our healthy eating plan, setting something like *"Follow the Think Lean Method 90% of the time"* can be a more realistic way to get into it and stay motivated.

This same principle applies for other goals we set that are not related to our body. For example, it may be part of our vision to be a more resilient person, and set goals such as these:

- *"Practice visualisation once a day"*
- *"Spend 15 minutes a day challenging my own beliefs"*
- *"Connect with at least one person every day"*

Attainable

For a goal to be attainable, it needs to be realistic and possible to achieve it. When it comes to body goals, we often have unrealistic expectations which set us up for failure and disappointment. Just think of how many people want to lose 10kg in 10 days, or lose 20cm in two months. These are unrealistic goals, and even if they are achieved, often result in the yo-yo effect as the weight comes straight back on afterwards.

Think Lean - **Developing clear goals**

To make your goals more realistic, here is a simple guideline – **aim for around 1kg weight loss every two weeks.** If you keep that up, you'd lose 26kg in a year, which is a lot! Anything above that is a bonus. Sounds a bit too slow? Keep in mind that this is for sustainable weight loss. The faster you lose weight, the harder it is to keep it off. Losing 1kg per week can be achieved, but you'd need a lot of discipline to keep it off and make it permanent.

> **Setting % targets**
>
> You can expect good results by following ACM 90% or more. Less than that can cause the free meals to stop you from losing weight. Think of targets this way:
>
> • 98% - one free meal per two weeks
> • 95% - one free meal per week
> • 90% - two free meals per week
> • 80% - four free meals per week

If you are aiming to put on weight (for those looking to put on muscle), about 1kg per two weeks is good guide as well to build lean muscle. More than that and you are probably putting on body fat as well, meaning you will need to cut body fat after a while.

This also applies to how closely we follow ACM. It would be unrealistic for us to just go for perfect 100% compliance with it. That means we are never allowed to eat anything off-diet, ever! Rather, start with something attainable, like *"Follow the Think Lean Method 80% of the time"*. That gives you four free meals a week – basically one every two days. Not bad for a big switch already! Then move it up to 85%, then 90% as you get better and manage more consistency for weight loss.

Setting attainable goals applies to everything else as well. If you are 20 years old and working in the mailroom and planning to be CEO in six months, you might want to consider how attainable that actually is. Attainable goals set us up for success and help us to get confidence in our ability to achieve our goals. If you have had trouble reaching goals in the past, start small and make them really attainable. As you get better, raise the bar and go for more!

Relevant (and congruent)

This is the absolutely crucial part of **clear goals**, and is a part that we often do not pay enough attention to. This is where we look at our body goal and compare it to other goals and our basic human needs to confirm that they are congruent and aligned. If our goals are in conflict with our needs or other goals, we will find it near impossible to stick to them, and not sticking to them can end up causing us a lot of distress and even result in depression.

> *For example, imagine Joe has a vision to be the biggest bodybuilder ever, but he has another vision to be a champion jockey, each with goals to achieve them. Now, jockeys need to be light so the horse can run faster, but bodybuilding will make Joe heavy.*

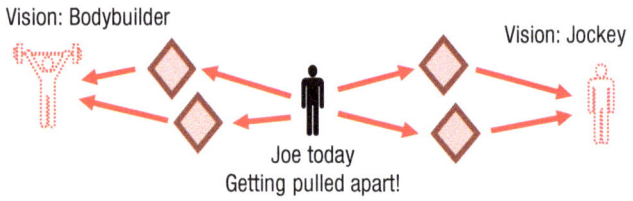

Conflicting goals prevent success

The goals to achieve these visions are completely at odds with one another, and can't be pursued at the same time. If he tries he'll end up not getting any success with either, resulting in great mental anguish for Joe as he is not getting any closer to any of his goals.

The diagram displays Joe's predicament. Joe is in the middle, with goals represented as the diamond shapes, and the outlines the misaligned visions he has of himself. He has to move in one direction or another, but any direction he goes moves him either away from the one or the other visions and goals. This is an extreme example of **conflicting goals**, but you'd be surprised how often we don't realise we have goals that oppose each other. Just think of wanting to lose weight but still wanting to enjoy lots of sugary and calorie-dense foods. These are two clearly opposing goals!

In contrast, when our goals align, it is an incredible experience as everything we do continuously supports each other. As the diagram below shows, if we have congruent goals and a vision, we can find multiple paths to success, since the goals work in support of one another! In this diagram the direction to move forward is clear, providing that crucial sense of control and orientation.

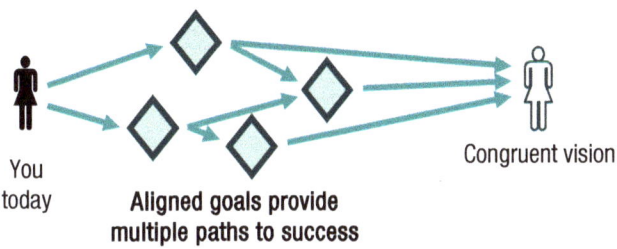

Aligned goals provide multiple paths to success

Having clear goals allows us to reach this state, but to reach it we also need to actually know what our other goals are. If we are unclear on our other goals, how can we align them? The keys here are to:

- Be aware of other goals
- Consider your goals in context of one another

By doing this, you can find where there is conflict and decide ahead of time how you will manage the conflict, or if goals need to be changed so that they better align. If you have a goal of losing 10kg, but you have another goal to take a big holiday that happens to be in the middle of it, then you'd need to decide how to handle it as those two goals could be at odds with each other. A holiday can easily result in some weight gain as we relax and eat more than usual. So do you postpone healthy eating during the holiday, or try to keep it going through it? You might have to reduce the overall weight loss target to keep it realistic if you realise you'll probably gain some weight during the holiday.

You may have other goals, like completing a major project at work and the project involves a lot of travel. Sticking to healthy eating and exercising can take extra preparation as you need to work out how you can still achieve your body goals when you don't have easy access to the right foods and equipment. It can definitely still be done, but you need to be prepared for it! Preparing for and resolving the natural conflict between these goals will prevent frustration and failure.

As the examples mentioned above, there is another component of congruence that is also crucial – **your goals must be congruent with your vision of yourself**. That means your goals must support the future vision of yourself and your values. Goals that conflict with your vision will result in procrastination as they will simply not be motivating.

> *For example, Claire loves her job and her vision is to be really successful at work, but she has also set a goal to spend loads of time with her family and friends. Because this goal conflicts with her vision, she might find it hard to get the motivation to actually spend time with them. She'd be at work most of the time, and thinking about work after hours to advance her career. Meanwhile, she communicates her goal to friends and family, so they have the expectation that she will spend more time with them, but she never does and everybody ends up frustrated and disappointed.*

The differences between goals

We've talked about conflicting goals and congruent goals, but there are also disconnected goals. Here are the differences:

- **Conflicting goals** – Moving towards one goal literally moves you further away from another goal, as in Joe's example
- **Disconnected goals** – Moving towards one goal doesn't move you further away or closer to the other goal. Like learning to play the piano doesn't help you be a better bodybuilder. There's nothing inherently wrong here, it is just that the goals do not work together
- **Congruent goals** – Here, moving towards one moves you closer to another. The goals support each other and success in one can give you greater success in another. Congruent goals are best for a fulfilling and resilient life

Being aware of our vision, and more importantly, **being honest with ourselves about what we really want**, allow us to spot these inconsistencies and deal with conflicts ahead of time. Doing this enhances our sense of control over our lives, as we essentially prevent crises before they arise! As you set your goals, be very conscious of relevance and congruence. Congruent goals and values hugely contribute to the fulfilment we feel from pursuing our goals!

Timeframe

We need to define the timeframe in which we want to accomplish the goal. Timeframes give goals more power, particularly for a goal like "Lose 10kg". Adding a timeframe changes a goal to something like "Lose 10kg in six months". We can then use it to work out that we need to lose around 1kg every two weeks to achieve the goal. This means we can now keep track of our progress and we know when we are on or off track to achieve our goal.

Without a timeframe, we would have no idea if we are on track, as we could always lose the weight next year, or the year after that! It sounds obvious once you think about it, but we so often set goals without timeframes and therefore never even feel the need to start working on it. We can always start next week, right? Putting in a timeframe gives us motivation to start working towards it now.

You can use timeframes to systematically shift towards healthy eating if you want to make a true lifestyle change. For example, as you complete each of the following goals, you move on to the next:

- *"Cut out all grains over two weeks"*, then
- *"Remove sugar and sugary drinks in the following two weeks"*, then
- *"Limit coffee to once per day in the morning over two weeks"*, then
- *"Start following Core ACM over the next month 80% of the time"*, then
- *"Do Core ACM 90% of the time for the next six months"*, and so on...

As you achieve one goal and move to the next, you continually improve your healthy eating habits. Making changes over time like this is much more sustainable and is more likely to result in strong new healthy habits. Of course, you can do it all in one big bang, but it takes more discipline to stick to it that way as it can be a big shock to your brain.

Setting solid and realistic timeframes for your goals gives them meaning and motivation and you can expect to get results in line with your efforts. Also, remember to write down the actual date you want to achieve it by! Once you have gone through all of the criteria above, you should have a goal that is something like this:

- *"Lose 10kg by the end of August"*
- *"Exercise three times a week for 30 minutes until the end of June"*
- *"Follow the Think Lean Method 80% of the time until October"*

> **Ongoing goals**
>
> As you become better at reaching your goals and staying consistent with healthy eating, you can set more general goals as well. For example, these days I only set general goals for myself around dieting, like *"Follow Complete ACM 97% of the time"*. There is no timeframe attached to it because I just do it permanently.
>
> If I wanted to achieve something in particular with my body, I'd set a clear goal again with a clear timeframe.

With body goals, as soon as one goal ends, set the next goal right away. For example, go from 80% to 85% for the next three months. This way you are constantly improving until you reach your goal body, at which point your goal changes to *maintain* your body by following ACM at whatever percentage you find works best. Set your goals for three months at a time. That will keep them fresh and motivating, since it's not too far away into the future.

Your task – *Write down your body goal!*

Use all the criteria above to set a clear goal for your body. Make it specific, measurable, attainable, relevant and congruent, and set a definite timeframe.

Just write it down anywhere for now, since next we need to identify other goals and then prioritise them.

Identifying goals

Once you have your body goal, it is important to also be aware of other goals you have so you can consider them in context with each other. As mentioned above, it is crucial for your goals to be aligned and congruent with one another. Here we need to dig a little deeper and look at all the other things in our life that is important right now and competes for our attention. We don't even have to look too far to find other goals. Some might not feel like goals, but instead seem more like obligations, though thinking of them as goals help to put them in context with one another. For example:

- **At work**
    - Do you have big projects you are working on?
    - Is your job demanding leaving little time for anything else?
    - Are you putting in extra effort to get a promotion or bonus?
    - Are you actively looking for a new job?
- **Family life**
    - Recently had a baby or have small children?
    - Is parenthood taking up lots of time?
    - Do you need to look after a sick or elderly family member?
    - New relationship? You might have to compromise on diets to make room for lots of eating out...
    - Do you want a new relationship?
    - Existing relationship needs some help and attention?
- **Friends, acquaintances and colleagues**
    - Do you have a goal to enjoy a lot of social events?
    - Is it really important to you to often go out with friends?
    - Do you have friends going through tough times and you are helping them through it?
- **Hobbies and side projects**
    - Do you have a hobby or side project that is important to you?
    - Do you play sports at a serious level?
    - Do you have something outside of work that is your true passion?
    - Are you aiming for personal development, like developing personal resilience, or other ways of improving yourself?
    - Do you have a goal of becoming more dependable and reliable, or working on another personal characteristic?

Think Lean - **Developing clear goals**

These are just some questions to get you thinking about what is happening in your life right now. Think of them all as goals to be completed – for each of them you can use the criteria for clear goals to define them as goals, just like your body and health goals. As you can see from the above, some of these can even be crises that need to be dealt with, as even crises present a goal in themselves – resolve the crisis!

Take some time to think through these and anything else that is taking up time in your life currently. Don't forget that leisure activities form part of our goals overall. If you really enjoy watching movies, going to concerts, have favourite TV programmes, or other things, these can be part of our goals as well. They might not be the most important goals, but if we neglect them we are neglecting our basic human need for pleasure.

You can always change what you take pleasure in, for example if you feel you have a TV habit that is taking up too much time, you can change that by limiting it and focusing on other activities. But don't just cut it out completely as your brain will fight back due to its need for pleasure. For now, just be honest with yourself about the most important things to you. After you write them down, we will prioritise them so we get real about what we spend our time on.

Your task – Write down your most important goals!

Now that you have thought through all these, write down all the big things that are important in your life. The big obligations, the big projects, the big events – write them down as goals. Try to follow the criteria for clear goals to make them more tangible and motivating.

4.3.4 Prioritise goals

So it has been a lot of fun setting big goals and identifying all the other things happening in our lives and writing those down as goals as well. But now, we need to make some tough choices – we need to prioritise these goals. Prioritising is different from congruent goals in that prioritisation shows which are more important than others while congruency means that the goals support and feed into each other.

Prioritising goals is a fundamentally important task, and is something we are intrinsically bad at doing. We tend to randomly prioritise goals as different situations come up, resulting in inconsistent actions and less consistency with our body goals. Since consistency is the most important contributor to success with healthy eating, we need to prioritise correctly so that we get that consistency!

The concept of prioritising is simple:

Audrey has two goals. One is to get a promotion, the other is to get lean. She prioritises them as follows:

- *First priority – Get a promotion*
- *Second priority – Get lean*

She usually does her meal preparation on Sundays for the week, but this Sunday a situation comes up at work and they are in desperate need for help. Now she has a choice – she can tell them she can't make it and disappoint them but get her meal prep done, or she can skip her meal prep and go help and potentially impress management.

Since she has clearly defined getting a promotion as her top priority, she decides to skip meal prep and help out as it works towards her goal. She gets through Monday by buying fast food and her healthy eating takes a bit of a hit, rearranges Monday night and does her meal prep then instead, and high fives herself for sticking to her priorities.

Here you can clearly see the benefit of having clear priorities set out. Prioritisation enables us to effectively make decisions in difficult situations and makes it easier for us to reach our most important goals. Once you have your goals prioritised, being a goal-driven person becomes extremely powerful – decisions become easier and you become more reliable to yourself.

- It becomes clear who you really are and what is really important to you
- It allows you to make a real commitment to achieve your goals as you realise your own power
- It also realigns your expectations, so when you make tough choices, you know why you did it and you have a greater appreciation for the result

This highlights an important concept that we need to accept to pursue our goals – **sacrifice**.

> **Important vs pressing tasks**
>
> It is important to know the difference between 'important' and 'pressing' tasks when it comes to prioritising what you do.
>
> Important tasks are those that align with your goals and support what you want to accomplish.
>
> Pressing tasks are often those that demand attention right away, but do not align with any goals – particularly not your own. Just think of how often at work something comes up that someone wants right away, but do not align to any of the other work you are trying to get done.
>
> At these times, let your goals be your guide and do not prioritise a pressing task just because someone wants it done sooner. Stay focused on your own goals and work on them first. If you have time after that, then you can help others. Remember – just because it is pressing, doesn't mean it is important!

Sacrifice

If we have some goals that are really important to us, but we have a great many other goals as well, we have to accept that there may need to be some sacrifices along the way. These sacrifices may be in the form of how effectively we reach some of our other goals, or we may even have to sacrifice other goals completely. Pursuing all goals at the same time essentially just ensures failure in nearly all of them.

For example, I would really like to learn the piano and the violin. At the same time, I have a great full time job, my health, diet and exercise is a big priority, and I have another big priority to write and bring useful ideas to people. To get any good at the piano and violin, I'd have to practice each for around an hour a day. That is a couple of hours that I really do not have available.

At the same time, being able to play the violin and piano is not congruent with any of my other goals, so it ends up so low on the priority list that I just sacrifice it completely and focus on more important goals instead.

It helps to remember that we really have limited time and attention available for goals, so the fewer goals we have, the more time we can spend on them. For example, someone who has a goal of becoming a champion chess player would set it as a solitary goal far above anything else. Nearly everything else is sacrificed for the goal, or at least aligned to it.

Singular goals can drive us to accomplish amazing feats, but it takes dedication and a lot of sacrifice. At the same time, sacrifice does not necessarily need to be a negative experience – instead, if the sacrifice is made for a powerful and motivating goal, it can be incredibly empowering and fulfilling as we know we are making the right choice for the right reason.

Every time I do not eat a slice of cake at a birthday party, I do not think to myself *"Oh, I'm missing out!"* Instead I think *"I am proud of myself for being able to stick to my goals"*. That totally changes how we feel about ourselves and about sacrifice, making it something positive instead.

Of course, there is one way to get around sacrifice, and that is efficiency.

Efficiency

How do we achieve more goals at the same time? By becoming more efficient at reaching them, of course! This is a big thing for reaching body goals, as it can seem like such a chore to prepare all those healthy meals all the time when we could just be buying fast food instead! Efficiency can play a big part here by becoming faster at preparing food.

> *For example, I make most of my food on a Sunday night in preparation for the week. That way, I end up only cooking a quick dinner each night, while breakfast, lunch and second lunch is all done for the next five days (yes I eat a second lunch). This saves me a lot of time during the week, allowing me more time to focus on other goals such as work and writing.*

Realistically, any repetitive activity is open for improved efficiency. As we cook specific recipes, we become better at timing our actions and how long it takes to do everything, meaning we get faster and faster. Up to a point, we can also physically move faster as well so that we get things done faster. We can also do multiple things at a time – like when I poach chicken or boil eggs, I throw them in, set a timer and then continue writing. When the timer is up, I put the next batch in and get back to writing again. This applies to anything we do:

> *I like to exercise, but I really dislike having to get dressed, drive to a gym and drive back. I think that is just a waste of time. Instead, I cancelled my gym membership, took the money I saved and used it to slowly purchase gym equipment to put in my unit. That meant I can easily do a workout whenever I like, and even do other things quickly while I work out. This is much more efficient for me and helps me achieve more goals at the same time.*

Take an active interest in performing tasks in a more efficient way. As you get better, you can take on more goals at the same time and achieve more of them. Your goals do not need to be perfect. You should come back to the list over time (I suggest every three months) and re-evaluate the goals to see if you are on the right track. Stick to only about five or so goals overall, as more than that will likely not get enough attention to be reached. If you feel they are all small goals and you can do more, then make them bigger!

Your prioritised list of goals is a powerful tool to use every day to guide your decisions and actions. It gives you the roadmap to actively pursue your goals every day. Even if times get really tough, you know what is most important and what to focus on. Feel like there is not enough time in the day to do everything? The prioritisation shows you what to do first! This will help make you a resilient person who is focused on reaching and achieving your most valued goals.

 ***Your task** – Prioritise your goals!*

Looking at your list of goals that you wrote down before, put a number next to each starting with number '1' as the most important and work down from there. This might take a few tries and also might need a bit of soul searching to decide what is really most important to you.

Once done, write down the top five (more if you really want) in the correct order, and pay particular attention to where your body goal ends up on the list. Is it near the top, middle, or bottom? The higher up it is, the more likely it is that you will reach that goal, as you will sacrifice other goals below it when times get tough. At the same time, don't just put your body goal on top for the sake of it. Be honest with yourself about what is most important to you.

4.3.5 Using habits to support goals

Now that we have our list of prioritised goals, we need to build new healthy habits to reach our goals for body and health. We also need to get rid of some old habits which are not useful to reaching our goals. First, it helps to understand habits.

Habits follow a simple pattern as shown below:

1. **Cue** – You are stressed, or bored (or whatever triggers it), and your brain searches through options to treat the feeling. *"Aha!"* the brain goes *"Let's eat something sweet. That always helps!"*
2. **Anticipate reward** – The brain releases dopamine in anticipation of the effect sugar has on the brain. The pleasure felt here makes anticipation hard to ignore
3. **Routine** – You just can't put aside the feeling, so you walk over to the vending machine and get a chocolate
4. **Reward** – Sweet, sweet dopamine and serotonin is released as you eat the chocolate, strengthening the neural network that supports this habit. Start again at #1

It's really not very complicated, but it can seem impossible to break bad habits. So how do we do it?

Change a habit in 21 days?

This is a phrase we hear often – so often, in fact, that many people and authors believe it to be true. Unfortunately, habits are too complicated to be overcome by a simple rule like that, and there is simply no evidence that 21 days is enough to make sufficient changes at a neural level in our brains to say that it is enough to overcome a habit[209].

If we think about it, some habits are formed over long periods and can be deeply rooted in childhood events. Other habits are more recent, or simply due to a misunderstanding of what needs to be done. Some habits can be changed really easily, while others take a while to properly change.

However there is hope – habits absolutely can be changed. First we have to recognise what kind of habit it is. Think of one of your dietary habits (maybe you often eat chocolate, sweets, chips, donuts, etc.) and ask yourself:

- How often do you eat it?
- How often do you think about it?
- How often do you want to eat it?
- When did this habit start – months, years, decades ago?
- How much does this habit work against your goals for your body?
- How often do you successfully resist it?
- What do you feel or think about when you eat it?

All of these answers give you clues as to how deep the habit runs, and how important it is to you. To be successful in really changing our habits, we have to recognise how deep our habits run, **and respect how powerful habits can be**.

This is where we often go wrong with trying to change deep habits. We think a short while of not doing it is enough, but just a few weeks is not enough to make a big enough change in our brains to get rid of it and we become complacent and we relapse. This kind of relapse can be disheartening, and we feel as if it's just not worth it, or we've tried everything and nothing works. This brings us to the golden rule of changing habits – **keep the same cue and reward, but change the routine.**

While it is incredibly hard to stop the cues from happening, it is far easier to change the routine following the cue. For example with our chocolate craving before, when you get a craving, instead of walking over to the vending machine, walk over to the kitchen and make a peppermint tea instead. Or reach for some chewing gum. Or keep some nuts or a sugar-free snack nearby and eat that instead. Or go for a walk. Or drink half a litre of water. The possibilities are endless!

This way you are working with your brain and the existing neural networks by making a small change, rather than trying to stop the neural network from functioning overall, which can be a daunting task.

Building new habits

Ok, so we have a way of breaking our old habits, but how about creating new healthy habits? Turns out, it is not so hard either!

There is one simple rule here – **start small**[210].

Committing to large goals and large changes can seem overwhelming and actually demotivate us, especially if we have had failures in the past. Want to build a new healthy habit quickly and effectively? Try this:

- Want to exercise more? Set a goal to exercise just five minutes every day for the next week. After that, increase to seven minutes. Then ten. This makes it easy and achievable, and slowly gets you into the rhythm of it
- Want to eat healthier? Aim to eat one healthy meal a day for a week. Then two the next week. Then three. Or start by first taking out grains, then sugar, etc. Making small changes are far more realistic than turning your entire diet upside down in one day

If you know you have trouble sticking to healthy eating, or have failed in the past, then take this advice and start small. Make small changes that add up over time to your true goals. This means you are building new neural networks over time, making them stronger every day. Soon, eating healthy will feel like a natural thing, and as it will align to your goals and it will be a fulfilling and rewarding process.

Committing to six months of healthy eating can seem huge. So how about instead just commit to making the next meal a healthy one. And then right after that meal, immediately commit to make the next meal a healthy one, and so on. Before you know it, you will have had a whole string of healthy meals, and you will see it in your body!

What to remember:
- Your vision defines personal characteristics that you want to develop in yourself
- Clear goals have SMART criteria – focus in particular on making your goals congruent with one another
- Prioritising goals gives you clarity when making difficult decisions so that you know what to fight for

4.4 Make it real

Now you can see how the whole Think Lean program fits together.

Each of the three keys flow into one another to create a virtuous circle:

Automatic Calorie Management provides you with the foods to eat to keep healthy and get your weight down to reach your goal body. This gives you that initial boost of confidence as you are starting to work towards your goals and achieving results.

Boost Your Brain gives you the techniques and nutrition to keep your brain working well, so you feel sharp, energetic and ready to face life and any challenge it brings.

Think Lean builds on your healthy brain by providing a method to help you become resilient, manage stress and bounce back from anything, driving your actions through clear goals to achieve a fulfilling lifestyle. This gives you the ability to follow the Think Lean Method as a lifestyle to maintain your ideal body in the long term.

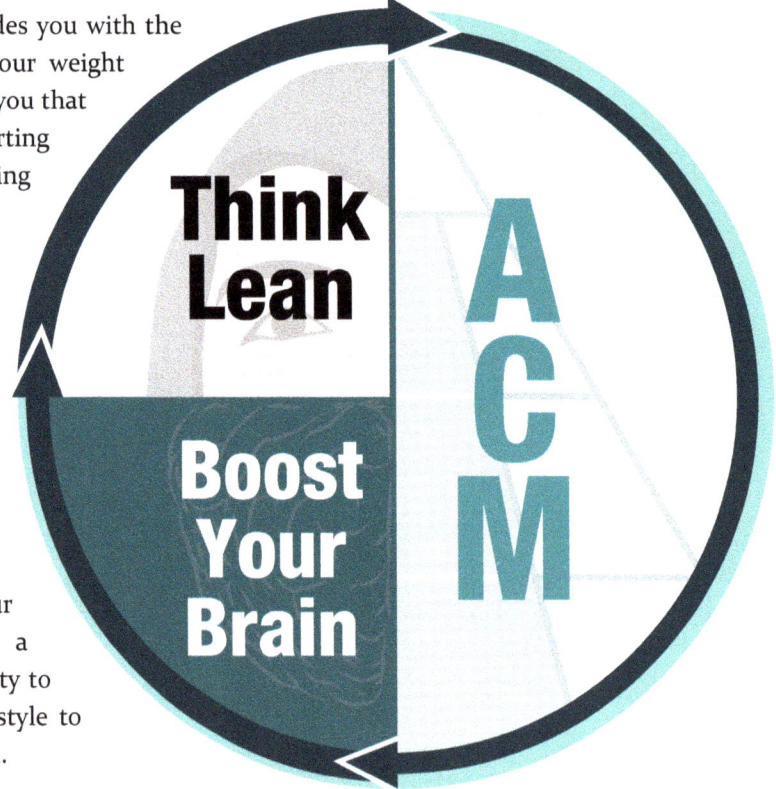

As we've seen from the evidence covering nutrition, neuroscience and psychology, we need all three these keys to be able to stick to healthy eating in the long term. If you commit to all three keys and build them into your life, you can achieve a state of mind that will change your life and allow you to create your goal body and stick to a healthy lifestyle for decades!

> You can make Think Lean part of your life through the simple steps set out along the way. All you need to do, is:
>
> 1. Develop and write down a **vision of yourself**
> 2. Identify and set **clear goals**
> 3. **Prioritise your goals** and write them down
>
> Once you have done this, **involve others** and share it with someone. Ask them to help you along the way, and hopefully you can do the same for them in return – maybe for a body goal, perhaps for another goal. All of this helps you towards one thing – **consistency**. If your body goal is important enough, you will do what you have to in order to stay consistent with healthy eating. Consistency is where the results come from!
>
> Now it is finally time to start eating healthy! Next is the **Think Lean Plan**.

Let's Get Started!

5 The Think Lean Plan

This is it! Now you know how ACM works, how to keep your brain in top condition, and how to stay consistent with healthy eating and reach your goals. All you need now is a clear plan so you can start eating right and put the method into action! This is what this plan below is all about – it gives you step-by-step instructions to get started on creating your goal body.

By now you must be ready to get started with healthy eating. Whether you are putting the full Think Lean Method into action, or even if you are just looking to make some small changes to your existing diet, you can make it happen with **six simple steps** in our Think Lean Plan:

1. *Set goals*
2. *Involve others*
3. *Clean up*
4. *Pick a meal plan*
5. *Think Lean and eat clean*
6. *Keep track*

Easy! The first four steps are designed to get you set up for success so that you can quickly put the method into action in as little as one afternoon. In fact, you can call this your Four Hour Life Makeover! Once you have ticked each of these, you can move on to steps five and six, which is all about living the Think Lean Method every day and keeping track of your success!

Get ready to make some changes so your journey can begin - let's get started!

5.1 Set goals

In the Think Lean section we went through the steps of setting clear goals to guide you on your journey to your goal body. We also prioritised the goals to make it clear just what fits in where so that you know what is most important to you. If your body goal is very important to you, then make sure it is high up on the list so that you can achieve it no matter what!

If you haven't set your goals yet, work through the steps in the *Developing clear goals* section. It is crucial to have a realistic and motivating body goal, as well as understand how it fits in with your other goals. Setting clear body goals is especially important if you have tried to lose weight in the past without any real or lasting results. Don't skip this step as it is crucial!

Setting clear goals should take less than an hour and is invaluable in your journey to achieve your body goal. Think of it as the first step in your Four Hour Life Makeover!

Of course, our goals change over time as our lives and situations change, so we will need to keep track of our goals and come back to them from time to time. Because of this, we will add our goals to the tracking sheet at the end of this section.

5.2 Involve others

By now you know how weight loss results can skyrocket when you involve others. Whether it is a friend, family, colleague, or someone else, they can help you stay on track even when things get tough (as they always do!). Even if it is just one other person, doing this with someone else will just be so much more rewarding. Better yet is if you can find someone to do the Think Lean Method with you as you can feed off each other's energy and passion to reach your goals!

When you talk to someone about your body goals, also tell them if there are other goals that are more important so they also know what your priorities are. Others are also great for tips on how to do things faster and easier, as you can tap into their experience and you can return the favour by sharing tips with them that helped you.

Even if you have tried diets before and failed, talk to people again and tell them what you are doing differently. For example, you can tell them about how:

- You have taken the time to identify and prioritise your goals
- You have set a clear goal for your body, prioritised it and made a commitment to achieve it
- You have a new eating plan that is proven to result in lasting weight loss

Involving someone else and sharing your journey is *highly* recommended, but you can also do it alone. Just be aware that you will need a lot more self-discipline if you will be doing it alone. Doing it with others is definitely easier, so even if it is just one person – **give someone a call now, tell them about your body goal and ask them to help keep you on track. Or better yet, ask them to join in!**

5.3 Clean up

Time for some action! We need to make some space for all the healthy foods that will help you reach your body goals. Where are we going to find space? Simple – by getting rid of all the bad foods hanging around! It is time for you to go around the kitchen, the pantry, and anywhere else that food might be hiding and throw out all foods that don't help you create your goal body.

Get a trash bag ready and let's go on a food hunt! Find the following and throw them out:

- **Grain products** – This is a big category, but we urgently need to get rid of this calorie-dense, carbohydrate-rich, high-GI foods that are no good for our health and hips! Look for:
    o Breads, bagels, biscuits and baked goods
    o Breakfast cereals (pretty much all of them are grains-based!)
    o Pasta, wraps
    o Flour, maize
- **Sugars** – The other big one. Sugar hides in so many products, so get rid of anything that contains sugar! Look for:
    o Bags of sugar, sugar pots (clean them all out!)
    o Sugary soft drinks
    o Honey
    o Sauces and salad dressings
    o Breads, cakes, cookies and most baked goods
    o Peanut butter, Nutella
    o Yoghurt with sugar
    o Cream
    o Some cheeses
    o Breakfast cereals
    o Fruit juices
    o Canned vegetables and fruit
    o Chocolate, fruit bars, breakfast bars, nut bars
    o Dried fruit
    o Sweets and candy
- **Alcohol** – If after that clean up you still have some beers and cruisers around – throw those out too! If you really want to keep some alcohol, keep red wine, champagne or less sweet white wines. Straight spirits are also better from a calorie perspective, but probably not from a mental health perspective

"But I don't want to waste food!" you say.

You mean it is just too much to bear to throw away that open pack of Oreos? You know, being able to throw out something that is bad for you is extremely empowering. Just give it a try! Throw away one thing and think about how that is not going to go on your hips now. Let you goals be your guide. If the foods do not support your goals, throw it out!

If you *really* do not want to throw it out, then give it to other people. Just do not eat it as a last quick 'hurrah' before healthy eating begins! If you do that, you'll only be making your goal harder to reach as you'll have to work off those biscuits as well.

Once you have it all bagged up, take it out of the house right now! A clean house supports a clean body and a clean mind! But there is one more thing we need to clean up...

Social media

It has become such a big part of our lives that we cannot underestimate how big a role social media plays in our ability to stay consistent with our diets. The main problem? Subscriptions to food pages that constantly bombard us with images of sugary treats! Go through your social media apps and start unsubscribing:

- Facebook
- Instagram
- Pinterest
- Twitter
- YouTube
- Tumblr

And any other apps and sites. If there is another channel (be it a website, TV channel, or anything else) that is tempting you through the day, remove it! It will make it so much easier if you are not tempted every now and then by pictures of sugary foods, so instead replace these by healthy eating and fitness motivation subscriptions instead. And subscribe to @ThinkLeanMethod on Facebook, Instagram, Pinterest or Twitter as well for more motivation!

5.4 Pick a meal plan

Now that the house and media is all cleaned up, we are ready to put some good foods in. You now need to know what to buy and work out what you will eat for the next few weeks. This part is key to put healthy eating into action and get you off to a flying start. The more prepared you are, the faster you will start to get results.

That bears repeating – **Preparation is key!**

What does it mean to be prepared with your diet? It means:

- You have a kitchen stocked with the right food
- You prepare meals in advance

- You have healthy snacks ready if you get hungry
- You know how to stick to healthy eating through upcoming work functions or social events

By now you should know if you are going with the Core ACM (no or little exercise) plan or the Complete ACM (regular exercise) plan. To make it easy for you to know what to shop for, take a copy of the **printable sheets of the food pyramid and detailed food lists** that support healthy eating included at the end of this section.

Remember to eat the foods in proportion to how large they are in the food pyramid – mostly meat and vegetables, some nuts, oil and dairy, and a bit of fruit every day or so. Remember to drink plenty of water as well. Water can help to overcome cravings and it replaces all those sugary drinks and juices that work against our health and hips!

Meal plans

Below are two ACM plans showing you a complete plan for 21 days each. The four plans are broken down as follows:

- **Variety Meal Plan**
    - Core ACM – Make only Core versions of each recipe
    - Complete ACM – Make the Complete version of one recipe per day
- **Low-effort Meal Plan**
    - Core ACM – Make only Core versions of each recipe
    - Complete ACM – Make the Complete version of one recipe per day

These two options give you templates that you can alter to suit your goals and your personality. Personally, I don't like to spend a lot of time on food and preparation, so I go for the low effort plans. I wanted to give you the same option in case you want to get great results with minimal effort.

Each plan has a balanced set of foods and is designed to give you all the vitamins and minerals for healthy living. This will support your body and brain, while providing large meals with low calories to keep you full while getting you lean.

Still, these are templates which mean that you can change them around as you need so that they suit your goals. A few examples:

- *If you don't like a particular type of meat or food, look through the recipes and swap it out*
- *If you want to lose weight faster, you can make the meal portions smaller*
- *If you are aiming to get more muscle definition from exercising, you can add in additional Complete ACM meals (up to six meals a day!)*

Also, if your goal is to follow ACM at a particular level then you'll have free meals every now and then. Plan out your free meals in advance so that you can prep meals accordingly and enjoy it guilt free! Remember the basic guidelines:

- 98% - one free meal per two weeks
- 95% - one free meal per week

- 90% - two free meals per week
- 80% - four free meals per week

My experience is that you need to follow it around 90% or more to start getting real weight loss results, but even at 80% you can still get great overall health and wellbeing benefits. Of course if your free meals are kept smaller, then you can still get great results at a good pace. For sustainable and lasting weight loss, aim for about a kilogram per two weeks. Faster than that and you are likely going to yo-yo and put it back on soon after.

We don't want a crash diet...

We want long-lasting, healthy lifestyle changes. The kind that will keep you feeling and looking great for years to come!

Print out the meal plan below that best suits your goal and modify as you need. This is all about you and getting you the right approach that will get you your goal body! Once you have your plan, head out to the shop and buy ingredients so you can start prepping healthy meals.

Variety Meal Plan

The structure of this meal plan is fairly simple – make breakfast around once every two days and have leftover breakfast the next day, while lunch is usually leftovers from dinner the night before. This way you always have something to take along to work, and you don't have to cook anything separate for lunch!

Most recipes can be converted between Core ACM and Complete ACM. Have a look on the recipes themselves for guidance.

* If you are on Core ACM, stick to only the Core ACM version of each recipe
* If you are on Complete ACM, make the Complete ACM version for one meal per day

Week 1

	Breakfast	Lunch	Dinner
Sunday	Salmon Eggs Benedict (page 171)	Grilled salmon with **Armenian Avo Salad** (page 189)	**Anytime Meatballs** (page 182) with **Veggie Spaghetti** (page 190)
Monday	Brain Boost Breakfast Salad (page 168)	Leftover **Anytime Meatballs** (page 182) with **Veggie Spaghetti** (page 190)	**Sicilian Sage Lamb** (page 174) with **Vaudeville Roast Veggies** (page 189)
Tuesday	Brain Boost Breakfast Salad (page 168)	Leftover **Sicilian Sage Lamb** (page 174) with **Vaudeville Roast Veggies** (page 189)	**Lemon Squeeze Salmon** (page 176) with grilled asparagus
Wednesday	3 egg omelette with mushroom and capsicum	Leftover **Lemon Squeeze Salmon** (page 176) with grilled asparagus	Three Spice Chicken (page 175)
Thursday	**Omega Quiche** (page 170) with spinach, tomato, olives and red onion salad with a **Balanced Vinaigrette** (page 202)	Leftover **Three Spice Chicken** (page 175)	**Three Keys Kebabs** (page 179) with steamed veggies or salad
Friday	Leftover **Omega Quiche** (page 170) with spinach, tomato, olives and red onion salad with a **Balanced Vinaigrette** (page 202)	Leftover **Three Keys Kebabs** (page 179) with steamed veggies or salad	Thai Beef Salad (page 177)
Saturday	Almond Pancakes (page 170) with Mixed berries	Leftover **Thai Beef Salad** (page 177)	Double Lemon Chicken (page 183) with **ACM Cauli Rice** (page 188)

The Think Lean Plan

Week 2 – Variety Meal Plan

	Breakfast	Lunch	Dinner
Sunday	Leftover **Almond Pancakes** (page 170) with Mixed berries	Leftover **Double Lemon Chicken** (page 183) with **ACM Cauli Rice** (page 188)	**Crusted Barramundi** (page 181) with **Sugar Snap Veggies** (page 191)
Monday	**Lean Morning Soufflé** (page 169) with Cos or rocket lettuce, crushed almond and pear slices	Leftover **Crusted Barramundi** (page 181) with **Sugar Snap Veggies** (page 191)	**Protein Punch Chicken Salad** (page 186)
Tuesday	Leftover **Lean Morning Soufflé** (page 169) with Cos or rocket lettuce, crushed almond and pear slices	Leftover **Protein Punch Chicken Salad** (page 186)	**Lemon Squeeze Salmon** (page 176) with **Lean Zucchini Salad** (page 188)
Wednesday	**Think Bacon Frittata** (page 168) with Iceberg lettuce, capsicum and onion slices	Leftover **Lemon Squeeze Salmon** (page 176) with **Lean Zucchini Salad** (page 188)	**Quick Steak** (page 185) with **Sugar Snap Veggies** (page 191)
Thursday	Leftover **Think Bacon Frittata** (page 168) with Iceberg lettuce, capsicum and onion slices	Leftover **Quick Steak** (page 185) with **Sugar Snap Veggies** (page 191)	**Clean Baked Chicken** (page 178) with **Lean Zucchini Salad** (page 188)
Friday	**Salmon Eggs Benedict** (page 171)	Leftover **Clean Baked Chicken** (page 178) with **Lean Zucchini Salad** (page 188)	**Anytime Meatballs** (page 182) with **Veggie Spaghetti** (page 190)
Saturday	**Almond Pancakes** (page 170) with Mixed berries	Leftover **Anytime Meatballs** (page 182) with **Veggie Spaghetti** (page 190)	**Lean Seafood Paella** (page 184) with **ACM Cauli Rice** (page 188)

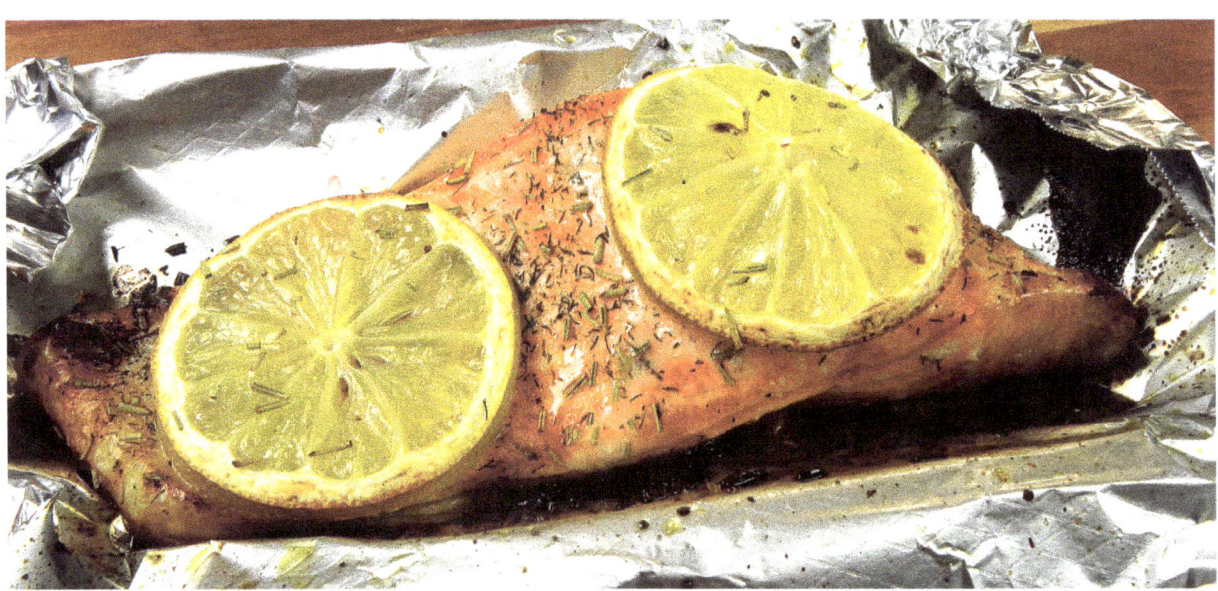

The Think Lean Plan

Week 3 – Variety Meal Plan

	Breakfast	Lunch	Dinner
Sunday	Leftover **Almond Pancakes (page 170)** with Mixed berries	Leftover **Lean Seafood Paella (page 184)** with **ACM Cauli Rice (page 188)**	**Poached Chicken Thyme (page 180)** with **Armenian Avo Salad (page 189)**
Monday	**Brain Boost Breakfast Salad (page 168)**	Leftover **Poached Chicken Thyme (page 180)** with **Armenian Avo Salad (page 189)**	**Three Spice Chicken (page 175)** with a light salad
Tuesday	Leftover **Brain Boost Breakfast Salad (page 168)**	Leftover **Three Spice Chicken (page 175)** with a light salad	**Three Keys Kebabs (page 179)** with steamed veggies or salad
Wednesday	**Omega Quiche (page 170)** with spinach, tomato, olives and red onion salad with a **Balanced Vinaigrette (page 202)**	Leftover **Three Keys Kebabs (page 179)** with steamed veggies or salad	**Lemon Squeeze Salmon (page 176)** with **Lean Zucchini Salad (page 188)**
Thursday	Leftover **Omega Quiche (page 170)** with spinach, tomato, olives and red onion salad with a **Balanced Vinaigrette (page 202)**	Leftover **Lemon Squeeze Salmon (page 176)** with **Lean Zucchini Salad (page 188)**	**Thai Beef Salad (page 177)**
Friday	**Think Bacon Frittata (page 168)** with Iceberg lettuce, capsicum and onion slices	Leftover **Thai Beef Salad (page 177)**	**Crusted Barramundi (page 181)** with **Sugar Snap Veggies (page 191)**
Saturday	Leftover **Think Bacon Frittata (page 168)** with Iceberg lettuce, capsicum and onion slices	Leftover **Crusted Barramundi (page 181)** with **Sugar Snap Veggies (page 191)**	**Porto Burgers (page 177)** with **Vaudeville Roast Veggies (page 189)**

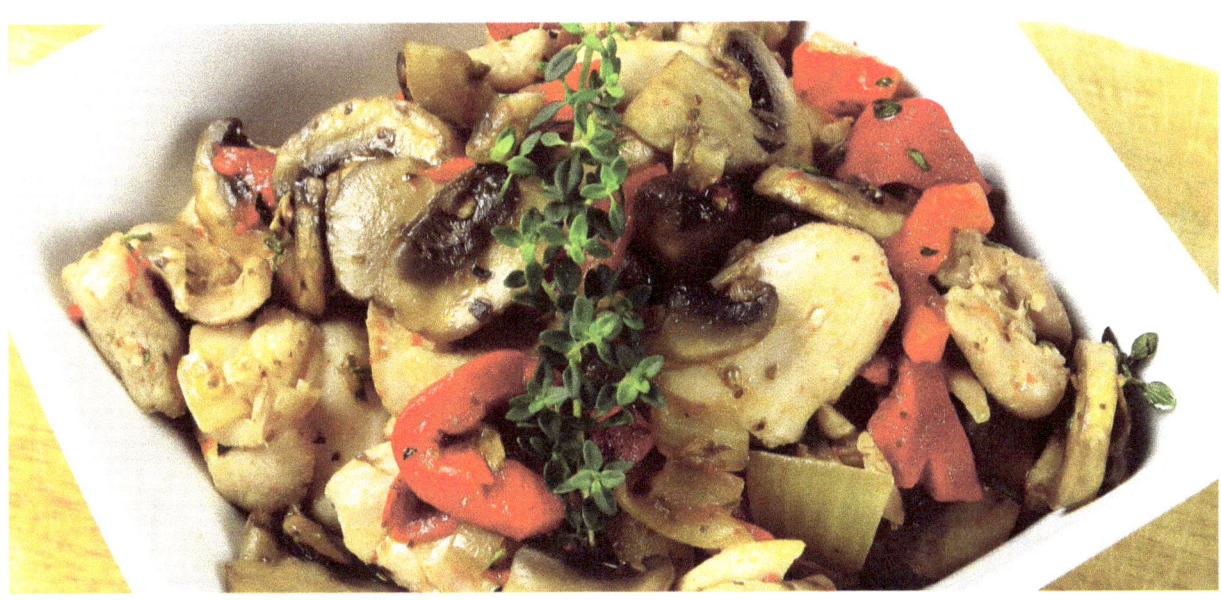

Low-effort Meal Plan

This meal plan is more my style since I really like to keep things simple and practical. By doing a bit of extra preparation on Sunday, both breakfast and lunch is sorted for the work week. Meanwhile, dinner only needs to be cooked every second day.

The great thing about this plan is that it becomes a habit and after a while living healthy is second nature. It is just so easy! Of course, you can always make substitutions if there are other foods you like more than the ones listed below. You can vary the weeks between different meats or other foods, use smoothies and protein shakes, or even add extra meals if you are bulking up. The possibilities are endless, so make it suit your goals and taste!

Most recipes can be converted between Core ACM and Complete ACM. Have a look on the recipes themselves for guidance.

- If you are on Core ACM, stick to only the Core ACM version of each recipe
- If you are on Complete ACM, make the Complete ACM version for one meal per day

Week 1

	Breakfast	Lunch	Dinner
Sunday	**Omega Quiche (page 170)** with spinach, tomato, olives and red onion salad with a **Balanced Vinaigrette (page 202)**	**Quick Steak (page 185)** with **Armenian Avo Salad (page 189)**	**Lemon Squeeze Salmon (page 176)** with **Lean Zucchini Salad (page 188)**
Monday	**Brain Boost Breakfast Salad (page 168)** (Hard boil 15 eggs and grill 250g of bacon on Sunday to prep for the week) Or bake a large frittata and vary the ingredients	**Poached Chicken Thyme (page 180)** (Poach enough chicken on Sunday for the week. Add 200g of frozen vegetables each day for lunch) Or make a large chicken bake with veggies and vary the ingredients	**Thai Beef Salad (page 177)**
Tuesday			Leftover **Thai Beef Salad (page 177)**
Wednesday			**Three Keys Kebabs (page 179)** with steamed veggies or salad
Thursday			Leftover **Three Keys Kebabs (page 179)** with steamed veggies or salad
Friday			**Crusted Barramundi (page 181)** with **Sugar Snap Veggies (page 191)**
Saturday	**Lean Morning Soufflé (page 169)** with Cos or rocket lettuce, crushed almond and pear slices	**Double Lemon Chicken (page 183)** with **ACM Cauli Rice (page 188)**	Leftover **Crusted Barramundi (page 181)** with **Sugar Snap Veggies (page 191)**

Week 2 – Low-effort Meal Plan

	Breakfast	Lunch	Dinner
Sunday	Leftover **Lean Morning Soufflé (page 169)** with Cos or rocket lettuce, crushed almond and pear slices	Leftover **Double Lemon Chicken (page 183)** with **ACM Cauli Rice (page 188)**	**Sicilian Sage Lamb (page 174)** with **Vaudeville Roast Veggies (page 189)**
Monday	**Brain Boost Breakfast Salad (page 168)** (Hard boil 15 eggs and grill 250g of bacon on Sunday to prep for the week) Or bake a large frittata and vary the ingredients	**Poached Chicken Thyme (page 180)** (Poach enough chicken on Sunday for the week. Add 200g of frozen vegetables each day for lunch) Or make a large chicken bake with veggies and vary the ingredients	Leftover **Sicilian Sage Lamb (page 174)** with **Vaudeville Roast Veggies (page 189)**
Tuesday			**Anytime Meatballs (page 182)** with **Veggie Spaghetti (page 190)**
Wednesday			Leftover **Anytime Meatballs (page 182)** with **Veggie Spaghetti (page 190)**
Thursday			**Crusted Barramundi (page 181)** with **Sugar Snap Veggies (page 191)**
Friday			Leftover **Crusted Barramundi (page 181)** with **Sugar Snap Veggies (page 191)**
Saturday	**Almond Pancakes (page 170)** with Mixed berries	**Sicilian Sage Lamb (page 174)** with **Vaudeville Roast Veggies (page 189)**	**Three Spice Chicken (page 175)** with a light salad

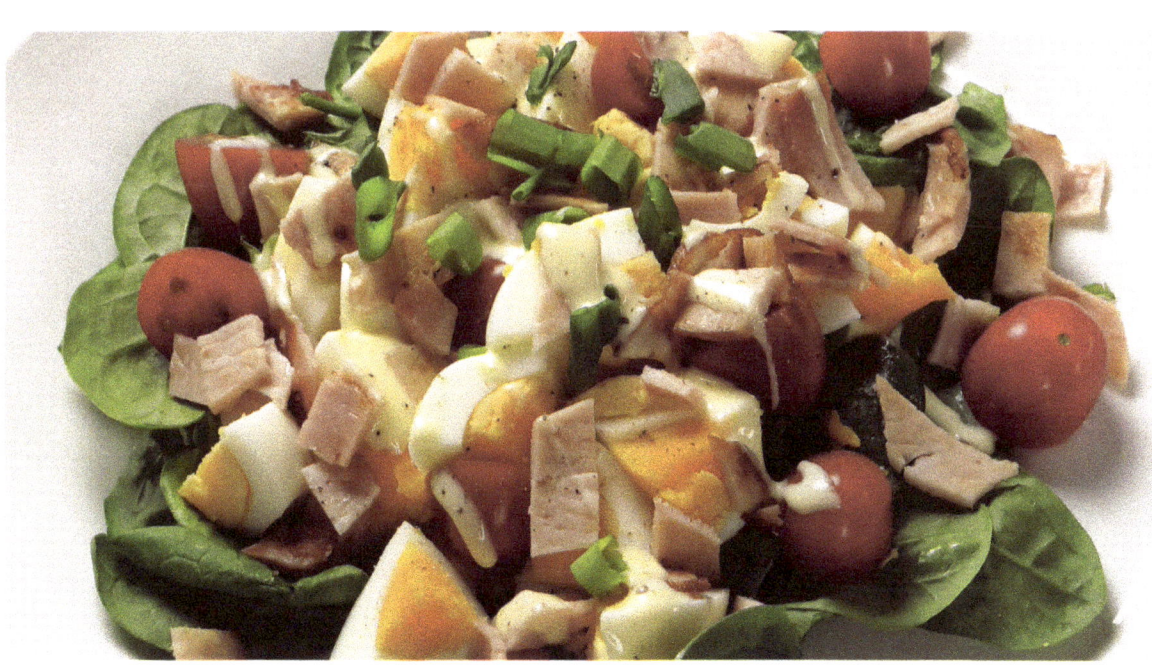

The Think Lean Plan

Week 3 – Low-effort Meal Plan

	Breakfast	Lunch	Dinner
Sunday	Leftover **Almond Pancakes (page 170)** with Mixed berries	Leftover **Sicilian Sage Lamb (page 174)** with **Vaudeville Roast Veggies (page 189)**	**Three Spice Chicken (page 175)** with a light salad
Monday	**Brain Boost Breakfast Salad (page 168)** (Hard boil 15 eggs and grill 250g of bacon on Sunday to prep for the week) Or bake a large frittata and vary the ingredients	**Poached Chicken Thyme (page 180)** (Poach enough chicken on Sunday for the week. Add 200g of frozen vegetables each day for lunch) Or make a large chicken bake with veggies and vary the ingredients	**Lemon Squeeze Salmon (page 176)** with **Lean Zucchini Salad (page 188)**
Tuesday			Leftover **Lemon Squeeze Salmon (page 176)** with **Lean Zucchini Salad (page 188)**
Wednesday			**Anytime Meatballs (page 182)** with **Veggie Spaghetti (page 190)**
Thursday			Leftover **Anytime Meatballs (page 182)** with **Veggie Spaghetti (page 190)**
Friday			**Lemon Squeeze Salmon (page 176)** with **Lean Zucchini Salad (page 188)**
Saturday	**Omega Quiche (page 170)** with spinach, tomato, olives and red onion salad with a **Balanced Vinaigrette (page 202)**	**Quick Steak (page 185)** with **Armenian Avo Salad (page 189)**	Leftover **Lemon Squeeze Salmon (page 176)** with **Lean Zucchini Salad (page 188)**

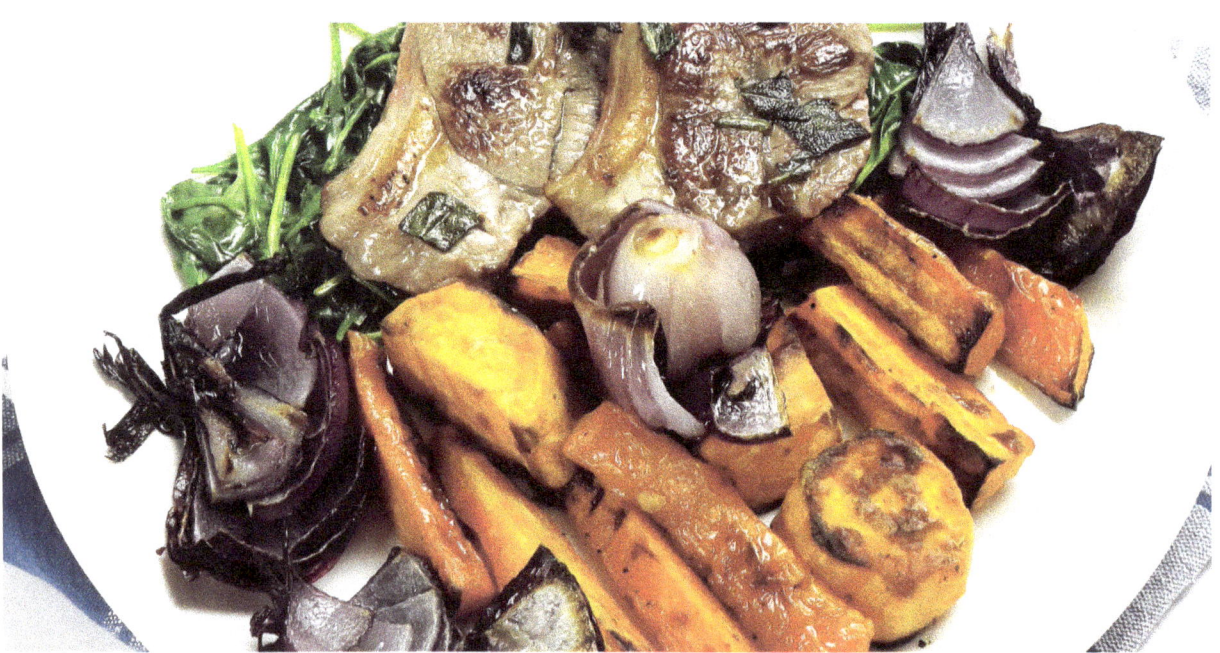

5.5 Think Lean and eat clean

So you've got your meal plan and your kitchen is stocked with healthy meals. Now comes the fun part of living it every day! When it comes to the day to day reality of eating healthy, remember to always be prepared. Keep your kitchen stocked with healthy food and keep unhealthy snacks away so that you do not get tempted.

Remember to bring in the lessons from the Boost Your Brain section:

- Get regular, good quality sleep
- Exercise at least three times a week
- Limit caffeine and alcohol
- Bring in any vitamin and mineral supplements if needed

As you pursue your body goals, keep working towards your other goals as well. Work on your personal resilience, your relationships, your work – anything that is important enough to you to make your list of goals. Anything worth doing takes time, so just focus on the next step. That way you will reach your personal vision in no time!

> **Live your goals!**
>
> I cannot stress this enough – **let your goals be your guide**. Live towards your goals and use them when you need to make decisions. This will help you constantly move forward and you will start to live a life of achievement that is truly fulfilling.

Sticking to your goals will make your goal body a reality and let you keep it too.

Think Lean, get lean, stay lean!

5.6 Keep track

We look at ourselves so often that it can be hard to notice real changes happening to our bodies. Sometimes it is also hard to remember just how well we are following our diets. That is why keeping track of our progress is key!

To do this, we need a tracking sheet! At the end of this section is a printable tracking sheet, showing the key concepts and a space to keep track of your progress.

5.6.1 How the tracking sheets work:

Each sheet is used to keep track of your goals and healthy eating for three months, so start by printing one for your first three months.

Step 1 – Write down your goals and vision of yourself
Write your goals down in prioritised order on the left-hand side, and your vision of yourself on the right. Your goals should support your vision, and represent steps along the way to become the person you really are.

The Think Lean Plan

Make sure your goals are clear, meaning that they are specific, measurable, attainable, relevant (this is especially important – they must be aligned and congruent to your vision and other goals), and they must have a timeframe.

Step 2 – Measure your progress

How do you really know if you are making progress? In three ways:

1. **Weigh yourself** – If your goal is to lose weight, then you need to weigh yourself, naturally! The tracking sheet has a spot for your starting weight. This is how much you weigh before starting the Think Lean Method at all. From there, weigh yourself every two weeks and put the number into the box on the sheet so you can see your progress

2. **Measure yourself** – Measure your waist at the start of your new healthy eating lifestyle, and then every two weeks as you weigh yourself and put the number into the box on the sheet so you can see your progress. If you do not have a measuring tape, get one from the supermarket, or any general goods store

   > **Weight and muscle**
   >
   > Note – If you are not overweight and are exercising, then you are likely to swap body fat for muscle. In that case, remember that **muscle is much denser than body fat**. This means that you might not see any change on the scale, but you will be getting leaner, tighter, and lose a dress size on the way!
   >
   > If you have a long way to go, the scale is the best way to measure. But if you weigh around 70kg or less, you'll be better off paying attention to the measurements than weight.

   a. If you have a lot of weight to lose, measure over your bellybutton to keep it consistent

   b. Later on as you get leaner, or if you don't have a lot of weight to lose, measure the smallest part of your waist while tensing your abdominal muscles (in other words, don't suck it in!)

3. **Photos** – Take some photos of your body at the start of your new lifestyle, and then again every three months as you complete a sheet. You can do this more often if you like, but it usually takes a few months of progress to see a real difference. In the meantime, weighing yourself and taking measurements will tell you what is happening with your body. For the photos, wear a bikini (or shorts for men) or something else that you would be happy to show others when you do your awesome before and after shots! In terms of poses, the following two are good:

   a. Feet shoulder width apart, stand up straight, arms by your sides and take a photo directly from the front

   b. Same pose as before and take a photo from the side while you look directly ahead

This schedule is pretty simple to keep to and the tracking sheet will remind you when to do each of these. Hopping on the scale and throwing a measuring tape around your waist takes 30 seconds, *so no excuses for not doing it!*

If you are very serious about developing a more muscular body, then I'd recommend taking more measurements, including biceps, chest, hips, thighs and calves. This is a bit more effort, but if you are that serious about seeing results in the right places, then I'm sure you won't mind a bit of extra work, right?

Step 3 – Track your day to day progress

The last step is ticking off your success each day. Many diets recommend keeping a food log as it helps to make you conscious of what you are eating. Food logs are great, but they take a lot of effort, so I've simplified this so you can do it in no time every day. The tracking sheet has a box for each day of the week and it simply works like this:

- If you stuck to healthy eating and your meal plan that day, **tick the box**
- If you didn't stick to the plan and had other foods that are not part of the pyramid, **don't tick the box**

You can't get any simpler than that!

If you had a planned free meal because you are doing it at 95% (for example), then you can still tick the box since it is all part of the plan and your current goals!

One important note here – if you had a single cookie (or something) that isn't part of the plan, then you can't tick the box, *but that does NOT mean the day is ruined and you might as well eat anything for the rest of the day!* Get back to healthy eating straight after. Don't wait until tomorrow. Get back on ACM and your plan right away.

Do not ever use the excuse that *"My diet is ruined today"*. If you hear yourself say those words, stop and think – if you eat more, you will just make you own journey harder tomorrow as you'll have to work off those extra cookies anyway in addition to the one you already had. You might not get to tick the box, but you can get back to healthy eating right after and make tomorrow easier. Do that, and you'll be proud of yourself that you got right back on the diet!

5.6.2 When you have completed a sheet

Celebrate! But do it in a way that doesn't involve food – buy yourself a dress, go rock climbing, go dancing, something you really enjoy.

Share your milestone with whoever is helping you or doing the Think Lean Method with you. Look over the results you got. How are you tracking towards your body goal? Are you going faster than expected, on track, or maybe a bit slower? If the results are not coming as fast as you want, look over how well you've been sticking to healthy eating and do some troubleshooting:

- If you have ticks in every box, are they all 100% honest?
- If there are gaps, try staying more consistent with healthy eating
- Are you fully sticking to all five rules of ACM?
- If you've been 100% consistent, then try switching to Core if you are on Complete
- If you are following ACM at 80% or 85%, move up higher to 90% or 95%
- Look at your free meals. If they are really big and really high in calories, they can prevent weight loss
- Try adding more exercise

Remember that we are all different and react differently to dieting. Some lose weight fast, while others take more effort. What is crucial as always is **consistency**. Make sure you stick to healthy eating and tweak it so you keep moving towards your goal.

> ## *Setting up a new sheet*
> This is important – when you have completed a sheet, go back over your vision and goals. Think about each one – have you achieved any of them? Are they all still important goals that are clear? Is the prioritisation still correct? Do they support your vision?
>
> Once you have gone through them, update them accordingly and write them down on a new sheet. **Do not just photocopy the old sheet!** It is important that you physically write (or type) them out again. This way you make sure you keep the goals current and relevant to what's happening in your life. Update them as needed and you're off for another three months of success!

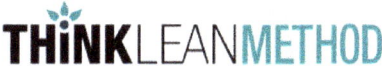

TRACKING SHEET

Personal resilience

Clear goals – Goals provide clarity in making both small and large decisions, directing your efforts to what you most desire.

Involve others – Your relationships with family, friends and work colleagues are crucial. Don't do it alone!

Embrace change – Each change is a challenge and a chance for you to improve yourself and move closer to your goals.

Realistic optimism – A grounded and realistic sense of hope for your future and your ability to reach your goals.

Look after yourself – Proper sleep, exercise and nutrition keeps you physically ready for anything.

Self-assured – Develop confidence and be centred within yourself.

Keys to brain health

Quality sleep – At least seven hours of quality sleep a day. Fight for your sleep!

Environment – Actively manage stress and take control of your life through clear goals!

Exercise – At least three sessions a week.

Healthy eating – Eat healthy, balanced meals with the right foods from the ACM food pyramid.

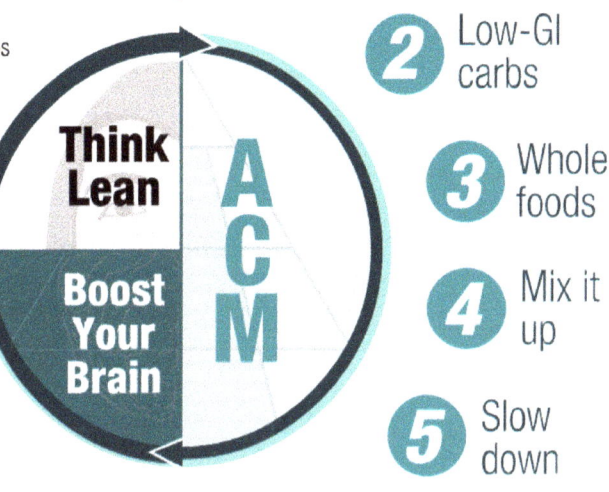

Five rules of ACM

1. Quality protein with every meal
2. Low-GI carbs
3. Whole foods
4. Mix it up
5. Slow down

Prioritised goals
Specific, measurable, attainable, **relevant** & timeframe

1. _____
2. _____
3. _____
4. _____
5. _____

Personal vision
Broad, positive characteristics to become

1. _____
2. _____
3. _____
4. _____
5. _____

	S	M	T	W	T	F	S	S	M	T	W	T	F	S	Weight / Waist	S	M	T	W	T	F	S	S	M	T	W	T	F	S	Weight / Waist
Month 1																															
Month 2																															
Month 3																															

☑ Tick each day that you stayed consistent with your eating plan.

Starting weight and waist measurement

Start date of this sheet

Next Steps!
→ Take new pictures
→ Start the next sheet

THINK LEAN METHOD

CORE Food Pyramid

Fruit

Stick to one a day or less

- Apples
- Apricots
- Avocados
- Bananas
- Blackberries
- Blueberries
- Cherries
- Cranberries
- Date
- Dragonfruit
- Grapefruit
- Grapes
- Guavas
- Kiwis
- Kumquat
- Lemons
- Limes
- Luquat
- Lychees
- Mandarins
- Mangoes
- Mangosteen
- Melons
- Mulberry
- Nectarines
- Olives
- Oranges
- Papayas
- Passionfruit
- Peaches
- Pears
- Pineapples
- Plums
- Pomegranates
- Raspberries
- Rhubarb
- Star fruit
- Strawberries
- Tangerines
- Watermelon

Vegetables

The more you eat, the better!

- Alfalfa seeds
- Amaranth
- Artichoke
- Asparagus
- Bamboo shoots
- Bell peppers
- Bok choi
- Broccoli
- Brussels sprouts
- Butternut squash
- Cabbage
- Carrots
- Cauliflower
- Celery
- Chicory
- Chilli
- Chinese broccoli
- Chinese cabbage
- Collard greens
- Cucumber
- Eggplant
- Fennel
- Gem Squash
- Green beans
- Green onions
- Jalapeno peppers
- Kale
- Leeks
- Lettuce (various)
- Mushrooms (various)
- Okra
- Onions
- Parsley
- Radishes
- Rhubarb
- Sauerkraut
- Scallions
- Seaweed
- Spaghetti squash
- Spinach
- Swiss chard
- Tomatoes
- Turnips
- Watercress
- Zucchini
- Daikon
- Snap peas

Nuts & Oils

Snacks & small amounts

Nuts

- Almonds
- Brazil nuts
- Cashews
- Chestnuts
- Coconut
- Hazelnuts
- Macadamia
- Peacan
- Peanuts
- Pine nuts
- Pistachio
- Wallnuts

Oils & Fats

- Butter
- Ghee
- Coconut oil
- Tallow
- Lard
- Avocado oil
- Almond oil

Dairy

One portion a day

- Milk (full cream)
- Cheddar
- Gouda
- Swiss cheese
- Cottage cheese
- Parmesan
- Edam
- Mozzarella
- Fat-free cheese
- Whey
- Yoghurt (sugar free)

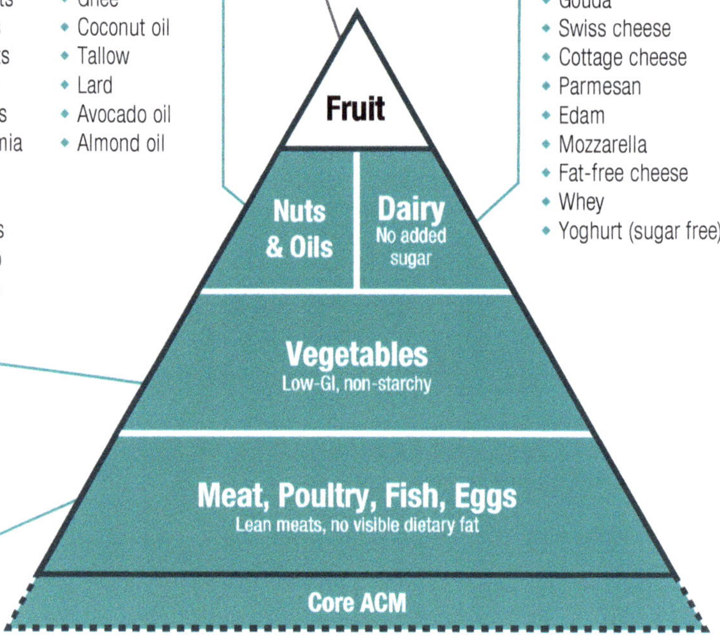

Fruit
Nuts & Oils
Dairy
No added sugar
Vegetables
Low-GI, non-starchy
Meat, Poultry, Fish, Eggs
Lean meats, no visible dietary fat
Core ACM

Meat, Poultry, Fish, Eggs

Eat most of - lean protein with every meal

Poultry

- Chicken
- Duck
- Goose
- Ostrich
- Quail
- Turkey
- All eggs

Lean cuts like:

- Breast
- Tenderloin

Meat

- Beef
- Kangaroo
- Lamb
- Pork
- Rabbit
- Veal
- Wild meat

Lean cuts like:

- 95% mince
- Sirloin
- Tenderloin
- Lean bacon

Fish

- Anchovy
- Herring
- John Dory
- Mackerel
- Mullet
- Octopus
- Salmon
- Sardines
- Snapper
- Squid
- Trout
- Tuna
- Whiting

Shellfish

- Clams
- Crab
- Lobster
- Mussels
- Oysters
- Prawns
- Scallops

Herbs & Spices

Use as much seasoning as you like!

- Angelica
- Anise
- Basil
- Bay leaf
- Caraway
- Cardamom
- Carob
- Cayenne pepper
- Celery seed
- Chervil
- Chili pepper
- Chives
- Cilantro
- Cinnamon
- Clove
- Coriander
- Cumin
- Curry
- Dill
- Fennel
- Fenugreek
- Galangal
- Garlic
- Ginger
- Horseradish
- Jasmine flowers
- Juniper berry
- Kaffir lime leaves
- Lavender
- Lemongrass
- Licorice
- Mace
- Marjoram
- Mint
- Mustard
- Nutmeg
- Oregano
- Paprika
- Parseley
- Pepper
- Peppermint
- Rosemary
- Saffron
- Sage
- Salt
- Sesame
- Star anise
- Tarragon
- Thyme
- Turmeric
- Vanilla
- Wasabi
- Wattleseed
- Za'atar

THINK LEAN METHOD

* This is not an exhaustive list! If you find foods that fit with the rules that are not on here, add them in!

THiNK LEAN METHOD
COMPLETE Food Pyramid

Fruit
Stick to one a day or less

- Apples
- Apricots
- Avocados
- Bananas
- Blackberries
- Blueberries
- Cherries
- Cranberries
- Date
- Dragonfruit
- Grapefruit
- Grapes
- Guavas
- Kiwis
- Kumquat
- Lemons
- Limes
- Luquat
- Lychees
- Mandarins
- Mangoes
- Mangosteen
- Melons
- Mulberry
- Nectarines
- Olives
- Oranges
- Papayas
- Passionfruit
- Peaches
- Pears
- Pineapples
- Plums
- Pomegranates
- Raspberries
- Rhubarb
- Star fruit
- Strawberries
- Tangerines
- Watermelon

Vegetables
Low-GI - The more the better!

- Alfalfa seeds
- Amaranth
- Artichoke
- Asparagus
- Bamboo shoots
- Bell peppers
- Bok choi
- Broccoli
- Brussels sprouts
- Butternut squash
- Cabbage
- Carrots
- Cauliflower
- Celery
- Chicory
- Chilli
- Chinese broccoli
- Chinese cabbage
- Collard greens
- Cucumber
- Eggplant
- Fennel
- Gem Squash
- Green beans
- Green onions
- Jalapeno peppers
- Kale
- Leeks
- Lettuce (various)
- Mushrooms (various)
- Okra
- Onions
- Parsley
- Radishes
- Rhubarb
- Sauerkraut
- Scallions
- Seaweed
- Spaghetti squash
- Spinach
- Swiss chard
- Tomatoes
- Turnips
- Watercress
- Zucchini
- Daikon
- Snap peas

Nuts & Oils
Snacks & small amounts

Nuts
- Almonds
- Cashews
- Coconut
- Hazelnuts
- Macadamia
- Peacan
- Peanuts
- Pistachio
- Wallnuts

Oils & Fats
- Butter
- Ghee
- Coconut oil
- Avocado oil
- Almond oil

Dairy
One portion a day

- Milk (full cream)
- Cheddar
- Gouda
- Swiss cheese
- Cottage cheese
- Parmesan
- Edam
- Mozzarella
- Fat-free cheese
- Whey
- Yoghurt (sugar free)

Legumes
Snacks & small amounts

- Black beans
- Broad beans
- Butter beans
- Chickpeas
- Edamame
- Kidney beans
- Lentils
- Peas
- Soy beans
- Split peas

Veggies
Starchy for fuel

- Beets
- Plantains
- Pumpkin
- Sweet corn
- Sweet potato
- Waterchestnuts
- Yam

Pyramid
- Fruit
- Nuts & Oils | Dairy (No added sugar) | Legumes
- Vegetables (Low-GI, non-starchy) | Veggies (Starchy)
- Meat, Poultry, Fish, Eggs (Lean meats, no visible dietary fat) | Fatty Meats (Visible dietary fat)

Complete ACM - Includes all Core ACM foods (regular exercise)

Meat, Poultry, Fish, Eggs
Eat most of - lean protein with every meal

Poultry
- Chicken
- Duck
- Goose
- Ostrich
- Quail
- Turkey
- All eggs

Lean cuts like:
- Breast
- Tenderloin

Meat
- Beef
- Kangaroo
- Lamb
- Pork
- Rabbit
- Veal
- Wild meat

Lean cuts like:
- 95% ground beef
- Sirloin
- Tenderloin
- Lean bacon

Fish
- Anchovy
- Herring
- John Dory
- Mackerel
- Mullet
- Octopus
- Salmon
- Sardines
- Snapper
- Squid
- Trout
- Tuna
- Whiting

Shellfish
- Clams
- Crab
- Lobster
- Mussels
- Oysters
- Prawns
- Scallops

Herbs & Spices
Use as much seasoning as you like!

- Angelica
- Anise
- Basil
- Bay leaf
- Caraway
- Cardamom
- Carob
- Cayenne pepper
- Celery seed
- Chervil
- Chili pepper
- Chives
- Cilantro
- Cinnamon
- Clove
- Coriander
- Cumin
- Curry
- Dill
- Fennel
- Fenugreek
- Galangal
- Garlic
- Ginger
- Horseradish
- Jasmine flowers
- Juniper berry
- Kaffir lime leaves
- Lavender
- Lemongrass
- Licorice
- Mace
- Marjoram
- Mint
- Mustard
- Nutmeg
- Oregano
- Paprika
- Parseley
- Pepper
- Peppermint
- Rosemary
- Saffron
- Sage
- Salt
- Sesame
- Star anise
- Tarragon
- Thyme
- Turmeric
- Vanilla
- Wasabi
- Wattleseed
- Za'atar

Meats
Fatty cuts for fuel

Poultry
- Drumstick
- Leg quarter
- Poultry with skin on
- Thigh

Meat
- New York Strip
- Porterhouse steak
- Ribeye steak
- Ribs
- T-bone steak
- Wagyu
- Chops
- Bacon

* This is not an exhaustive list! If you find foods that fit with the rules that are not on here, add them in!

6 Easy Recipes

Time to start eating! The recipes here show you some examples of simple yet delicious recipes using the foods included in the Think Lean food pyramid. After all, eating healthy doesn't need to feel like a diet! You'll notice that the portion sizes are fairly large and include a healthy amount of protein to help you feel full and satisfied after every meal. The recipes are split up as follows:

- **Breakfast**
- **Mains** (for both lunch and dinner)
- **Side Dishes** (for the Mains)
- **Snacks**
- **Sauces and Dips**

Nearly all of the recipes are suitable for both Core and Complete ACM, or can be converted between the two by swapping ingredients. This means that even if you are Core ACM, you still have a full variety of meals to choose from! Naturally, you are not limited to these recipes! You can convert nearly any existing recipe to the Think Lean Method by replacing ingredients with those that are on the Think Lean food pyramid.

Especially for all you culinary experts out there – this section is focused on *easy* recipes, which means nothing in here is particularly complicated. If you really love cooking and are used to doing all kinds of fancy things in the kitchen, then I encourage you to take some of your favourite recipes and convert them to Think Lean instead. Given that you can make a great tasting soufflé with Think Lean goes to show that you can convert nearly any recipe to this diet!

For everyone else who might not have a great deal of time to spend in the kitchen (like me), these easy recipes are for you. They are simple, easy, and they taste great. This is all about being practical so that you can follow it day after day, making it easy to turn this into a long-term healthy lifestyle. So use all of this as a template and turn it into your own lean eating lifestyle. Make it work for *you*!

Conversion tables

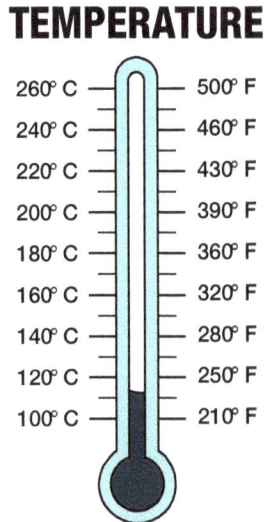

TEMPERATURE

260° C	500° F
240° C	460° F
220° C	430° F
200° C	390° F
180° C	360° F
160° C	320° F
140° C	280° F
120° C	250° F
100° C	210° F

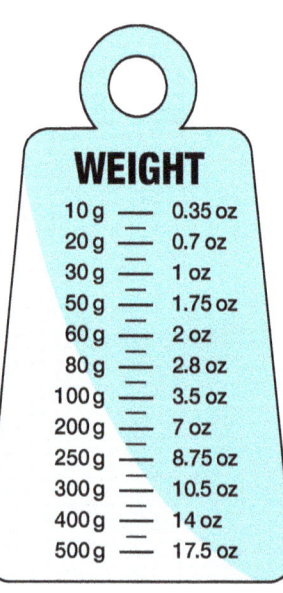

WEIGHT

10 g	0.35 oz
20 g	0.7 oz
30 g	1 oz
50 g	1.75 oz
60 g	2 oz
80 g	2.8 oz
100 g	3.5 oz
200 g	7 oz
250 g	8.75 oz
300 g	10.5 oz
400 g	14 oz
500 g	17.5 oz

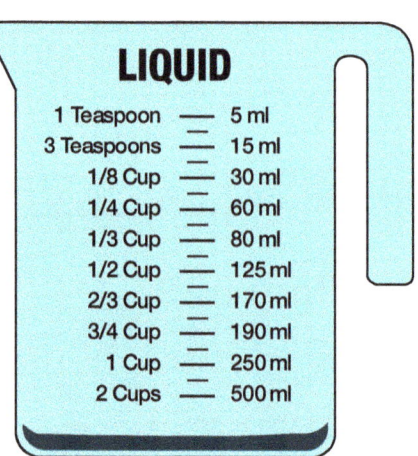

LIQUID

1 Teaspoon	5 ml
3 Teaspoons	15 ml
1/8 Cup	30 ml
1/4 Cup	60 ml
1/3 Cup	80 ml
1/2 Cup	125 ml
2/3 Cup	170 ml
3/4 Cup	190 ml
1 Cup	250 ml
2 Cups	500 ml

Breakfast

Think Bacon Frittata *168*

Brain Boost Breakfast Salad *168*

Lean Morning Soufflé *169*

Almond Pancakes *170*

Omega Quiche *170*

Salmon Eggs Benedict *171*

Creamy Coconut Smoothie *172*

Natasha's Lean Green Smoothie *172*

Orange Blast Smoothie *172*

Super Veg Smoothie *172*

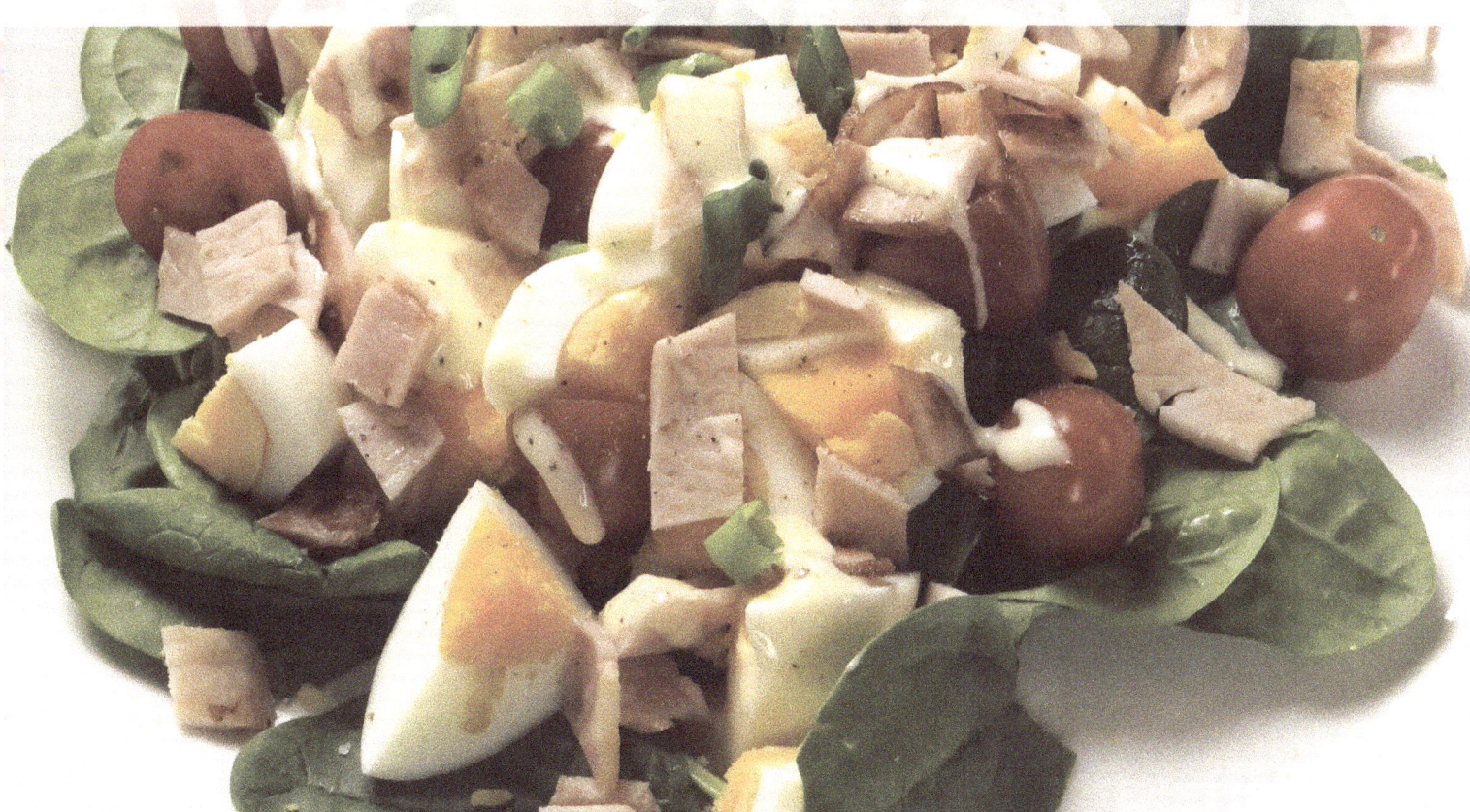

Think Bacon Frittata

Prep time: **10 mins** - Cook time: **25 mins** - Servings: **2 to 3**

This trusty Italian dish is great for using up leftover ingredients as you can put just about anything in them.

Ingredients: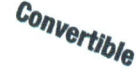

- 6 fresh eggs
- 100g bacon, diced (use short cut with fat removed for **Core ACM**, or leave fat on for **Complete ACM**)
- 2 tomatoes, sliced (200g)
- 1 zucchini, diced (150g)
- 50g Swiss cheese, grated
- 1 bunch chives, chopped (20g)
- ¼ teaspoon salt
- Pinch of pepper

Method:

1. Preheat the oven to 175° / 350°F
2. Combine all the ingredients except the tomato and 10g of cheese in a bowl and stir until mixed
3. Pour the mix into an oven-proof pan
4. Arrange the tomatoes on top and sprinkle the remaining cheese
5. Place in oven and bake for about 25 minutes or until golden brown

Serve with a crisp lettuce or simple salad and save some for breakfast the next day.

*Mix it up by using **Poached Chicken Thyme (page 180)** instead or ham instead of bacon, and try different vegetables as well.*

Brain Boost Breakfast Salad

Prep time: **5 mins** - Cook time: **15 mins** - Servings: **2**

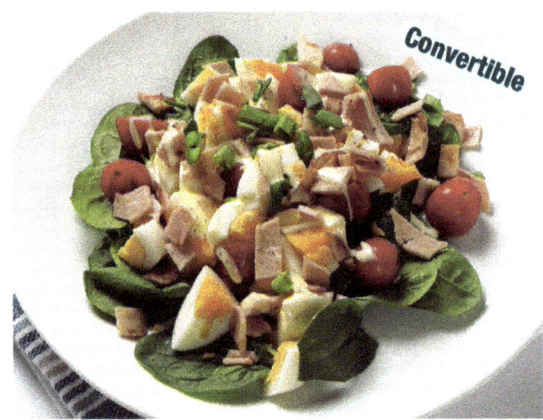

Ingredients:

- 6 fresh eggs
- 100g bacon (use short cut with fat removed for **Core ACM**, or leave fat on for **Complete ACM**)
- 60g sweet solanato or cherry tomatoes
- Two handfuls of spinach (about 60g)
- 1 tablespoon **Macadamia Mayonnaise (page 200)**
- ¼ teaspoon butter
- Pinch of salt and pepper
- Chives for garnish, chopped

Method:

1. Bring a saucepan of water to the boil and boil eggs for 10 minutes
2. In a skillet over medium-high heat, fry the bacon in butter
3. Cube the bacon and eggs and combine remaining ingredients to serve

If you are making this in larger quantities to take to work over a few days, do not add mayonnaise until the day you take it out and always use fresh mayonnaise. Also, take it easy on the mayo, as it is still calorie dense!

Lean Morning Soufflé

Prep time: **20 min** - Cook time: **8-15 mins** - Servings: **3 to 4**

A cheese soufflé is a great breakfast treat and can actually be made with all healthy ingredients! This recipe works for both Core and Complete ACM, and creates a lovely and fluffy soufflé that melts in your mouth!

Ingredients:

- 4 eggs, separated into yolks and whites
- 30g butter
- ¼ cup coconut flour
- 1 ¼ cup milk
- 50g cheddar cheese, grated
- ¼ teaspoon salt
- ¼ teaspoon pepper
- ¼ teaspoon oregano

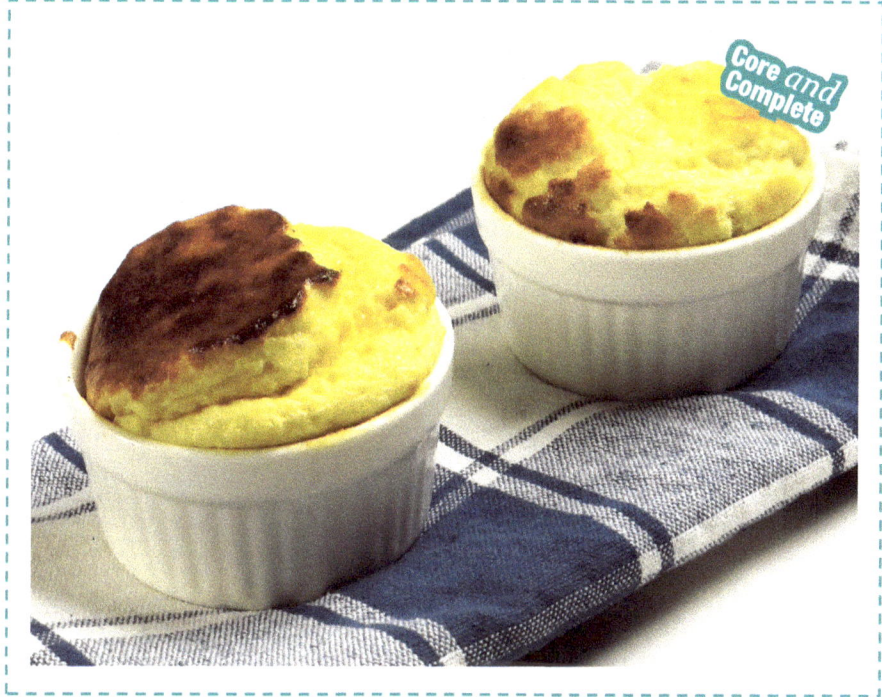

Method:

1. Preheat the oven to 200° / 390°F along with a baking tray
2. Rub the inside of 4 ramekins with butter and dust the buttered areas with coconut flour
3. Over medium heat, melt the butter in a saucepan and then add the flour. Mix until thick
4. Remove from heat and add half the milk. Stir until mixed, then add the rest of the milk over heat for about 10 minutes until boiling and starting to thicken
5. Remove from heat, add the cheese, spices and egg yolks. Stir until even, then set the saucepan aside
6. Use a mixer to whip the egg whites in a bowl until soft peaks form
7. Put ¼ of the whipped egg whites into the saucepan and fold into the mix
8. Add in the rest of the egg whites and mix. Pour equal amounts into three or four ramekins
9. Put ramekins on the hot baking tray and bake for 10 minutes until golden brown and risen

Serve with a crunchy salad with cos or rocket lettuce, crushed almond and a few pear slices. The cheese, egg and milk in them make them very filling, so you won't have trouble feeling full after one of those and a salad side dish!

Almond Pancakes

Prep time: **7 mins** - Cook time: **15 mins** - Servings: **2 to 3**

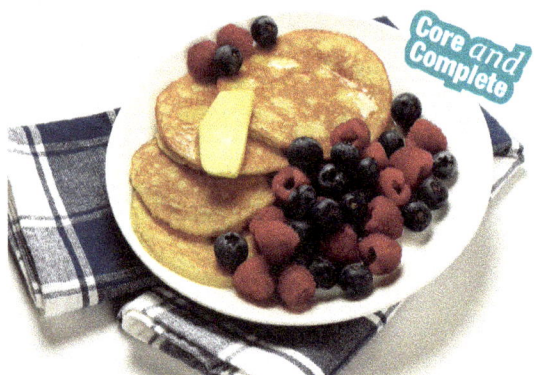

Ingredients:

- 1 cup almond flour
- 2 eggs (room temperature)
- ¼ cup water (sparkling water for extra fluffy pancakes)
- 1 tablespoon melted coconut oil
- ¼ teaspoon salt
- ¼ teaspoon butter
- ¼ teaspoon vanilla extract
- *Optional – 1 tablespoon sweetener (xylitol, erythritol, or equivalent stevia)*

Method:

1. Combine all the ingredients (except the butter) in a mixing bowl and blend
2. Bring a non-stick pan up to medium heat and pour pancakes that are slightly larger than your spatula (not much larger, otherwise the edges of the pancake will break)
3. Flip when bubbles form on the uncooked side, or after 3 minutes

Serve with butter and berries (as your one serving of fruit for the day), or sugar-free yoghurt. Add blueberries, raspberries, banana or lemon into the pancake mix for more variety.

Omega Quiche

Prep time: **10 mins** - Cook time: **35 mins** - Servings: **3 to 4**

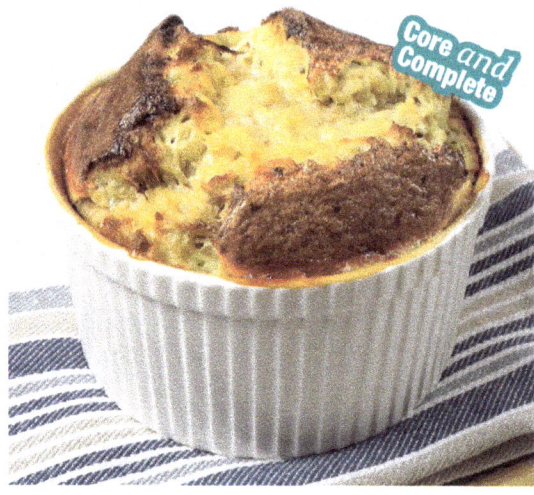

Ingredients:

- 4 fresh eggs
- 200g smoked salmon, shredded (or canned salmon or tuna in brine)
- 50g cheddar cheese, grated
- 10g parmesan cheese
- 1 cup coconut cream
- 1/4 cup coconut flour
- 1/4 brown onion, chopped
- 1/2 teaspoon salt
- Pinch of pepper

Method:

1. Preheat the oven to 170° / 340°F
2. Lightly beat the eggs in a bowl
3. Mix the salmon, cheeses, flour, onion and salt in the bowl and mix until evenly coated
4. Heat the coconut cream on low heat in a saucepan for 2 minutes and mix into the other ingredients
5. Pour mix into three medium or four smaller ramekins
6. Bake in oven for 30 minutes or until golden brown (longer for larger ramekin)

Salmon Eggs Benedict

Prep time: **5 mins** - Cook time: **10 mins** - Servings: **2**

What better than a great comfort dish like eggs benedict to treat yourself with after a long week? This is a tasty and healthy way to get some quality protein and omega 3!

Ingredients:

- 4 fresh eggs (fresher eggs stay together better when poaching)
- 1 tablespoon white vinegar
- 100g smoked salmon
- 2 handfuls of lettuce
- Pinch of chives, chopped
- **Today's Hollandaise Sauce (page 200)**

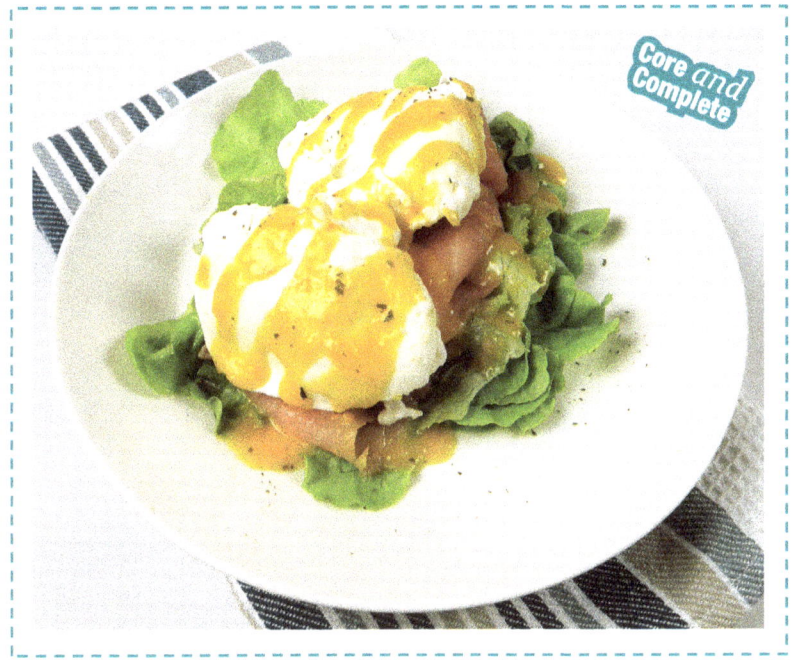

Method:

1. Boil a large saucepan of water and vinegar. Turn down to a gentle simmer
2. Crack the eggs into separate small bowls or ramekins
3. Stir the simmering water to form a vortex and gently slip in an egg from the ramekin into the middle of the vortex
4. Move the first egg to the side and repeat step 3 for another egg
5. Cook each eggs for 4 minutes for a runny yolk, or 6 minutes for a more solid yolk
6. Remove the two eggs and cook the next two using steps 3 and 4
7. Place salmon on a bed of lettuce, place poached eggs on top and drizzle with Hollandaise sauce
8. Garnish with pinch of chives

Serve with grilled asparagus for an extra vegetable hit. Mix it up by replacing the salmon with bacon (keep fat on for **Complete ACM***, or remove fat for* **Core ACM***).*

Smoothies

Creamy Coconut Smoothie

Prep time: **5 mins** - Serving: **1**

Get some protein with your smoothies like this delicious and simple recipe.

Ingredients:

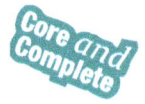

- 1 cup coconut cream
- 1 cup sliced mango
- ½ banana (together with mango as your one fruit serving for the day)
- 30g whey protein isolate powder (vanilla flavoured or flavourless)
- 4 ice cubes

Method:

1. Mix together and blend

Natasha's Lean Green Smoothie

Prep time: **8 mins** - Serving: **1**

Ingredients:

- ½ cup coconut water
- ½ cup almond milk (unsweetened)
- 1 to 2 handfuls of green leafy vegetables (kale, baby spinach, etc.)
- 1 pinch sunflower seeds
- 1 pinch pumpkin seeds
- 1 teaspoon LSA
- 1 teaspoon goji berries
- 1 teaspoon chia seeds
- 1 teaspoon maca powder
- *Optional – 1 banana (as your one fruit serving for the day)*

Method:

1. Mix together and blend

Orange Blast Smoothie

Prep time: **5 mins** - Serving: **1**

Ingredients:

- 1 cup coconut water
- 2 carrots (150g)
- 2 peaches (as your one fruit serving for the day)
- 30g whey protein isolate powder (vanilla flavoured or flavourless)
- 4 ice cubes

Method:

1. Mix together and blend

Super Veg Smoothie

Prep time: **5 mins** - Serving: **1**

Ingredients:

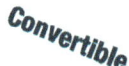

- 4 roma tomatoes
- ½ cucumber
- 1 stalk celery
- ½ beet (**Complete ACM** only, remove for **Core ACM**)
- 2 carrots (150g)
- Handful of romaine lettuce leaves
- ½ clove garlic

Method:

1. Mix together and blend

Mains

Sicilian Sage Lamb 174

Three Spice Chicken 175

Lemon Squeeze Salmon 176

Porto Burgers 177

Thai Beef Salad 177

Clean Baked Chicken 178

Three Keys Kebabs 179

Poached Chicken Thyme 180

Crusted Barramundi 181

Anytime Meatballs 182

Double Lemon Chicken 183

Lean Seafood Paella 184

Quick Steak 185

Protein Punch Chicken Salad 186

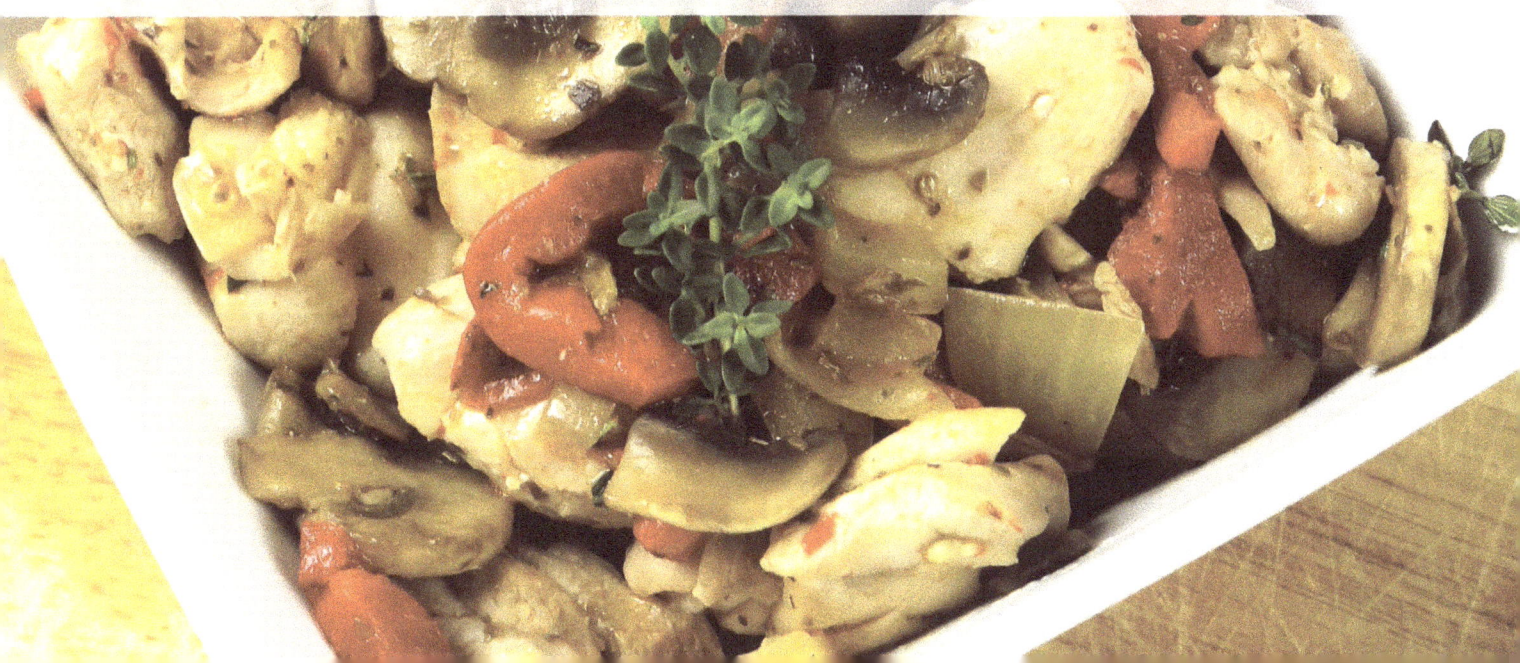

Sicilian Sage Lamb

Prep time: **5 min** - Cook time: **6 mins** - Servings: **2 to 3**

This is one of those meals where it can be hard to believe you can eat something so delicious while on a diet! The Sicilians have been eating spinach for over a thousand years, and it's easy to see why when you experience how the bed of spinach brings out the flavour of the lamb and sage! The Complete ACM version is a great post-workout meal to help you refuel, while the Core ACM version is perfect for any time.

Ingredients:

- 500g lamb steaks (lean cuts for **Core ACM**, regular cuts for **Complete ACM**)
- 4 handfuls spinach (about 100g)
- 6 fresh sage leaves, chopped
- ¼ teaspoon butter
- ½ teaspoon salt flakes
- **Vaudeville Roast Veggies (page 189)**

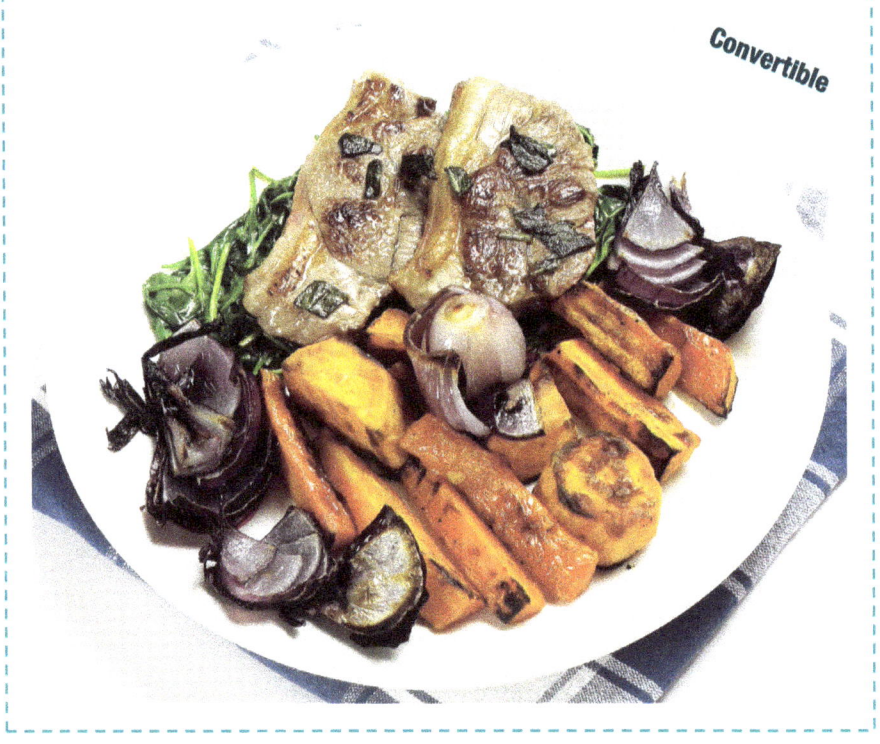

Method:

1. Bring a pan up to high heat
2. As it heats up, lightly sauté the spinach and set on plate for lamb to rest on
3. When the pan is hot, melt butter, lay down the chopped sage leaves and put the lamb steaks on top of that and season with salt
4. For a 2.5 cm (1 inch) thick steak, grill for 2.5 minutes for medium rare. Another 30 seconds each side for well done
5. Turn and grill another 2.5 minutes for medium rare (only turn once!) and season with the rest of the salt
6. Remove from heat and let sit for 2 minutes to drain remaining blood

Serve over spinach with **Vaudeville Roast Veggies (page 189)**. *For the Core ACM version, remember to change the sweet potato from the roast veggies to something like zucchini, or another veg that is on the Core ACM food list.*

Three Spice Chicken

Prep time: **10 mins** - Cook time: **20 mins** - Servings: **2 to 3**

This quick and easy dish is one of my favourites. The spices and mushroom create a fantastic aroma while the roast capsicum adds an extra kick of flavour. Eat one serving for dinner and take the other half to work the next day for lunch.

Ingredients:

- 500g chicken, strips (breast for **Core ACM**, thigh for **Complete ACM**)
- 500g mushrooms, sliced
- 200g roasted capsicum, sliced into thin strips (if you buy pre-roasted, make sure it has no added sugars)
- ½ brown onion, chopped
- ½ teaspoon butter
- ½ teaspoon fresh rosemary, chopped
- ½ teaspoon fresh thyme, chopped
- ½ teaspoon oregano
- ½ teaspoon salt flakes

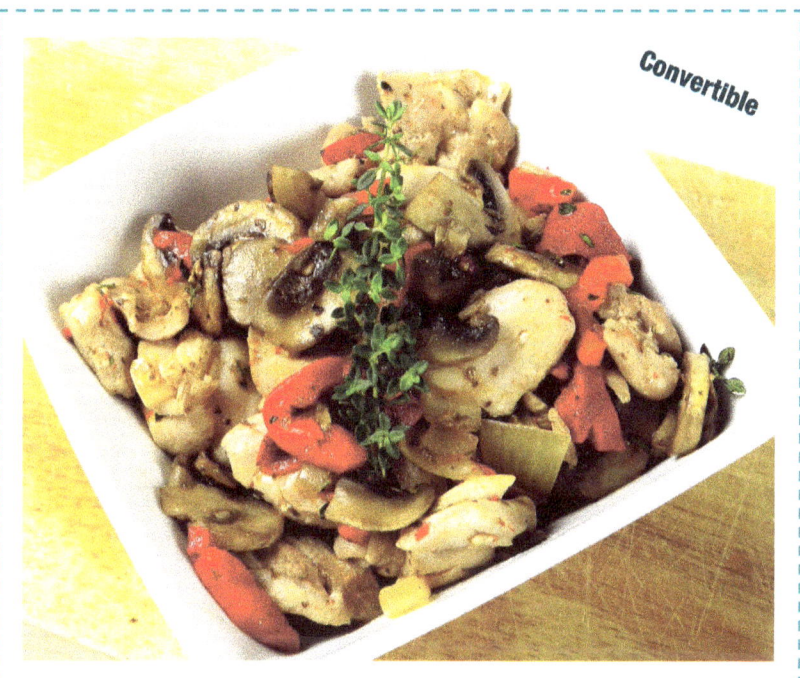

Method:

1. Bring a wok and a skillet up to high heat
2. Add ½ teaspoon butter to the wok and sauté the capsicum and onion
3. Add ½ teaspoon butter to the skillet and brown the chicken
4. After 7 – 10 minutes or when the onion is transparent, add the mushrooms to the wok
5. When the mushrooms are cooked and chicken is brown, use a slotted spoon to add the chicken into the wok
6. Add the salt and spices and cook for another 5 minutes until the chicken is coated by the other ingredients

*Serve on its own or with **ACM Cauli Rice (page 188)**.*

Lemon Squeeze Salmon

Prep time: **5 mins** - Cook time: **12-15 mins** - Servings: **2**

Grilling salmon on a stove is easy, but baking it can be even easier with less clean up! This simple recipe is quick and extremely versatile – swap any herbs or spices with your favourites. What's great about it is that once served, everyone can squeeze out more lemon juice from the slices on top to suit their own tastes.

Ingredients:

- 300g salmon fillets with skin
- 1 teaspoon fresh lemon juice
- 1 lemon, sliced
- ½ teaspoon salt flakes
- ¼ teaspoon rosemary
- ¼ teaspoon dill
- ¼ teaspoon butter

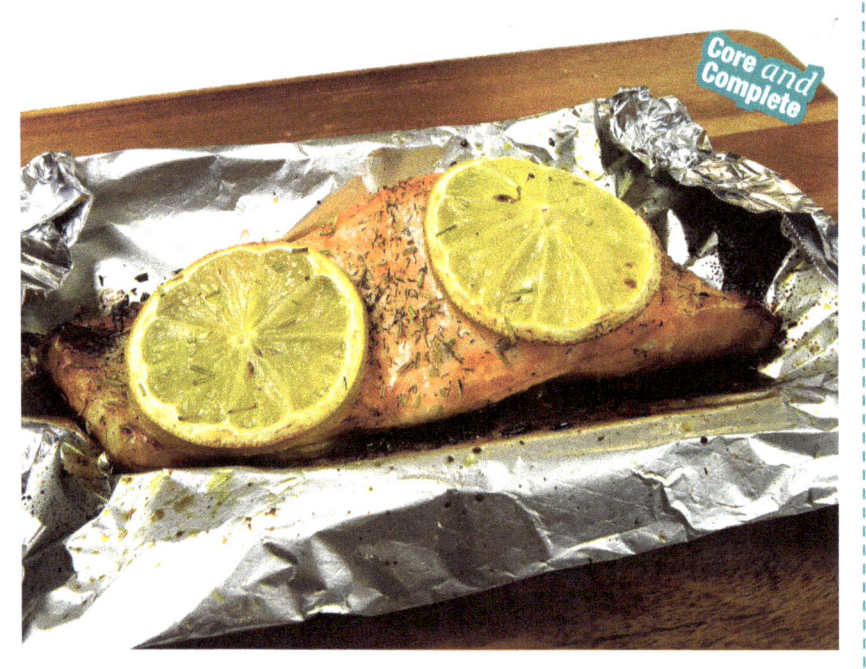

Method:

1. Preheat the oven to 230° / 450°F
2. Fold foil into a 'bath' for the salmon to lie in (this helps to minimise clean up afterwards)
3. Run hands over the salmon to check for bones and remove if necessary
4. Rub the spots where the salmon will lie with butter
5. Place salmon skin down on top of the buttered spots
6. Pour lemon juice over the salmon fillets, and top with rosemary, salt and dill
7. Put two slices of lemon on top
8. Put in middle of oven with top exposed and bake for 12-15 minutes

Serve with **Lean Zucchini Salad (page 188)** *or grilled asparagus.*

Leaving the top of the salmon exposed creates a lovely brown and crisp exterior. Mix it up by adding broccoli, zucchini and carrots below the salmon and wrap in baking paper to create Salmon en Papillote.

Porto Burgers

Prep time: **5 mins** - Cook time: **15 mins** - Serving: **1**

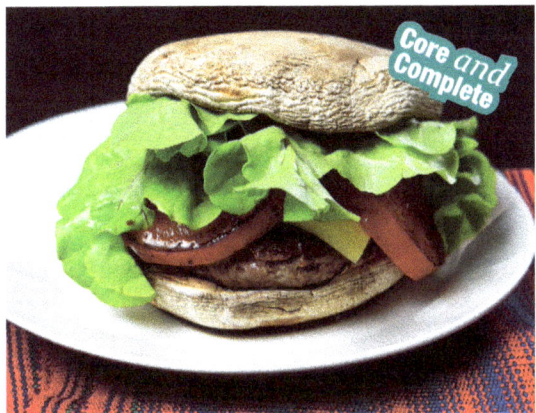

Ingredients:

- 2 large Portobello mushrooms
- 100g lean mince
- 1 tomato, sliced
- 2 lettuce leaves
- 1 cheddar cheese, sliced
- ¼ teaspoon butter
- Pinch of salt
- Pinch of thyme

Method:

1. Pre-heat the oven to 175° / 350°F
2. Bring a skillet to medium-high heat
3. Place mushrooms stem side up on a baking tray with foil and cook for 12 minutes in the oven
4. Mix salt and thyme into mince and press into a flat patty about as large as the mushrooms
5. Cook patty until no pink remains
6. Lightly sauté two or three tomato slices
7. Take mushrooms out of oven and place stem side down on a drip tray for 5 minutes to dry
8. Combine all ingredients into a burger

Serve with **Complete Sweet Fries (page 195 Complete ACM** *only) or steam vegetables (for both* **Core ACM** *and* **Complete ACM***).*

Thai Beef Salad

Prep time: **5 mins** - Cook time: **15 mins** - Servings: **2**

This salad turns a traditional high-sugar Thai meal into a healthy dish that supports you getting a lean body and healthy mind. Simple changes are all it takes!

Ingredients: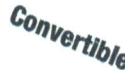

- 400g **Quick Steak (page 185)**
- 2 cups bean sprouts, chopped
- ½ cup mint leaves
- ½ cup cilantro leaves
- 2 green onions, chopped
- 1/4 teaspoon salt
- Pinch of pepper
- 8 large iceberg lettuce leaves to serve
- **Thai Chilli Sauce (page 202)**

Method:

1. Prepare the steaks and sauce as per respective recipes
2. Combined green onions, bean sprouts, mint and cilantro
3. Slice the steaks into thin strips
4. Add steaks to salad mix, top with sauce, salt and pepper, and toss lightly
5. Serve over iceberg lettuce leaves

Mix it up by using other meats, like lamb or chicken. Remember to use lean meats if you are on **Core ACM**.

Clean Baked Chicken

Prep time: **5 mins** - Cook time: **25 mins** – Servings: **2 to 3**

Ingredients:

- 500g chicken breast (both **Core ACM** and **Complete ACM**)
- 1 clove garlic, crushed and chopped
- ¼ teaspoon butter
- ¼ teaspoon rosemary
- 2 fresh rosemary sprigs
- ¼ teaspoon oregano
- ¼ teaspoon salt
- Pinch of pepper

Method:

1. Preheat the oven to 220° / 430°F
2. Line a baking tray with foil and rub the foil with half the butter
3. Sprinkle half the salt, pepper, oregano and rosemary on the butter where the chicken will sit
4. Splay the chicken breasts onto the foil and cover with the rest of the spices as well as the crushed garlic and rosemary sprigs
5. Bake for 25 minutes, or until juices run clear when cut
6. Bring a wok up to high heat

Serve with steamed veggies or with **Lean Zucchini Salad** *(page 188).*

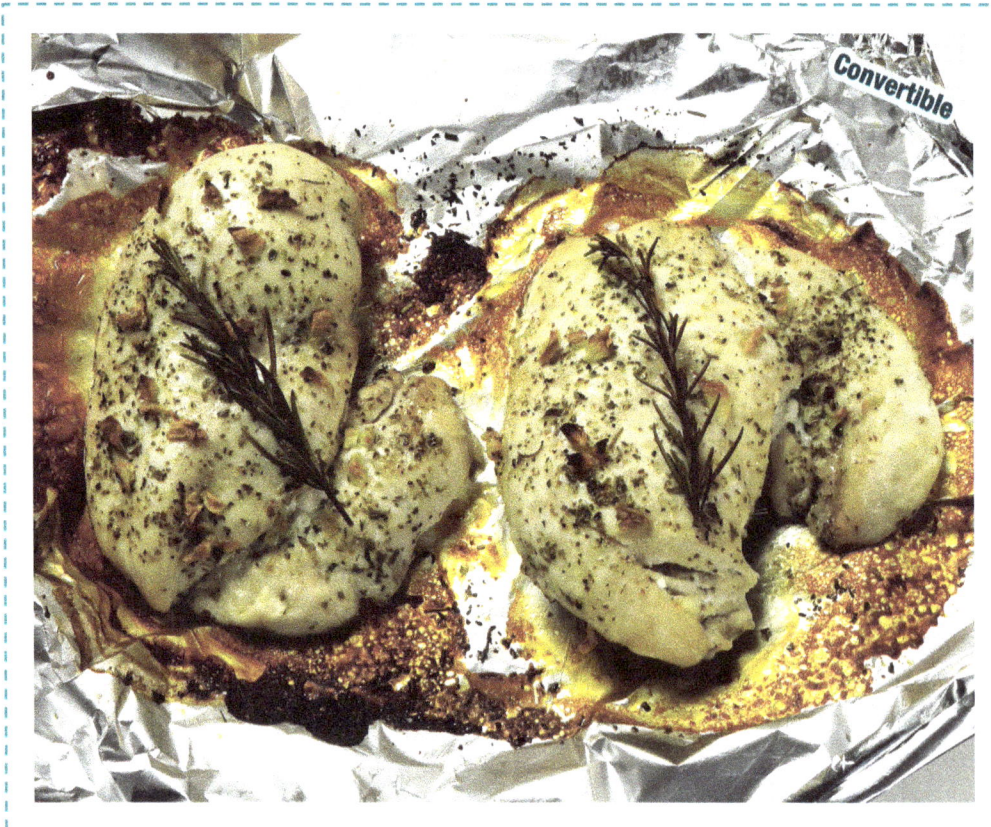

Three Keys Kebabs

Prep time: **10 mins** - Cook time: **16 mins** - Servings: **2 (4 to 6 kebabs)**

Kebabs are great over a grill or if you have a large enough frying pan, but even if you don't have those, you can make them in the oven as well! These are extremely versatile and you can mix and match meats and veggies – just make sure you stick to the ACM rule and food lists!

Ingredients:

- 500g beef, cubed (lean meat for **Core ACM**, ribeye for **Complete ACM**) Get the butcher to cube it for you to save some time
- 1 zucchini, sliced
- 1 yellow capsicum, large chunks
- 1 red capsicum, large chunks
- 1 red onion, large chunks
- **Lemon Vinegar Marinade (page 201)**

Method:

1. Marinade the cubed beef for at least an hour before baking
2. If you are using wooden skewers, soak them in water for an hour before using
3. Preheat the oven to 200° / 390°F
4. Thread the skewer through all the ingredients, producing 4 to 6 kebabs
5. Space evenly on a baking tray lined with aluminium foil
6. Put in upper rack of oven, bake for 8 minutes, turn, and bake another 8 minutes until brown

Serve with steamed veggies or salad.

Mix it up by using different meat, like lamb or chicken with your favourite marinade. If you are using lean meats for **Core ACM***, be careful not to overcook as it can become dry quickly.*

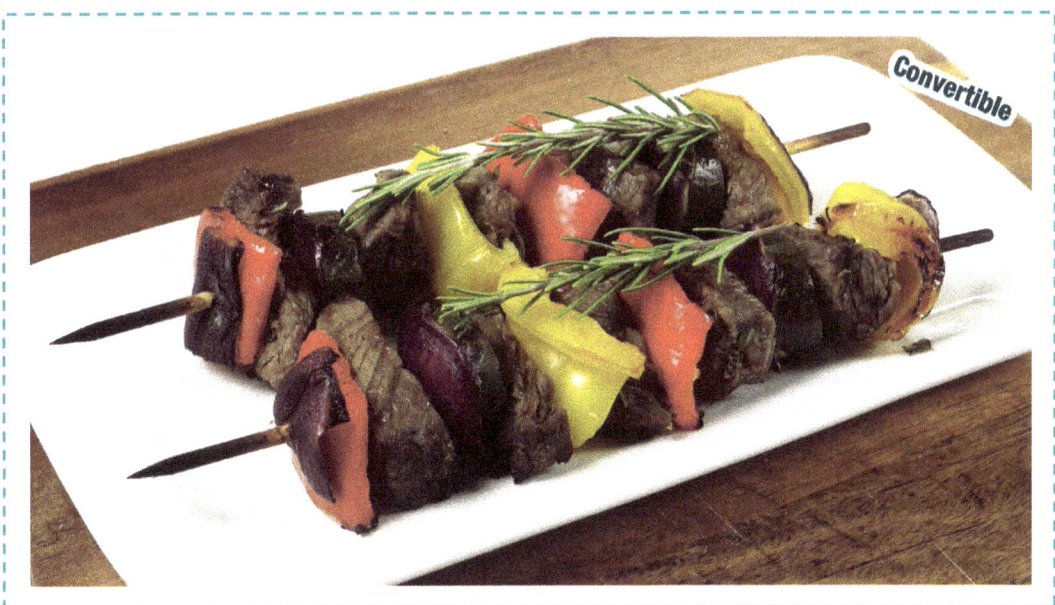

Poached Chicken Thyme

Prep time: **5 mins** - Cook time: **30 mins to 2 hours** - Servings: **2 to 3**

Definitely one of the easiest ways to cook chicken – poaching can produce melt-in-your-mouth results if you cook if for longer, or with shorter cooking times you can produce a firm chicken that is great for salads.

Ingredients:

- 500g chicken (breast for **Core ACM**, thigh for **Complete ACM**)
- 500ml chicken stock
- 250ml water
- 4 fresh thyme sprigs
- 1 teaspoon green onion, chopped

Method:

1. Add the water and chicken stock to a saucepan over medium to high heat
2. Add the chicken along with the herbs. Make sure the chicken is fully covered by the liquid
3. Bring to a boil, then reduce heat to a simmer and cover with a lid
4. Simmer until done
    a. Firm chicken breast – simmer for 30 minutes
    b. Soft chicken breast – simmer for 2 hours
    c. Firm chicken thigh – simmer for 20 minutes
    d. Soft chicken thigh – simmer for 1.5 hours
5. For longer cooking times, remove with a slotted spoon so that it doesn't fall apart

Serve with any vegetable mix or as part of a **Protein Punch Chicken Salad (page 186)**.

Mix it up by using different spices and herbs, or by using chicken on the bone. You can also cook turkey and duck this way as well. The longer you leave it in, the more melt-in-your-mouth it becomes, but be careful not to leave in too long, otherwise it will become a chicken soup!

Crusted Barramundi

Prep time: **15 mins** - Cook time: **15 mins** - Servings: **2**

This is a great dish for entertaining friends while still keeping it healthy! If you keep an eye on the oven, you can catch the spot where the macadamias just to make a nice brown crust on top, giving it that extra delicious look!

Ingredients:

- 4 barramundi fillets (or other white fish)
- 1/2 cup Macadamia Nuts
- 1/2 cup dried shredded coconut
- 1 tablespoon butter
- 1 tablespoon parsley, chopped
- 1 tablespoon chives, chopped
- 1 teaspoon fresh lemon juice
- 1/4 teaspoon salt
- Pinch of pepper

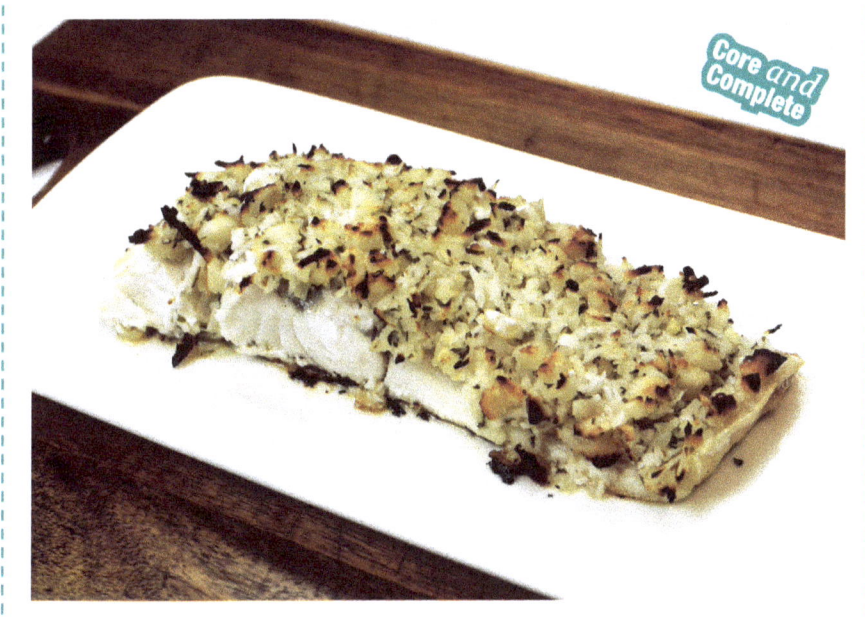

Method:

1. Preheat the oven to 180° / 360°F
2. Mix the macadamia, coconut, parsley, salt, pepper and lemon juice in a bowl
3. Line a baking tray with foil and rub with butter
4. Lay the barramundi fillets on the foil and scoop the seasoning mix evenly over the fillets
5. Bake for 15 minutes on the lowest tray until fish is cooked. If the nuts on top are not going brown after 12 minutes, move the tray up to the top element of the oven for the last 3 minutes

Serve with **Veggie Spaghetti (page 190)** or **Vaudeville Roast Veggies (page 189)**.

Anytime Meatballs

Prep time: **10 min** - Cook time: **15 mins** - Servings: **2 to 3**

Sometimes all it takes to turn a traditional recipe into something healthy that promotes weight loss and health, is a simple ingredient switch. In this traditional recipe, we replace olive oil with a smaller amount of coconut oil, while everything else stays the same to create juicy and flavourful healthy meatballs.

Ingredients:

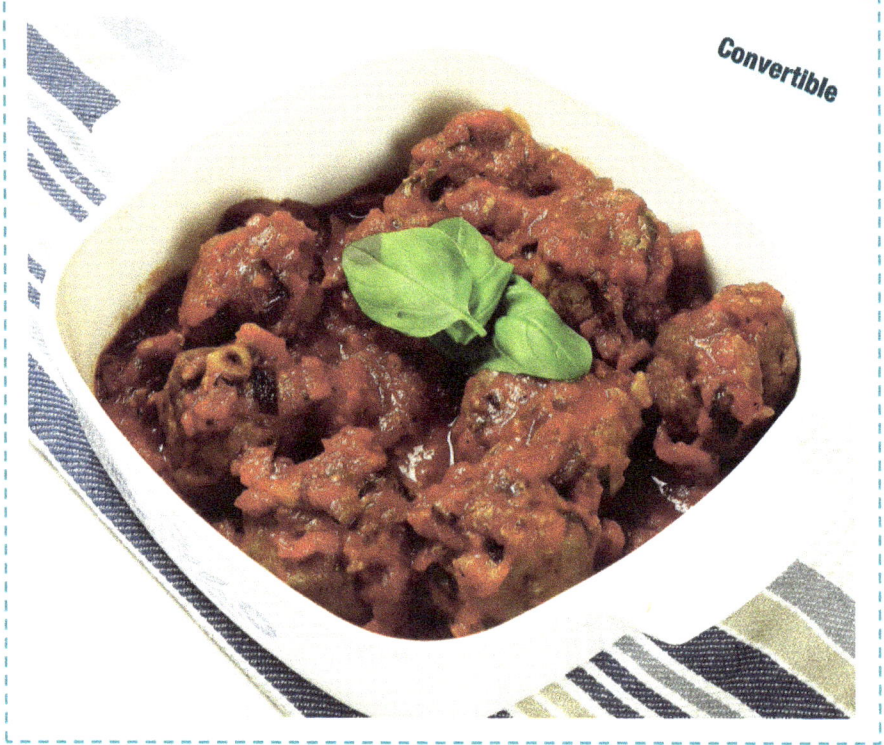

- 500g mince (lean mince for **Core ACM**, normal mince for **Complete ACM**)
- 2 tablespoons coconut oil
- 1 clove garlic, crushed and chopped
- ½ red onion, chopped
- 1 egg yolk
- ½ teaspoon salt
- **Italian Tomato Sauce (page 201)**

Method:

1. Preheat the oven to 175° / 350°F
2. Mix all the ingredients together with the mince
3. With the palms of your hands, separate and roll into about 9 or 10 golf sized balls
4. Place in an oven-proof container and bake for 10 minutes or until cooked through
5. Turn over meatballs, add Italian Tomato Sauce to container and bake with lid on for another 5 minutes

Serve with **Veggie Spaghetti** *(page 190).*

Mix it up by using different meats such as lamb or pork. Using lean beef can result in it drying out more quickly, so be careful not to overcook.

Double Lemon Chicken

Prep time: **5 mins** - Cook time: **10 mins** - Servings: **2 to 3**

This is my favourite kind of recipe – super fast, healthy and tasty! I often make one of these when I'm in a rush and need some leftovers for the next day. I usually eat it with steam vegetables, so within 15 mins, dinner is on the table!

Ingredients:

- 500g chicken (breast for **Core ACM**, thigh for **Complete ACM**)
- Zest from one lemon
- 1 teaspoon lemon juice
- ½ teaspoon salt
- ¼ teaspoon cracked pepper
- ½ teaspoon fresh thyme, chopped

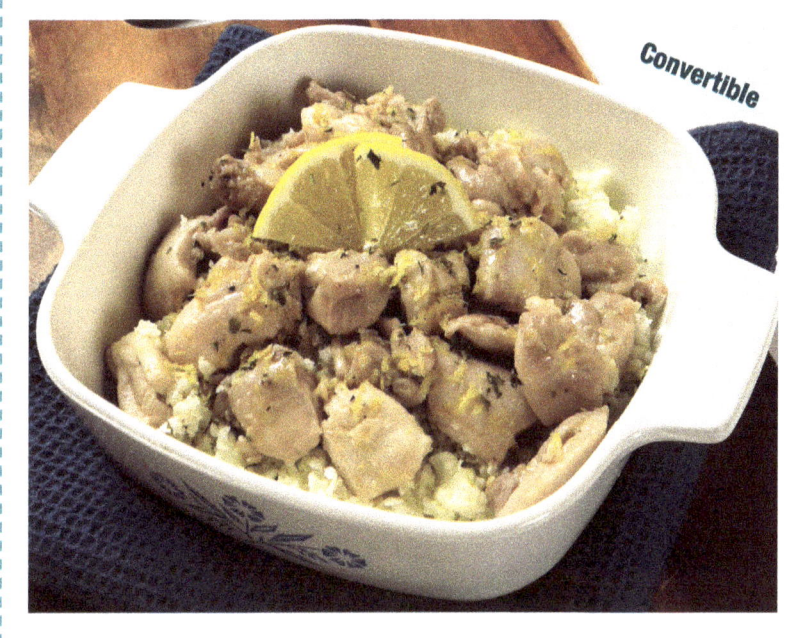

Method:

1. Bring a wok up to high heat
2. Slice the chicken into strips or chunks
3. Add ½ teaspoon butter to the skillet and brown the chicken
4. Add the lemon juice when the chicken is almost done cooking
5. While the chicken is cooking, zest one lemon and mix the salt, pepper and chopped thyme with the lemon zest
6. Spread the spices over the chicken when it is brown and mix until evenly spread
7. Scoop out chicken and serve. If there is any sauce left, let it stand until thick and pour over the served dish

*Serve with steam vegetables, or on a bed of **ACM Cauli Rice (page 188)**.*

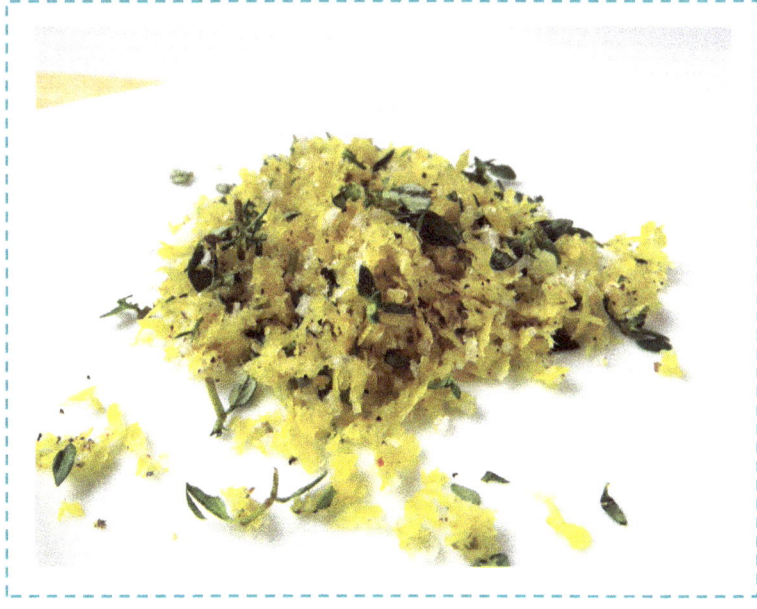

Lean Seafood Paella

Prep time: **30 mins** - Cook time: **30 mins** - Servings: **4 to 6**

A Spanish paella is a great weekend feast for the family. Traditional paella calls for a lot of rice and vegetable oil, so all we need to do is swap a few things around and you can still enjoy a hearty paella as before!

Ingredients:

- 400g fresh mussels
- 1 chicken breast, strips
- 200g scallops
- 200g large shrimp, peeled and deveined
- 1 head cauliflower
- 1 cup tomatoes, skinned and grated (or canned tomatoes)
- 1 cup chicken stock
- 1 large onion, chopped
- 2 tablespoons parsley leaves, chopped
- 3 tablespoons coconut oil
- 1/2 teaspoon bay leaf, crushed
- 1/2 teaspoon paprika
- 1/4 teaspoon salt
- Pinch of saffron threads
- Pinch of pepper
- 2 quartered lemons to serve

Method:

1. Grate the cauliflower to a rice-like consistency (see **ACM Cauli Rice** recipe for more detail on **page 188**)
2. Bring 1.5 cups of water to a boil in a saucepan with a lid. Turn down heat to a simmer, add the mussels and close the lid to steam. Steam for 4 to 5 minutes until mussels have opened. Remove from heat and set aside
3. Heat the coconut oil in a paella pan over medium to high heat in an outdoor grill with a closable lid. Wood or charcoal fires work best. Brown the chicken strips and season with salt and pepper. Remove the chicken from the pan and set aside
4. Add onion to the pan, close the grill and cook for about 5 minutes. Stir occasionally. Add the paprika, saffron and bay leaf. Cook for 30 seconds
5. Add the grated tomato, salt and pepper, and cook until starting to thicken. Add the chicken stock and cauliflower rice and stir until mixed. Flatten the cauliflower rice evenly around the pan
6. Drain chicken and mussels. Arrange the scallops, shrimp, chicken and mussels on the cauliflower rice. Close the grill and cook until shrimp is pink and cooked through

Quick Steak

Prep time: **1 min** - Cook time: **5 mins** - Servings: **2 to 3**

This steak is so simple that it really doesn't need a recipe. Why include it then? Simply because when I started eating properly many years ago, I did actually need a recipe to make something as basic as a steak! Also, I want to show that a lot of what I actually eat is extremely simple recipes like this one. It takes no time to make, is tasty and healthy!

Ingredients:

- 500g steaks (lean meats like sirloin or rump for **Core ACM**, fatty meats like ribeye, porterhouse or New York strip for **Complete ACM**)
- ¼ teaspoon butter
- ½ teaspoon salt flakes

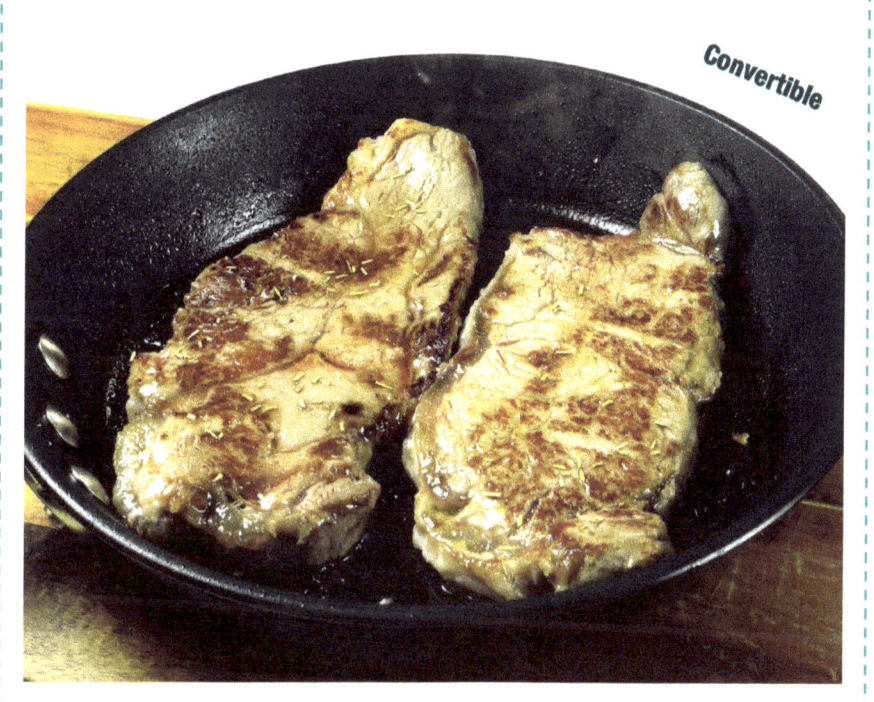

Method:

1. Bring a pan up to high heat. Just as it starts to smoke is a good indicator it is ready
2. Spread the butter over it when ready. It should make a nice sizzle and the butter should start to go brown after a few seconds
3. Lay the steaks down away from you (to avoid splashing) and spread salt over them
4. For a 2.5 cm (1 inch) thick steak, grill for 2.5 minutes for medium rare. Another 30 seconds each side for well done
5. Turn and grill another 2.5 minutes for medium rare (only turn once!) and season with salt
6. Remove from heat and let sit for 2 minutes to drain remaining blood. Serve while hot

Serve with **Vaudeville Roast Veggies (page 189)**, steamed veggies, or use to create a steak salad.

Mix it up by cooking different meats and using additional seasoning and marinades. You can use this same technique to cook salmon, lamb, pork, just about anything. This simple technique is ideal if you are new to cooking at home.

Protein Punch Chicken Salad

Prep time: **7 mins** - Cook time: **5 mins** - Servings: **2 to 3**

Ingredients:

- 500g **Clean Baked Chicken (page 178)**
- 2 handfuls of lettuce
- 2 eggs
- 50g cheddar cheese, cubed
- 100g cherry tomatoes, halved
- 100g bacon with fat cut off
- ¼ teaspoon butter

Method:

1. Fry bacon over medium-high heat with butter. Dice and add into mix
2. Hard boil eggs for 10 minutes in boiling water in a saucepan. Dice and add into mix
3. Cut chicken into bite-sized chunks
4. Combine all ingredients and serve

This salad can seem like a lot of work if you are making it on its own, but I tend to boil a lot of eggs each Sunday evening for the week, and then use leftover baked chicken and bacon from other dishes to throw this salad together.

As far as you can, try to avoid adding mayonnaise or other sauces as they tend to be calorie-dense. If you do use some, use it very sparingly, only to enhance the taste. If you notice weight loss slowing, try to cut out the sauces.

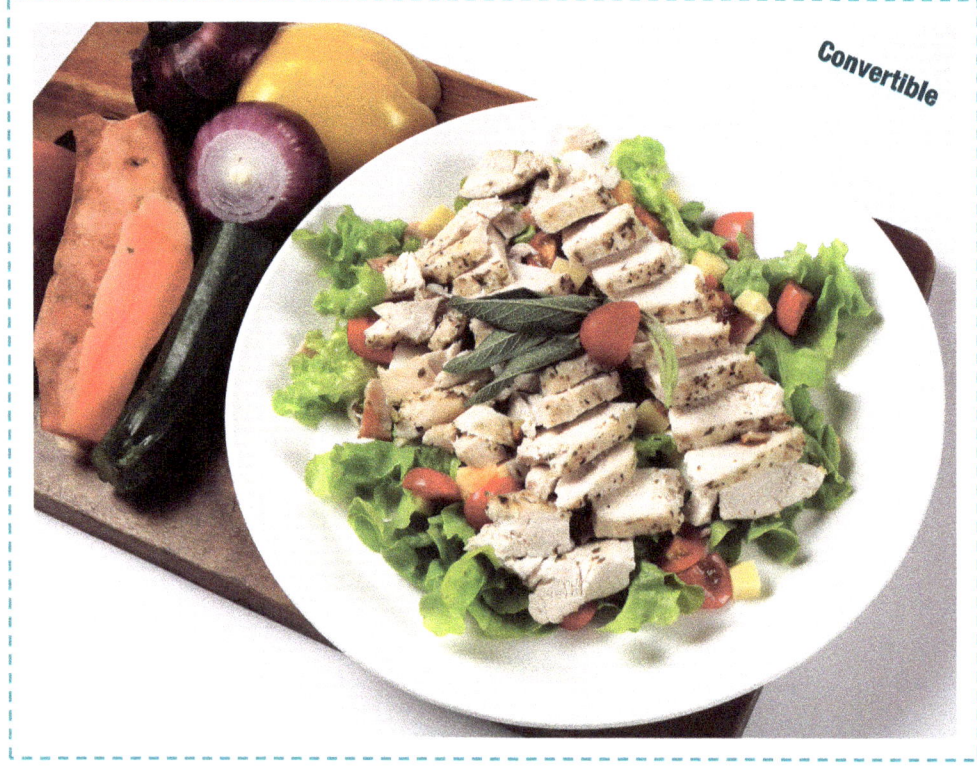

Side Dishes

Lean Zucchini Salad *188*

ACM Cauli Rice *188*

Vaudeville Roast Veggies *189*

Armenian Avo Salad *189*

Veggie Spaghetti *190*

Focus Fries *190*

Sugar Snap Veggies *191*

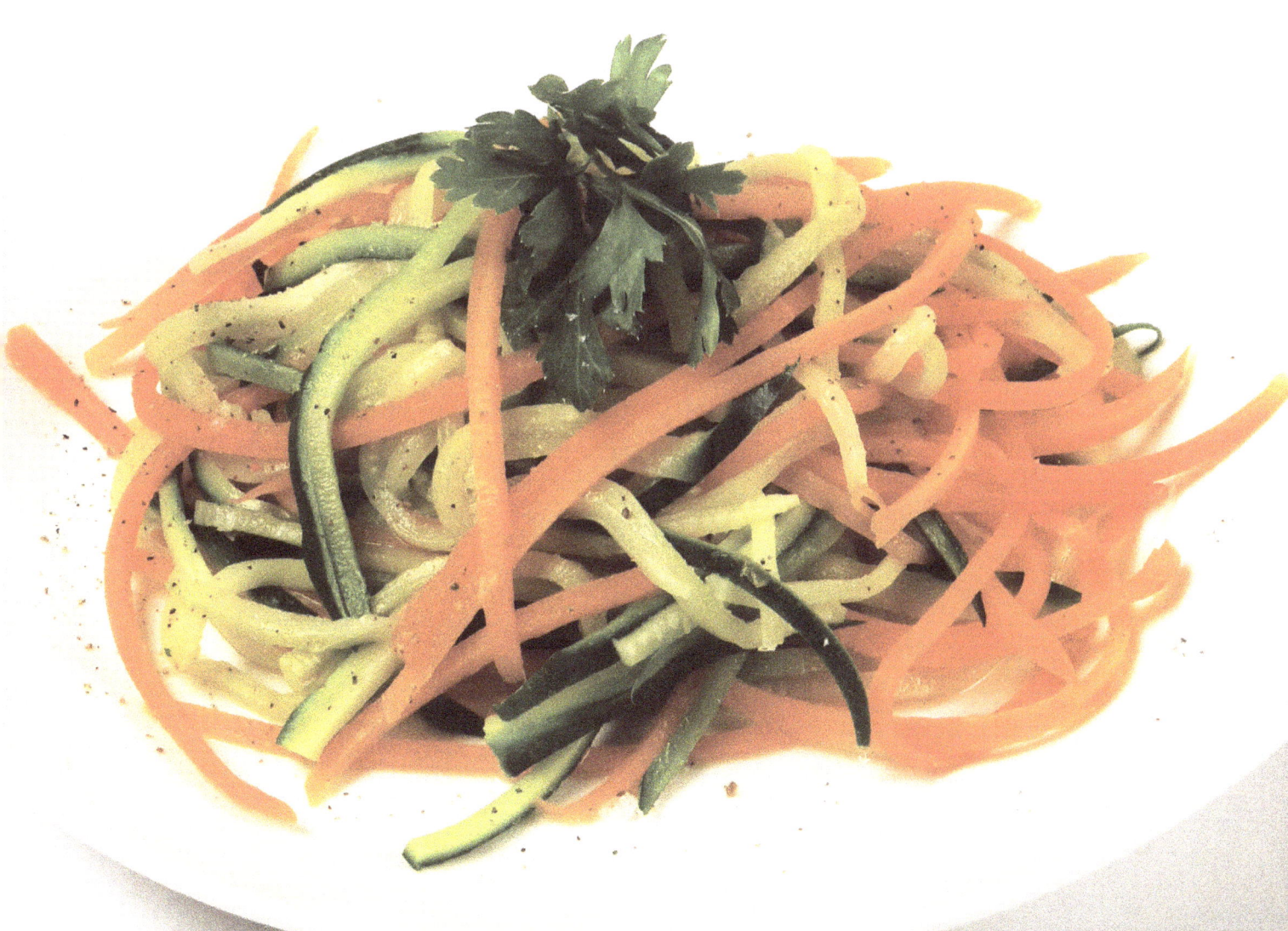

Lean Zucchini Salad

Prep time: **5 mins** - Cook time: **10 mins** - Servings: **2**

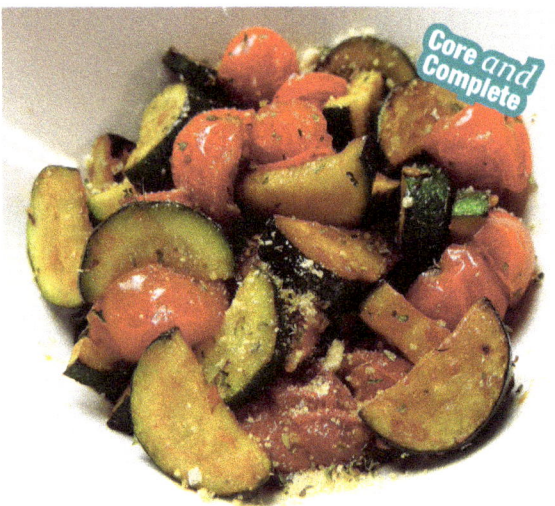

Ingredients:

- 2 zucchinis, sliced and halved (350g)
- 400g cherry tomatoes, halved
- 1 teaspoon parmesan cheese
- ¼ teaspoon butter
- ¼ teaspoon oregano
- ¼ teaspoon salt
- ¼ teaspoon parsley

Method:

1. Bring a wok up to medium-high heat and melt the butter
2. Add zucchini and cook for 5 minutes
3. With the zucchini soft, add the tomatoes and grill for another 2 minutes
4. Add oregano and salt
5. Remove from heat and serve garnished with parsley and parmesan

*Serve with **Lemon Squeeze Salmon (page 176)**.*

ACM Cauli Rice

Prep time: **5 mins** - Cook time: **4 mins** - Servings: **2**

This is a fantastic substitute for usual rice and is a great way to get in more veggies each day. Cauliflower doesn't have much flavour in general, so it really takes on the flavour of what you put on it very well!

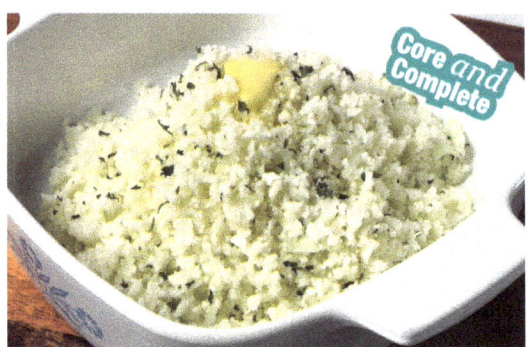

Ingredients:

- ½ head of cauliflower
- ¼ teaspoon parsley

Method:

1. Cut out the stems of the cauliflower until you have chunks that can fit into a food processor. Use the shredder blade to cut into size of rice
2. If you don't have a food processor, leave the stems in and use a grater to cut into rice size (don't grate the stems, it is for grip only)
3. Mix with parsley and cook in microwave for 4 minutes

*Serve with **Double Lemon Chicken (page 183)** or with any dish where you would have used rice in the past*

Mix it up with extra spices, like garlic salt, fresh chives, thyme, or any favourite herbs that you like!

Vaudeville Roast Veggies

Prep time: **5 mins** - Cook time: **20 mins** - Servings: **2 - 3**

The best part of these veggies is the red onions that takes on a sweet taste after roasting. Love these!

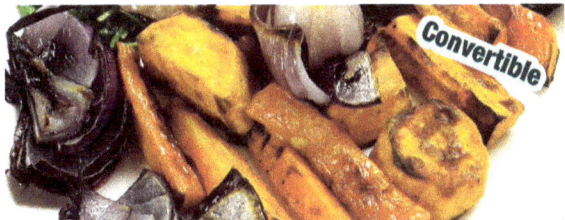

Ingredients:

- 2 red onions, quartered
- 2 large carrots, large chunks (300g)
- 200g sweet potato, cubed (for **Complete ACM** version or 350g zucchini for **Core ACM**)
- 2 tablespoons coconut oil
- ¼ teaspoon salt
- ¼ teaspoon pepper

Method:

1. Preheat oven to 220° / 430°F
2. Heat the coconut oil in a bowl in the microwave for about 30 seconds until melted
3. Add the salt and pepper to the oil and toss the vegetables in the oil
4. Lay vegetables on a baking foil lined tray
5. Roast for 8 minutes, turn and roast for another 8 minutes or until golden

Serve with **Sicilian Sage Lamb (page 174)**.

Mix it up by using your favourite vegetables. Remember to leave out the sweet potato if you are on **Core ACM**, *or leave out the zucchini if you are on* **Complete ACM**. *Though it is still amazing either way!*

Armenian Avo Salad

Prep time: **10 mins** - Servings: **2**

Get a taste of Armenia with its native almond trees with this versatile salad! It can be the base of many options depending on your goal. Whether you are on Core or Complete ACM, this salad is for you!

Ingredients:

- 1 avocado, peeled with stone removed, roughly chopped
- 1 English cucumbers, thinly sliced
- 2 handfuls of rocket lettuce or kale
- ½ cup mint leaves
- ½ cup almonds, chopped or crushed into slightly smaller pieces
- **Balanced Vinaigrette (page 202)**

Method:

1. Chop the lettuce or kale into bite-sized pieces
2. Place the vinaigrette at the bottom of the serving bowl
3. Put all the other ingredients on top. Toss lightly to coat evenly in the vinaigrette

Serve with **Lemon Squeeze Salmon (page 176)** or on its own as a snack. Mix it up by using different ingredients. Try one of these variations:

- *For super low calories, skip the vinaigrette*
- *For your fruit serving of the day, try adding some pomegranate or orange slices*
- *For a bit more crispy tang, add in some chopped red and yellow peppers*
- *For a healthy calorie boost, add in some crumbled feta and black olives*

Veggie Spaghetti

Prep time: **3 mins** - Cook time: **2 mins** - Servings: **2 to 3**

These are an excellent substitute for where you would have used spaghetti in the past. Plus, they take even less time to make than real spaghetti!

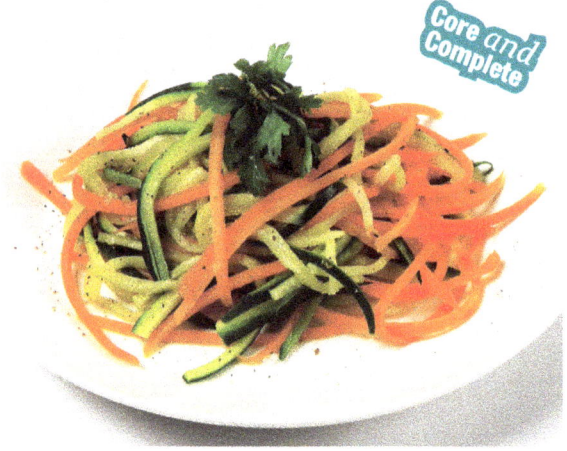

Ingredients:

- 2 large zucchinis (350g)
- 2 large carrots (300g)
- Pinch of salt
- Pinch of pepper

Method:

1. Bring a saucepan with water to a gentle boil
2. With a julienne slicer, cut the carrot and zucchini into thin, spaghetti-like strips
3. Add the carrot to the water first with salt and pepper, and boil for 1 minute
4. Add the zucchini and boil for another minute
5. Drain and rinse with cold water to preserve their texture

Serve with **Anytime Meatballs (page 182)**.

The thin strips are super juicy. Leave out any herbs and spices for a great, clean taste.

Focus Fries

Prep time: **6 mins** - Cook time: **20 mins** - Servings: **2**

Stay focused on your goals with this healthy anytime snack! These are tasty, healthy, easy to make, yet extremely low in calories, with a hit of protein to boot! Just overall the perfect side dish that also doubles as a snack for later.

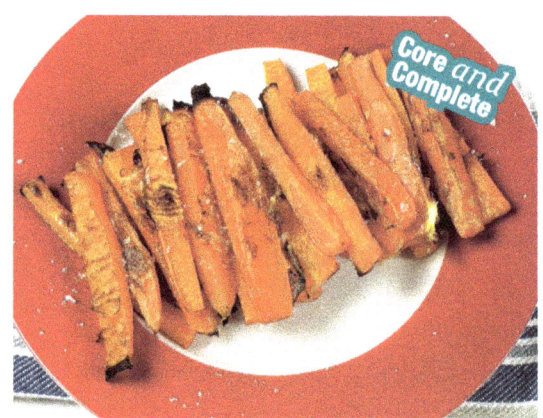

Ingredients:

- 2 large carrots (300g)
- 1 egg white
- Pinch of salt
- Pinch of pepper

Method:

1. Preheat the oven to 200° / 390°F
2. Cut the carrot into fries roughly 1cm thick
3. Put the egg in a bowl and toss the carrots to coat in egg white
4. Space the fries evenly on a baking tray lined with foil
5. Dust with salt flakes and pepper
6. Bake for 10 minutes, turn over and bake for another 10 minutes until lightly browned and fluffy

Sugar Snap Veggies

Prep time: **5 mins** - Cook time: **12 mins** - Servings: **2**

Baking vegetables with coconut oil brings out amazing flavours and aromas. This simple recipe is a sure way to get anyone to eat more healthy foods!

Ingredients:

- 300g sugar snap peas
- 1 zucchini (200g)
- 2 carrots (250g)
- 2 tablespoons coconut oil
- ¼ teaspoon salt
- ¼ teaspoon pepper

Method:

1. Preheat oven to 220° / 430°F
2. Top the sugar snap peas, cut the zucchini into thick strips and the carrot into thinner strips (this allows it to get ready along with the other ingredients)
3. Heat the coconut oil in a bowl for about 20 seconds on medium in microwave until melted
4. Toss the veggies in the coconut oil and spread on a baking tray lined with baking paper
5. Sprinkle salt and pepper and roast for 12 minutes until golden brown

Serve with slices **Quick Steak (page 185)***, or other meat dish.*

For best weight loss results, always try to use as little oil as possible. Even if the veggies look a little dry, it is just because the coconut oil seeps into them a bit and they will still taste fantastic!

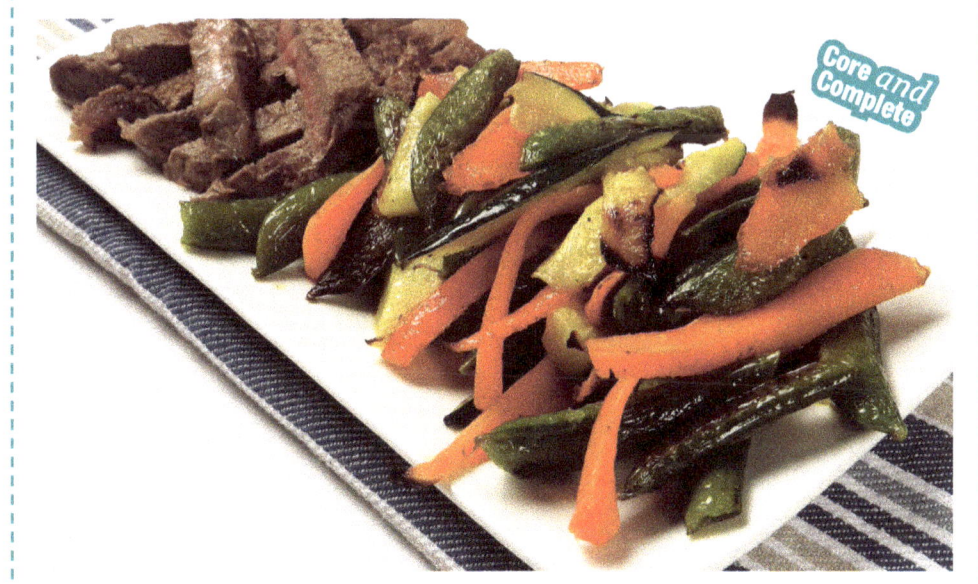

Snacks

Salmon & Camembert Bites 194

Bonus Breadsticks 194

Complete Sweet Fries 195

Lean Strawberry Soufflé 196

Simple Snack Ideas 197

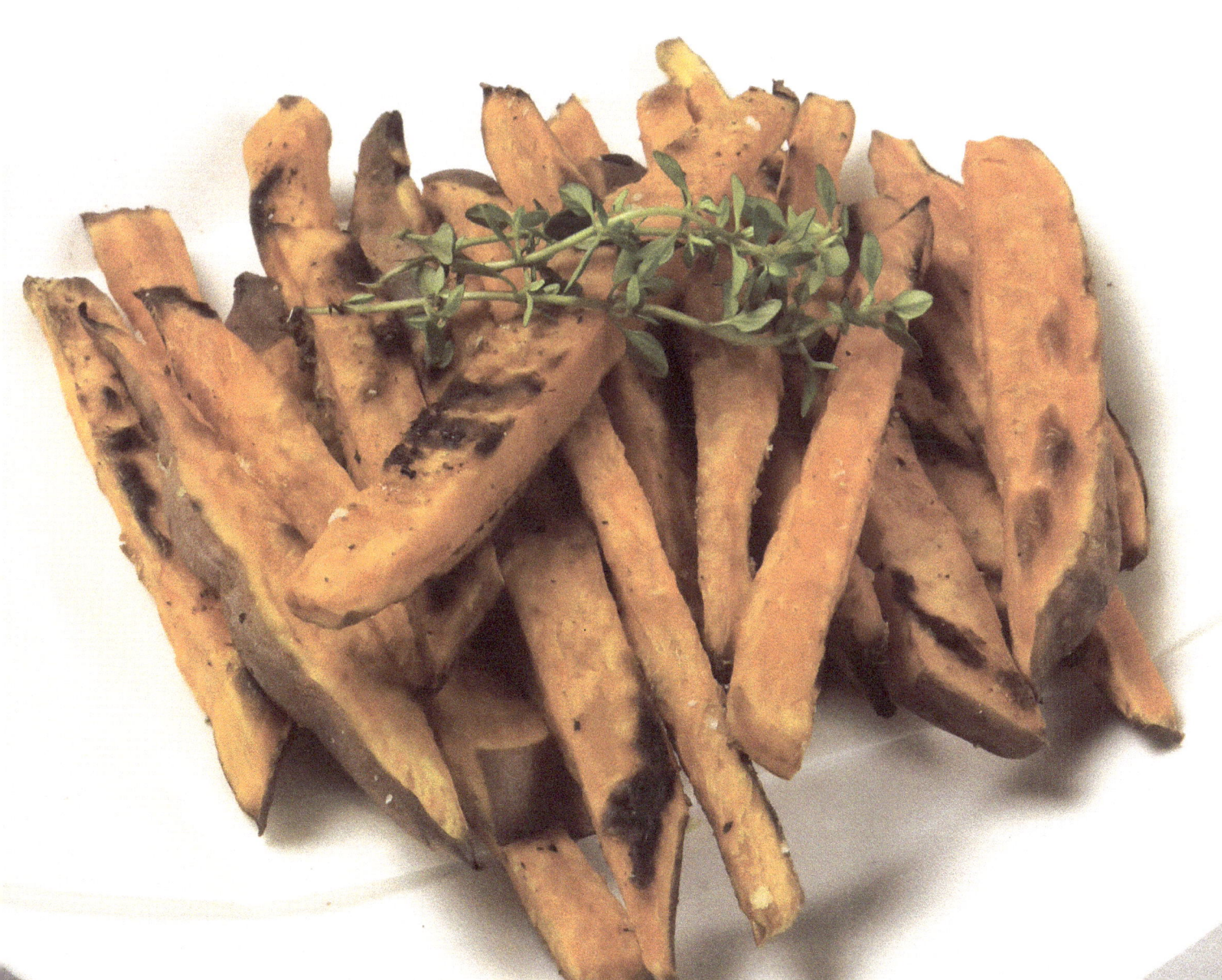

Salmon & Camembert Bites

Prep time: **5 mins** - Servings: **3**

Sometimes I make these when I need something really quick to eat, or they are great for guests as well. Cucumber is a healthy and clean substitute for crackers, so try these out next time!

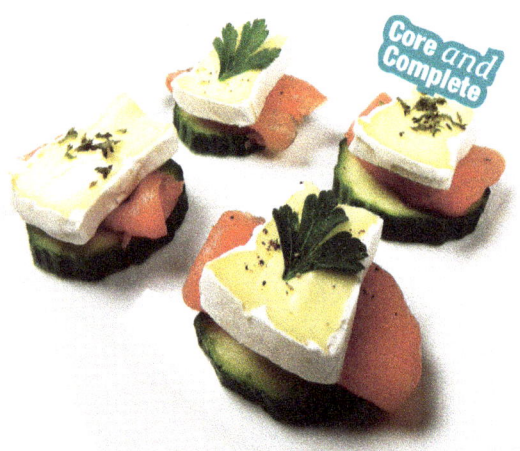

Ingredients:

- 1 English cucumber
- 150g smoked salmon
- 100g camembert cheese
- Small bunch fresh parsley
- Pinch of pepper
- Pinch of chives

Method:

1. Slice the cucumber and camembert in similar sized slices
2. Fold a piece of salmon, but on top of cucumber and place cheese on top
3. Garnish with fresh parsley and pepper, or with chives

Mix it up by using brie or other cheeses. Add some olives and avocado too!

Bonus Breadsticks

Prep time: **10 mins** - Cook time: **10 mins** - Servings: **2 to 4**

This snack is great for parties as finger food, or to keep for later as a snack between meals.

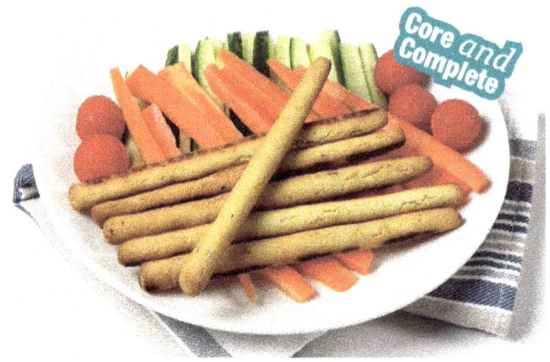

Ingredients:

- 1 cup almond flour
- 1 medium egg
- 1 tablespoon melted coconut oil
- Pinch of salt
- Pinch of garlic salt
- ¼ teaspoon parsley
- ¼ teaspoon baking soda

Method:

1. Preheat the oven to 170° / 340°F
2. Combine all the ingredients in a mixing bowl and mix by hand or with stand mixer on low until dough forms
3. Divide the dough into 6 to 8 even parts and roll into 20cm long sticks
4. Place evenly on a baking tray lined with baking paper
5. Bake for 5 minutes, turn, and bake for another 5 minutes

Serve with strips of carrot, cucumbers and cherry tomatoes for a great healthy option when entertaining guests.

Complete Sweet Fries

Prep time: **6 mins** - Cook time: **20 mins** - Servings: **2**

These fries are fantastically tasty, but don't eat more than 1 serving in a day as the combination of fat and starches can hold back weight loss. If you are exercising a lot, these are a great way to get a carbohydrate boost!

Ingredients:

- 400g sweet potato (**Complete ACM** only)
- 1 tablespoon coconut oil
- ½ teaspoon salt flakes
- ¼ teaspoon cracked pepper
- ¼ teaspoon cumin

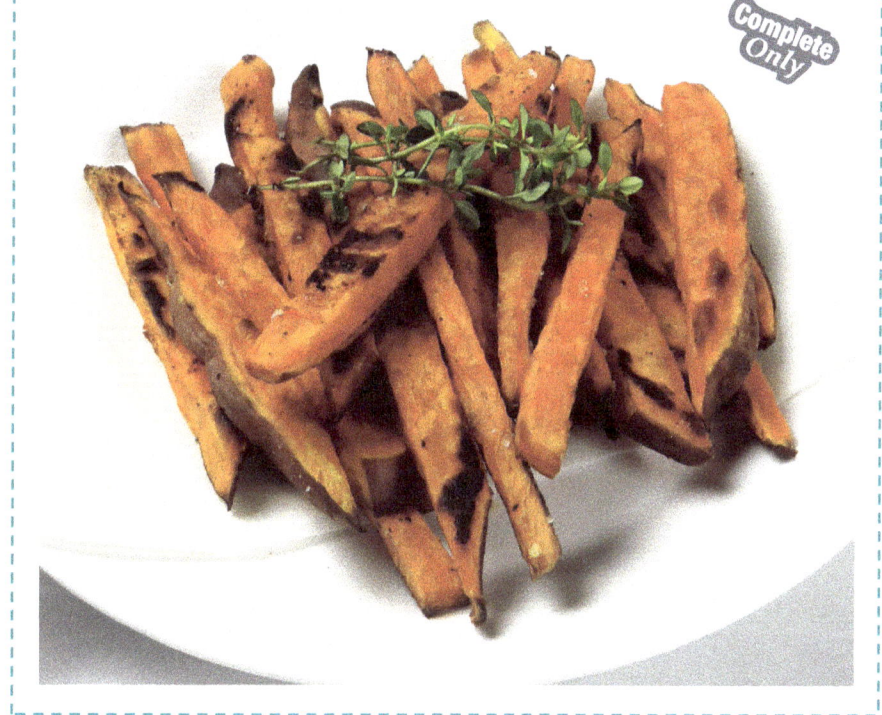

Method:

1. Preheat the oven to 200° / 390°F
2. Cut the sweet potato into fries roughly 1cm thick. Leave the skin on for extra fibre
3. Hold the coconut oil in your hands until melted, then rub the oil onto the fries
4. Space the fries evenly on a baking tray lined with baking powder
5. Dust with salt flakes, pepper and cumin
6. Bake for 10 minutes, turn over and bake for another 10 minutes until lightly browned and puffy

Serve as a side dish at parties or with **Porto Burgers** *(page 177).*

Lean Strawberry Soufflé

Prep time: **20 min** - Cook time: **8-15 mins** - Servings: **4**

I generally never eat dessert, but a traditional vanilla soufflé with strawberries is my absolute favourite. By swapping a few ingredients, this version tastes just as good as the original (although maybe slightly less photogenic). After all – why give up your favourite treat if you can just make it healthy instead?

Ingredients:

- 2 eggs, separated into yolks and whites
- 15g butter
- 10g coconut flour
- ½ cup milk
- ½ teaspoon vanilla extract
- 3 tablespoons sweetener (I find granulated xylitol works best)

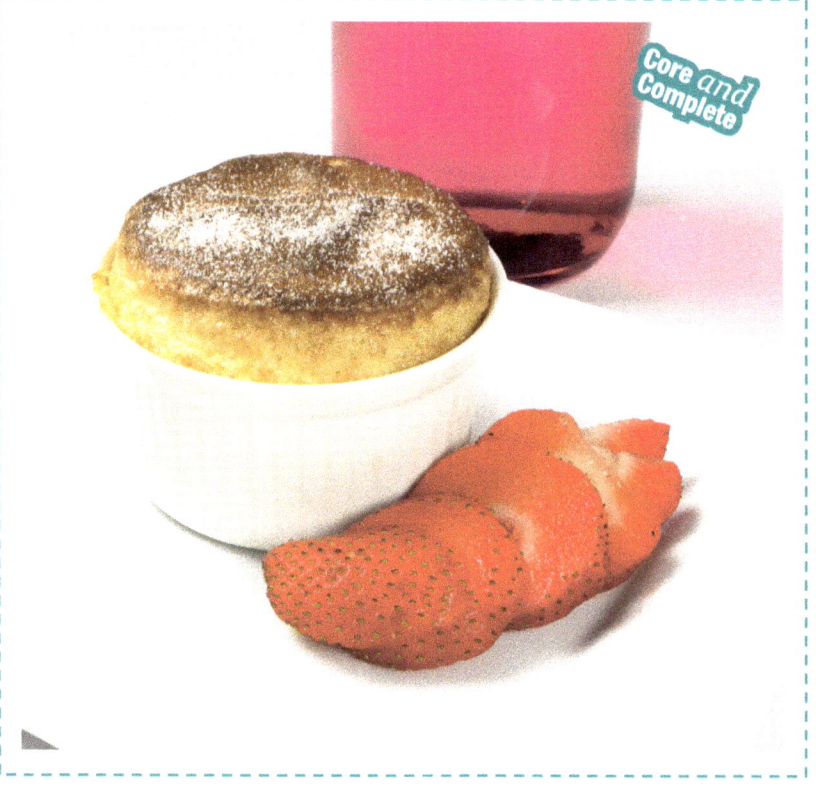

Method:

1. Preheat the oven to 180° / 360°F along with a baking tray inside
2. Rub the inside of 4 ramekins with butter in an upwards direction and dust the buttered areas sweetener
3. Heat the milk for 40 seconds in a microwave on high
4. Over medium heat, melt the butter in a saucepan and then add the flour. Mix until thick
5. Remove from heat and add half the milk. Stir until mixed, then add the rest of the milk over heat for about 10 minutes until boiling and starting to thicken
6. Remove from heat and add the vanilla extract and stir in the egg yolks one by one. Pour into a new bowl and set aside
7. Use a mixer to whip the egg whites in a separate bowl until soft peaks form
8. Put ¼ of the whipped egg whites into the other ingredients and fold into the mix
9. Add in the rest of the egg whites and mix until even. Pour equal amounts into the ramekins
10. Put ramekins on the hot baking tray and bake for 10 minutes until golden brown and risen

Serve with sliced strawberry and a bit of fine sweetener on top. Experiment with your oven to see what works best. I find with mine that only switching on the bottom element and putting the baking tray on the bottom works best.

Simple Snack Ideas

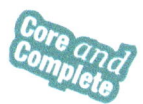

Who said snacks need to be hard? Sometimes we forget about the **really** simple snacks that are still healthy and support our body goals. These are simple snacks you can pack and leave in your bag for whenever.

Mixed Nuts

Prep time: **1 min** - Servings: **10**

Mixing nuts give you more taste variety and keeps in interesting. Use whichever nuts you like!

Ingredients:

- 250g cashews
- 250g macadamia nuts

Method:

1. Mix and put in ziplock bags for later

Veggie Sticks

Prep time: **3 mins** - Servings: **2 to 4**

Ingredients:

- 1 large carrot
- 2 celery sticks
- ½ cucumber

Method:

1. Cut all the ingredients into similar sized sticks and put in individual ziplock bags for later
2. Leave in fridge until the day you plan to use it

Egg Whites

Prep time: **1 min** - Cook time: **10 mins** - Servings: **4**

Ingredients:

- 6 fresh eggs
- ¼ teaspoon salt
- ¼ teaspoon pepper

Method:

1. Bring water to boil in a saucepan and boil eggs for 10 minutes
2. Let eggs cool, then peel, cut in quarters and remove yolks

Season with salt and pepper and put in 4 ziplock bags for later

Canned Tuna

Prep time: **1 min** - Serving: **1**

Keep close a few cans of flavoured tuna in brine as a healthy protein snack through the day!

Ingredients:

- Canned tuna or salmon (Only use fish kept in brine, as the oils used are unhealthy and too high in calories as well)

Method:

1. Not that you need instructions, but open and eat on its own or with some lettuce (no sauce for snacks!)

Sauces & Dips

Today's Hollandaise Sauce 200

Macadamia Mayonnaise 200

Lemon Vinegar Marinade 201

Italian Tomato Sauce 201

Thai Chilli Sauce 202

Balanced Vinaigrette 202

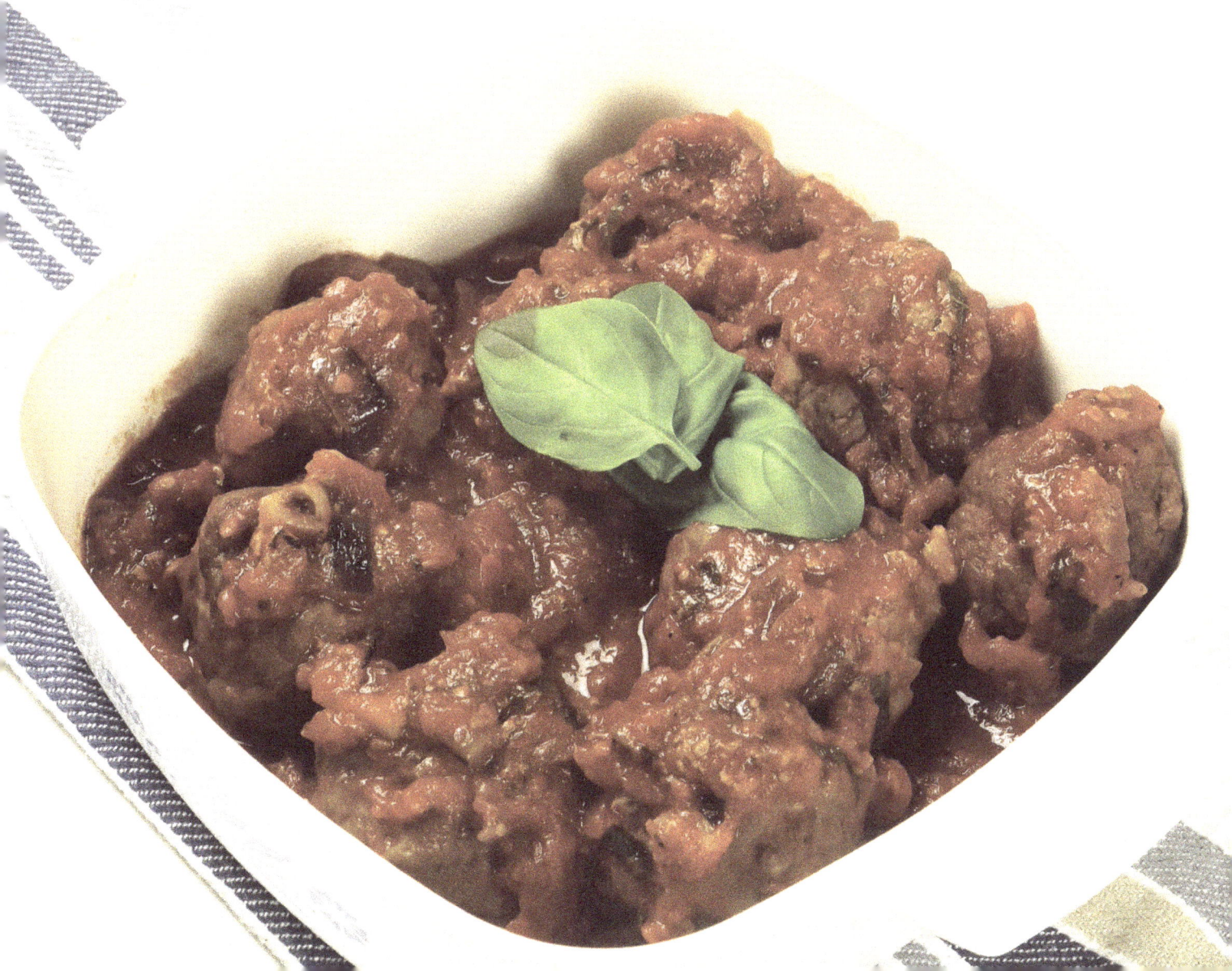

Today's Hollandaise Sauce

Prep time: **15 mins** - Servings: **2**

Homemade hollandaise is a great treat for a lazy Sunday breakfast, especially over eggs benedict. This coconut version is a fantastic twist on the traditional Hollandaise sauce.

Ingredients:

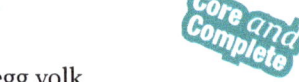

- 3 tablespoons coconut oil or butter
- 2 egg yolks
- 1 tablespoon white vinegar
- 1 tablespoon lemon juice
- ½ teaspoon salt
- Pinch of cayenne pepper

Method:

1. Bring a litre of water to the boil on in a saucepan and turn down to simmer
2. Melt the butter or coconut oil in a heat-proof bowl over the simmering water, then set aside
3. Put the egg yolks and vinegar in a heat-proof bowl
4. Whisk over the simmering water until the yolks start to cook and the mixture becomes stringy
5. Remove from heat and very slowly add the coconut oil or butter. Adding it slowly gives it time to emulsify and produces a more consistent sauce
6. Add in the salt and cayenne pepper

Serve over **Salmon Eggs Benedict (page 171)**, *over salmon or grilled asparagus.*

Macadamia Mayonnaise

Prep time: **10 mins** - Servings: **4**

Making mayonnaise at home can be tricky, but using this method is incredibly easy and is really fast as well!

Ingredients:

- 1 large egg yolk
- ¾ cup macadamia oil
- 1 teaspoon lemon juice
- ¼ teaspoon salt
- Pinch of cracked pepper

Method:

1. Put all the ingredients together in a glass jar that is around the same width as an immersion blender (this is the easiest way!)
2. Put all the ingredients together in the jar and wait for the egg yolk to settle in the bottom
3. Hold the immersion blender at the bottom of the jar and blend for about 30 seconds, then slowly move the blender up to catch all the oil and remaining ingredients
4. Blend until the mixture resembles mayonnaise

Serve with snacks or with **Brain Boost Breakfast Salad (page 168)**.

Mix it up by adding in different spices and fresh herbs.
*Note, as this contains raw egg, do not store for long and ensure that you sterilise the jar first. Keep refrigerated and use within a few days.

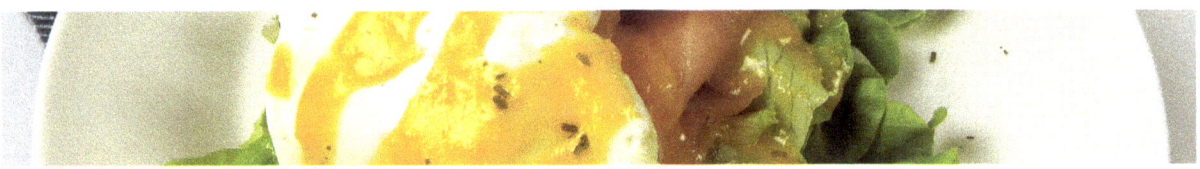

Lemon Vinegar Marinade

Prep time: **10 mins** - Marinade time: **1 hour**

This is a simple low calorie, fresh and sugar-free marinade with a great herb taste. Marinade overnight for extra flavour.

Ingredients:

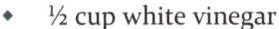

- ½ cup white vinegar
- 2 tablespoons fresh lemon juice
- 1 clove garlic, crushed and chopped
- 1 teaspoon fresh lemon thyme, chopped
- ½ teaspoon salt
- ¼ teaspoon pepper

Method:

1. Combine all ingredients in a mixing bowl
2. Mix meat into marinade and coat evenly
3. For overnight marinading, put all ingredients and meat into a bag and seal

Use with **Three Keys Kebabs (page 179)**, or other meats.

When making your own marinades, remember to stay away from olive oils and other plant oils (except coconut), as plant oils tend to be loaded with omega 6.

Italian Tomato Sauce

Prep time: **10 mins** - Cook time: **10 mins** – Servings: **2 to 3**

Tomato sauces are incredibly healthy while still being as tasty as always. With this recipe, you can make large batches of sauce to save for later.

Ingredients:

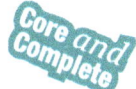

- 500g canned peeled tomatoes
- 1 teaspoon butter
- ½ red onion, finely chopped
- 1 garlic clove, crushed and chopped
- ½ teaspoon oregano
- ½ teaspoon salt
- ¼ teaspoon pepper

Method:

1. Melt the butter in a saucepan over medium heat
2. Sauté the onion with garlic in the saucepan
3. Remove the saucepan from heat to cool slightly, then add the canned tomatoes and pat back on heat
4. Bring to a simmer and break up the tomatoes with the sharp end of a spatula
5. Add oregano, salt and pepper, and simmer for about 7 minutes or until it becomes a thick sauce

Serve over **Anytime Meatballs (page 182)**.

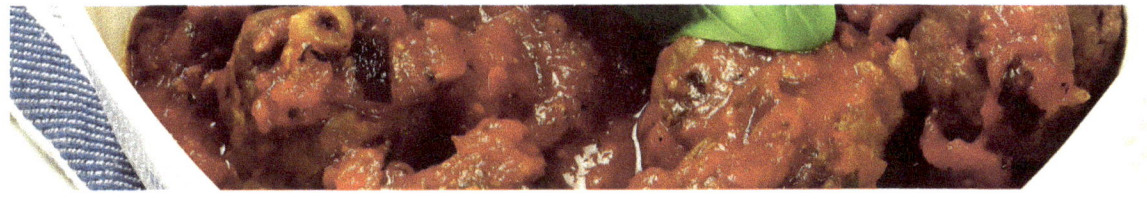

Thai Chilli Sauce

Prep time: **10 mins** – Marinade time: **1 hour**

The problem with Thai food is that it usually is loaded with sugar. After all, that is why it tastes so good! We can get around that with just a bit of sweetener.

Ingredients: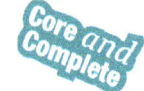

- 2 red chillies
- 5 cilantro roots
- 2 garlic cloves
- 10g fresh ginger
- 3 tablespoons fish sauce
- 3 tablespoons lime juice
- 1 heaped tablespoon sweetener (xylitol, erythritol, or equivalent stevia)

Method:

1. Chop all the ingredients into smaller pieces
2. Combine in a blender and blend until finely chopped with small pieces still visible

Use with **Thai Beef Salad (page 177)**, or other meats.

You can leave out the sweetener if you don't want to use any, though do not substitute for honey or another form of 'natural' sugar.

Balanced Vinaigrette

Prep time: **2 mins** - Servings: **2 to 3**

Most vinaigrettes are made with olive oil which have far too much omega-6. This version has balances omega-3 to omega-6 to keep your levels balanced, while still tasting great!

Ingredients: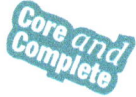

- 2 tablespoon macadamia oil
- 1 tablespoon white wine vinegar
- Pinch of salt
- Pinch of pepper

Method:

1. Put all the ingredients together in a bowl
2. Whisk together with a balloon whisk for about 30 seconds to 1 minute until it starts to emulsify

Serve over **Armenian Avo Salad (page 189)** or any other salad.

Mix it up with one of these variations:

- *Try apple cider vinegar instead of white wine vinegar*
- *Add a teaspoon of wholegrain mustard*
- *Or add a teaspoon of fresh finely chopped red onion and ¼ teaspoon finely chopped garlic*
- *Replace the vinegar with lemon juice and add a teaspoon lemon zest for a lemon vinaigrette*

Keep experimenting!

Appendices

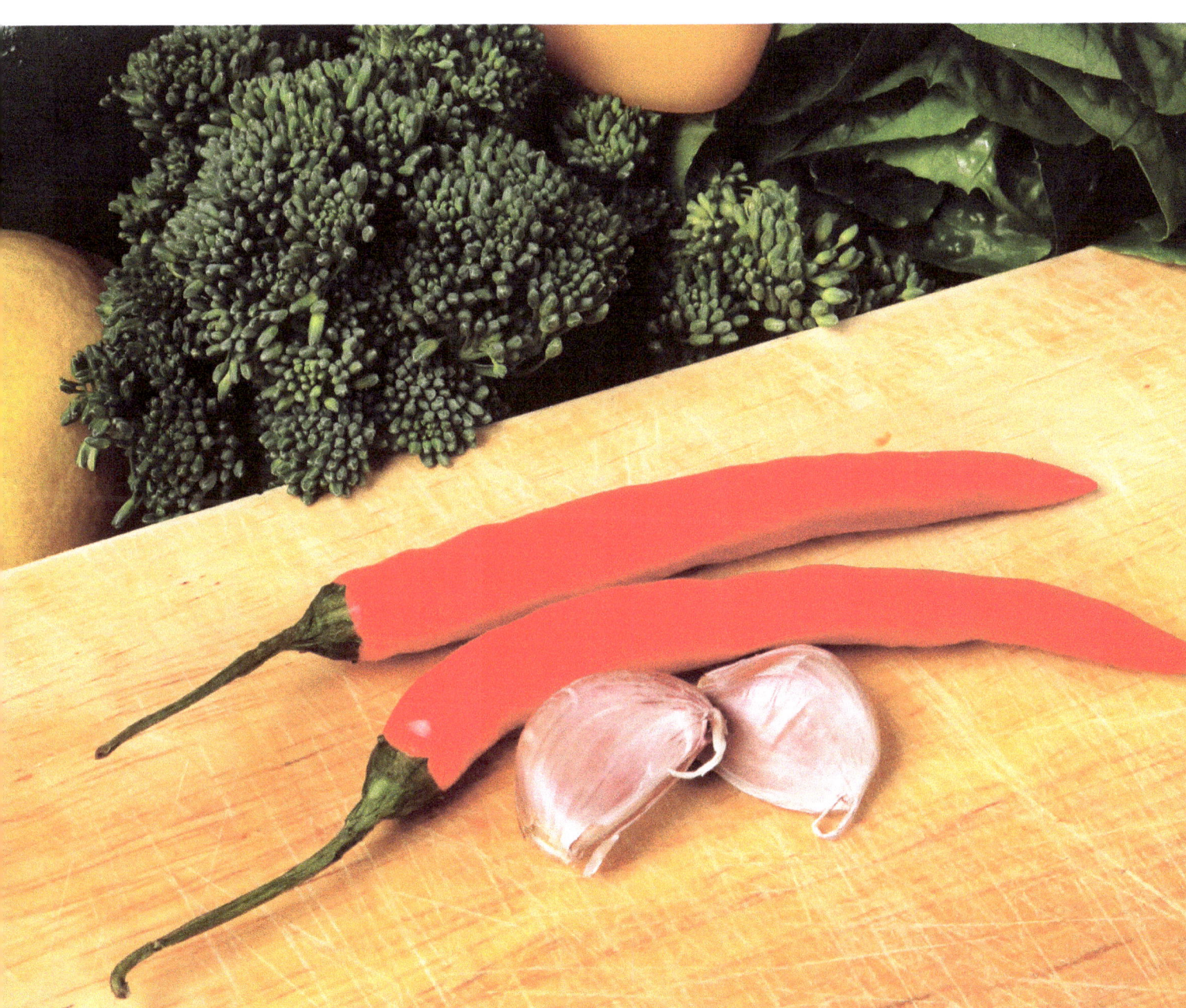

Appendix A – Vitamins

This appendix sets out a more detailed analysis of the individual vitamins with a summary of what they are, what they do and the effects of having too much or too little. Each vitamin is also shown against an average score of which food sources they are mostly found in as compared to our recommended daily intake.

Vitamin A

What is it

This includes a set of compounds, including retinol, retinal, retinoic acid, and provitamin A carotenoids, such as alpha-carotene, beta-carotene and gamma-carotene. It is a fat soluble vitamin, meaning they are stored for longer periods in the body.

Vitamin A sources (averaged)
RDI: 700mcg
Upper Limit: 3000mcg

	Red meat & poultry	Fish	Dairy products	Legumes & nuts	Vegetables	Fruit	Grains	Sweets
Serving size (g)	100	100	50	30	100	100	100	100
Vitamin A	4%	10%	9%	-	122%	4%	-	-

What does it do

As the names of the compounds imply, vitamin A is very important for vision by forming retinal. It is also important for the immune system, as well as maintaining skin health. High doses of vitamin A are sometimes prescribed for acne, though high doses come alongside a number of side effects. Research has highlighted specific advantages of carotenoids, such as:

- **Alpha-carotene**, while not as popular as beta-carotene, has come to light in a recent long-term study where it showed that increased intake is linked to longevity through lowering the risk of death through cardiovascular disease, cancer, and many other causes[211]. This is thought to take place through its action as an antioxidant, preventing cell death from free radicals
- **Beta-carotene** is also a powerful antioxidant which can help to protect the brain which is particularly vulnerable to oxidative damage. A study was conducted that showed long-term supplementation of beta-carotene helped to maintain brain function and prevent cognitive decline[212]

The beta-carotene example is a reminder of why we need to get on a healthy lifestyle and **maintain** it. It is no use to finally clean up your diet in old age, since by then the damage may already be done and a diet change is not always going to reverse it!

And yes, carrots are an excellent source of carotenes...

Deficiency

In the developing world, vitamin A deficiency causes hundreds of thousands of people to go blind each year. As a fat soluble vitamin, very low-fat diets can result in a vitamin A deficiency as effective absorption requires dietary fat intake. Adequate zinc and iron intake is needed for proper vitamin A absorption.

> **It's all connected!**
>
> This highlights the interactive nature of vitamins, minerals and macros - as you can see here, vitamin A is dependent on both dietary fat and minerals. This reminds us why it is important to have balanced healthy eating habits, but also to balance the right macros and micros.

Early signs include difficulty to see in the night, and can lead to a depressed immune system. Effects of a deficiency can be severe if untreated, so seek medical advice quickly if you experience these symptoms.

Overdose

If you continuously take in around five times the recommended dose of vitamin A, you may start to experience nausea, irritability, headaches, hair loss, drowsiness, and a long list of other effects. Too much vitamin A can also lead to brittle bones as it competes with vitamin D for receptors. Just another reminder of why we need to get the right balance in our diets!

Vitamin B1 (Thiamine)

What is it

Also called Thiamine, this is part of a number of B complex vitamins. It is water soluble and is only synthesized by bacteria, plants and mushrooms.

Vitamin B1 sources (averaged) RDI: 1.1mg Upper Limit: N/A	Red meat & poultry	Fish	Dairy products	Legumes & nuts	Vegetables	Fruit	Grains	Sweets
Serving size (g)	100	100	50	30	100	100	100	100
Vitamin B1	8%	17%	-	18%	6%	3%	28%	-

What does it do

nervous system, and is used by all living organisms. Its role in the brain is to help synthesise the neurotransmitters acetylcholine and GABA, without which you could suffer serious neurological disorders. It is also needed to metabolise carbohydrates, dietary fats and proteins and myelin production (a component of neurons).

Deficiency

Deficiency in B1 can be serious, possibly resulting in a coma or death. There are various foods that contain **thiaminase**, which breaks down B1 and can cause a deficiency. These foods include raw shellfish and raw freshwater fish such as carp. Other foods can have anti-thiamine effects, such as tea and coffee. Alcoholism and persistent vomiting can also add to a vitamin B1 deficiency. Alcohol requires B1 to be metabolised, but is not found in alcoholic beverages, meaning that binge drinking can result in a deficiency.

Symptoms of deficiency include:

- Confusion and speech difficulties
- Loss of muscle coordination
- Shortness of breath
- Fatigue, apathy, irritability, depression
- Memory impairment
- Slow reflexes
- Involuntary eye movements
- Tingling in hands or feet

There is actually a massive list of symptoms of B1 deficiency, along with a number of syndromes. Why so many effects? Because B1 is a crucial **brain food**, and since our brains regulate the majority of functions in our bodies, if we don't treat it right, a great many things can go wrong!

Overdose

Being a water soluble vitamin, currently there is no upper limit for B1 with little evidence for adverse effects. High levels of supplementation can result in negative effects, but with the kind of natural foods Think Lean advocates, this is highly unlikely to happen.

The importance of B1 has resulted in Australia and New Zealand mandating enrichment of bread with the vitamin. That is why you will see in the charts that grains contain large amounts of B1. While this has helped to eliminate B1 deficiency to a large degree, it comes with the negative effects of grains, so we still prefer to focus on unrefined natural sources such as fish, nuts and vegetables.

Vitamin B2 (Riboflavin)

What is it

Also called riboflavin, vitamin B2 is a water soluble vitamin and has an orange colour that you often see in vitamin supplements.

What does it do

It is needed to metabolise macro fuels and ketones, without which your body will be unable to draw enough energy from the foods you eat. It is also needed to convert vitamin B6 into its bioactive form and helps to maintain healthy skin.

Vitamin B2 sources (averaged) RDI: 1.1mg Upper Limit: N/A	Red meat & poultry	Fish	Dairy products	Legumes & nuts	Vegetables	Fruit	Grains	Sweets
Serving size (g)	100	100	50	30	100	100	100	100
Vitamin B2	23%	27%	9%	4%	8%	4%	15%	-

Deficiency

Low levels of B2 usually show up through some common symptoms:

- Cracked lips
- Cracked corners of the mouth
- Sore throat
- Redness and swelling in the mouth
- Scaly skin, particularly around the groin

This usually happens alongside other vitamin deficiencies, and since it is regularly excreted through urination, it can be a common deficiency. Similar to B1, a deficiency can be as a result of binge drinking as alcohol also reduces B2 levels along with B1.

Overdose

Since it is actively excreted, the most common symptom of overdose is bright yellow urine. One study investigated if high doses of B2 would help with migraine treatment. The doses were over 300 times the recommended dose, and recorded no ill effects[213]. Also, the study showed that high levels of B2 helped to reduce migraine length by half after around three months of high doses.

Vitamin B3 (Niacin)

What is it
Continuing with the B vitamins, B3 is also known as niacin and includes nicotinamide and nicotinic acid. Like all B vitamins, it is also water soluble, though B3 is more prone to overdose than the ones we've looked at so far.

Vitamin B3 sources (averaged) RDI: 14mg Upper Limit: 35mg	Red meat & poultry	Fish	Dairy products	Legumes & nuts	Vegetables	Fruit	Grains	Sweets
Serving size (g)	100	100	50	30	100	100	100	100
Vitamin B3	43%	44%	-	4%	4%	5%	17%	-

What does it do
It is important for catabolism of macros, as well as cell signalling and DNA repair. Damage to DNA, in particular preventing damage to the telomeres at the ends of DNA strands are key to slowing down the ageing process. Longer telomeres indicate healthier DNA strands, allowing the strand to survive more cell divisions. B3 helps to keep the telomere length from shortening, thereby helping to keep us younger for longer.

Deficiency
There used to be much higher occurrence of deficiency in B3, particularly for people on a corn-based diet with little balance overall. Since then, there is now mandatory B3 supplementation for corn-based products. These days it is more often alcoholism that causes deficiencies, slowing down the metabolism and impacting brain functions[214].

- Slow metabolism
- Skin sensitivity to the sun
- Diarrhoea
- Delirium
- Poor concentration
- Irritability, apathy, depression
- Fatigue

> **Boost Your Brain!**
> We've seen in a few vitamins now what a powerful effect they can have on our mindset, even leading to tiredness and depression. Imagine trying to keep a lean figure and going about your life while contending with a malnourished brain! This is why it is so important for us to keep our brains healthy, address any imbalances and build a solid foundation from which we can be successful in life!

Overdose
Our bodies are not as quick to get rid of excess B3, making us more likely to get too much of it. High doses can result in skin flushing, dry skin and liver damage. Fortunately, you need to take about 60 times the recommended intake to risk this happening, which is equivalent to eating about 15 kg of chicken per day! So unless you are taking high doses of B3 supplementation, healthy eating will keep you from getting too much.

Vitamin B5 (Pantothenic acid)

What is it
Also known as pantothenic acid, B5 is water soluble like all B vitamins. It is a component of Coenzyme A and is essential to most forms of life. Likewise it is found in most food sources, particularly in fish, beef and poultry.

Appendices - Vitamins

What does it do
Like the B vitamins before, it is needed to metabolise dietary fats, carbohydrates and proteins.

Vitamin B5 sources (averaged)
RDI: 4mg
Upper Limit: N/A

	Red meat & poultry	Fish	Dairy products	Legumes & nuts	Vegetables	Fruit	Grains	Sweets
Serving size (g)	100	100	50	30	100	100	100	100
Vitamin B5	23%	36%	3%	6%	8%	8%	10%	-

Deficiency
Since vitamin B5 is so common in food sources, it is very rare to have a deficiency. Symptoms are quickly reversed by intake of larger amounts of B5. These include:

- Fatigue
- Irritability, apathy
- Slow metabolism
- Muscle cramps
- Numbness
- Restlessness

Overdose
Massive doses are needed to experience any side effects and even then, the effects are mild. Because of that, there is no upper limit set for B5.

Vitamin B6 (Pantothenic acid)

What is it
B6 includes pyridoxine, pyridoxamine, pyridoxal and their respective 5' phosphates, and is a water soluble vitamin.

Vitamin B6 sources (averaged)
RDI: 2.4mg
Upper Limit: 50mg

	Red meat & poultry	Fish	Dairy products	Legumes & nuts	Vegetables	Fruit	Grains	Sweets
Serving size (g)	100	100	50	30	100	100	100	100
Vitamin B6	16%	17%	-	4%	6%	5%	5%	-

What does it do
Vitamin B6 is important for amino acid metabolism and as you might remember from the Protein section, amino acids are crucial for every cell in the body. B6 also helps us metabolise dietary fats and to be able to derive energy from excess proteins, which is helpful in a high-protein diet.

B6 is also important for our mental states. It aids the biosynthesis of five key neurotransmitters, some of which you have likely heard of:

- **Serotonin** – It is important for appetite, mood and sleep regulation. Most anti-depressants work via Serotonin
- **Dopamine** – The well-known 'reward' chemical that plays a key role in motivation
- **Epinephrine** – Better known as **adrenaline** which is important for our fight-or-flight response
- **Norepinephrine** – Also called **noradrenaline**, which is stress hormone that affects the amygdala in the brain, controlling our attention
- **Gamma-aminobutyric acid (GABA)** – Helps to decrease neural activity, preventing neurons from firing too much (runaway thoughts, unable to stop thinking about something)

From the quick descriptions it should be clear that these are some of the most important chemicals in our brains, critical for a healthy mind and body.

Deficiency

Being another vitamin that is crucial to brain health, too little B6 can result in:

- Neural damage (neuropathy)
- Confusion
- Drowsiness
- Skin conditions such as cracked mouth corners and dermatitis

Overdose

Similar to other B vitamins, you would need to do some serious supplementation of B6 to get any negative effects, while natural sources are unlikely to ever provide too much. Taking too much in supplementation form over a long period can result in irreversible neural damage. So in the same way that too little can cause brain damage, so can too much. As always, it is all about balance!

Choline

What is it

Choline is usually included with the other B vitamins. It can be manufactured by the body itself, but is often not able to synthesise enough on its own, thus needing adequate intake through diet.

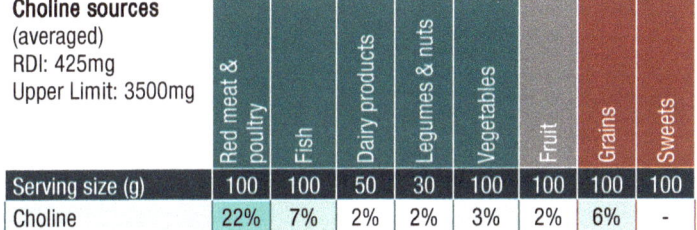

What does it do

Choline is needed to synthesise the neurotransmitter acetycholine which is important for the nervous system and lowering the heart rate. A 2011 study has shown that supplementation of choline helps cognitive function and improves memory[165], provided that choline is concurrently taken in higher doses. This is why the **nootropic** (smart drugs) movement is interested in it and many people take it as a supplement to improve their brain function.

While supplementation is one route, eggs are a major natural source of choline. Eating four eggs a day already puts you over the RDI, and with some chicken or beef added in as well, you naturally reach the levels of choline that you can get through nootropics.

It is also involved in aiding the signalling that happens within the cells of our bodies, as well as transporting dietary fats and cholesterol.

Deficiency

Too little choline has been shown to cause liver disease, neurological disorders, memory loss, muscle damage, and result in heart disease[215]. It is estimated that a significant portion of the population do not get enough choline in their diets. Insufficient intake can have long-term consequences. For example it has been shown that choline supplementation during late stages in pregnancy when the baby's memory centre is being formed, can cause permanent brain changes that have long-term improvement in memory function[215].

Overdose

An upper limit is set at about seven times the RDI, meaning you'd have to take a lot to start feeling negative effects. Symptoms of having too much choline include sweating, fishy body odour, diarrhoea and vomiting.

Vitamin B9 (Folate)

What is it
Also known as folate, B9 is water soluble and while not biologically active itself, it converts into dihydrofolic acid which is an important compound for our bodies.

What does it do
B9 is needed to synthesise, repair and methylate DNA. We need our cells to divide to keep on living, and without B9, cells cannot divide. It is also needed to create red blood cells, and thus is important to prevent anemia.

Its role in brain function through assisting the production of serotonin and dopamine has also lead to studies showing that B9 supplementation is useful in treating depression alongside other antidepressants[216].

Deficiency
Deficiency generally shows up first through the symptoms of anemia:

- Weakness
- Fatigue
- Irritability
- Palpitations

During periods of rapid cell division, such as during pregnancy, sufficient B9 is crucial to prevent the foetus developing neural tube defects (NTD) which can cause permanent brain damage to the foetus.

Overdose
Only through supplementation are you likely to get too much B9. In this case, if there is also a B12 deficiency present, a deficiency in B9 can result in neurological disorders. Overall if you stick to a natural healthy eating plan, you should not have to worry about toxicity.

Vitamin B9 sources (averaged) RDI: 400mcg Upper Limit: 1000mcg	Red meat & poultry	Fish	Dairy products	Legumes & nuts	Vegetables	Fruit	Grains	Sweets
Serving size (g)	100	100	50	30	100	100	100	100
Vitamin B9	3%	4%	1%	13%	16%	6%	17%	-

Vitamin B12 (Cobalamin)

What is it
The last of our B vitamins, B9 is also called cobalamin and is still a water soluble vitamin. B12 is interesting as it does not occur in plant foods, with meat and dairy being the source for normal intake.

What does it do
B12 is important for the brain through the synthesis of fatty acids in myelin. Since our brains are made almost entirely of fats, it's easy to see why this is an important function. Because of that, B12 is important for normal brain function, but also normal blood function as well and DNA synthesis.

Vitamin B12 sources (averaged) RDI: 2.4mcg Upper Limit: N/A	Red meat & poultry	Fish	Dairy products	Legumes & nuts	Vegetables	Fruit	Grains	Sweets
Serving size (g)	100	100	50	30	100	100	100	100
Vitamin B12	45%	415%	10%	-	-	-	1%	-

Deficiency

Given that is it generally only found in animal products, it presents a problem for **vegans** who do not consume any animal products. Vegetarians have less difficulty, as they can obtain a sufficient amount through dairy products. For vegans, B12 fortified foods are needed possibly alongside B12 supplements as well. As it is a water soluble vitamin, it is regularly flushed from the system and thus needs to be constantly included in the diet.

B12 deficiency can cause anemia and neurological disorders such as mania and psychosis. Symptoms of B12 deficiency include:

- Weakness
- Fatigue
- Poor concentration
- Slow reflexes
- Depression
- Poor memory
- Mania (extended periods of irritability)
- Psychosis (delusions, hallucinations, catatonia)

Overdose

Currently there is no evidence of negative effects of too much B12, even through supplementation. This is a good thing, since even just 100g of tuna contains 400% of our daily requirement.

Vitamin C (Ascorbate)

What is it

Finally moving on from the B vitamins, we come to vitamin C. Vitamin C is the last water soluble vitamin and is also known as ascorbate.

Vitamin C sources (averaged)
RDI: 45mg
Upper Limit: N/A

	Red meat & poultry	Fish	Dairy products	Legumes & nuts	Vegetables	Fruit	Grains	Sweets
Serving size (g)	100	100	50	30	100	100	100	100
Vitamin C	2%	-	-	1%	103%	50%	-	-

What does it do

It has a role in collagen synthesis which is a key protein used in connective tissues. It is also involved in the synthesis of the neurotransmitters dopamine and norepinephrine. It has a role as an antioxidant, helping to prevent oxidative damage.

Deficiency

The most commonly known effect of a lack of vitamin C is scurvy. Scurvy is a deadly disorder that eventually results in death if untreated. In the middle ages, many sailors on long trips died on the seas due to scurvy, with ships sometimes losing 90% of their crew due to vitamin C deficiency.

Since vitamin C is mainly found in vegetables and also in fruits, diets low in these can result in vitamin C deficiency. Symptoms include:

- Fatigue
- Weakness
- Shortness of breath
- Bone pain
- Rough skin

Appendices - Vitamins

- Bruising
- Gum disease
- Loose teeth
- Jaundice
- Neuropathy

Overdose

Vitamin C is well tolerated and easily cleared out of the system with little evidence of negative effects in larger doses other than occasional indigestion. Some people use megadoses of vitamin C in an attempt to help with certain ailments, but mostly these results have been contradictory and thus does not provide us with any real evidence for using it in higher doses beyond RDI.

Vitamin D

What is it

Vitamin D, the sunshine vitamin, is a fat soluble vitamin that does not commonly appear in food. Our main mechanism to obtain it is through exposure to sunshine.

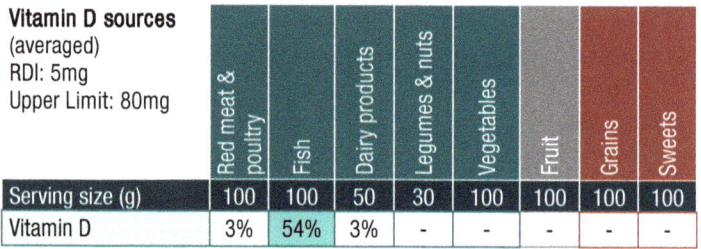

What does it do

Vitamin D plays a key role in calcium absorption and maintaining calcium balance in the body, making it important to maintain bone health. It is also needed for the immune system through the expression of vitamin D receptors.

Deficiency

Our indoors lifestyle has resulted in a large number of people having vitamin D deficiency, even in a country like Australia with so much sunshine! Part of the issue is that the use of sunscreen actually blocks the majority of vitamin D production[217]. This presents obvious problems for health authorities who have been bombarding us with messages to wear sunscreen to prevent skin cancer.

Arguably the drive to prevent skin cancer has become so overprotective that it is resulting in mass vitamin D deficiency. Our skin developed through millions of years of evolution, so the drive to prevent skin cancer to some extent is putting us off balance. It seems reasonable to conclude that there is such a thing as "safe sun exposure". What exactly this is, we don't have any real guidance for, but a guideline for this may be the amount of sun exposure that does not result in you getting sunburn (without using sunscreen).

Vitamin D deficiency is closely related to rickets and osteoporosis. Symptoms include:

- Muscle aches and weakness
- Muscle twitching
- Fragile bones
- Low bone mineral density

Adding to that, a recent study has also shown that deficiency is linked to higher rates in mortality[218].

Overdose

Vitamin D has relatively low toxicity and given that most foods do not contain it, you will generally have to be getting tons of sun exposure and supplementation to achieve an overload. For example, you'll need to take about 16 average vitamin D supplement pills every day for a while to build up an overdose. Given that it is a fat soluble vitamin, it can stay stored for months, so recovering from an overdose can take a month or more. Symptoms of too much Vitamin D include dehydration, decreased appetite, irritability and muscle weakness.

Vitamin E

What is it

Vitamin E consists of eight fat soluble compounds. It is mainly found in plant and animal fats and oils, and exists itself as yellow coloured oil.

Vitamin E sources (averaged)
RDI: 7mg
Upper Limit: 300mg

	Red meat & poultry	Fish	Dairy products	Legumes & nuts	Vegetables	Fruit	Grains	Sweets
Serving size (g)	100	100	50	30	100	100	100	100
Vitamin E	6%	13%	5%	2%	9%	10%	18%	-

What does it do

As a fat soluble antioxidant, vitamin E embeds itself in cell walls, protecting the cells themselves from oxidative damage. It also helps to prevent the oxidation of polyunsaturated fats and plays a role in proper immune and brain function. It plays a role in vitamin A absorption and helps to protect against the effects of too much vitamin A.

Deficiency

A deficiency in vitamin E can be due to diet, or other causes such as coeliac disease or alcoholism. There are usually few outward signs of deficiency that you can look for. Eventual effects include:

- Nerve damage
- Neuromuscular disorders
- Red blood cell destruction
- Eye damage

Overdose

Too much vitamin E can be dangerous as it can prevent blood from clotting. This, in combination with blood thinners can result in massive bleeding. High doses also interfere with vitamin K absorption and can lead to a K deficiency.

Vitamin K

What is it

The last of our vitamins, this is another fat soluble vitamin. It is synthesised by plants and mainly makes its way into our diets through leafy green vegetables.

Vitamin K sources (averaged)
RDI: 60mcg
Upper Limit: N/A

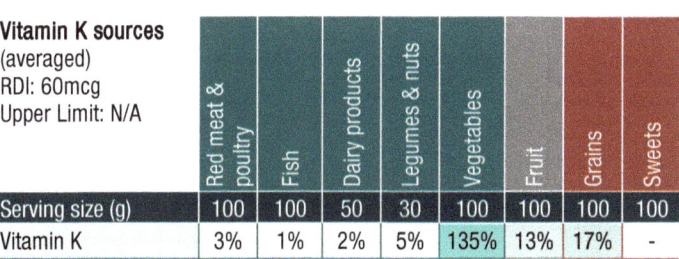

	Red meat & poultry	Fish	Dairy products	Legumes & nuts	Vegetables	Fruit	Grains	Sweets
Serving size (g)	100	100	50	30	100	100	100	100
Vitamin K	3%	1%	2%	5%	135%	13%	17%	-

What does it do

Vitamin K is needed for the development of clotting agents, helping to prevent excessive bleeding.

Deficiency

As vitamin K conversion takes place in the liver, forms of liver damage and surgery can result in a deficiency, along with long-term antibiotic use. Overall, deficiency is very rare as it usually makes its way into our diet through various food sources. Symptoms of deficiency include:

- Bruising
- Excessive bleeding (nose, stomach, skin)
- Stomach pains
- Cartilage calcification

Overdose

There is currently no evidence of too much vitamin K being toxic. As such, there is no upper limit set for it.

Appendix B – Minerals

As with the vitamin appendix, this appendix sets out a more detailed analysis of the individual minerals with a summary of what they are, what they do and the effects of having too much or too little. Each mineral is also shown against an average score of which food sources they are mostly found in as compared to our recommended daily intake.

Calcium

What does it do

Calcium has a key role in building stronger and denser bones. The vast majority of calcium is stored in the bones and teeth, with the rest used for critical functions such as neurotransmitter release. Calcium is key for a long and active life, especially later in life. Intake of calcium while young affects bone density in old age, so start eating healthy today to live a long and healthy life!

Calcium sources (averaged)
RDI: 1000mg
Upper Limit: 2500mg

	Red meat & poultry	Fish*	Dairy products	Legumes & nuts	Vegetables	Fruit	Grains	Sweets
Serving size (g)	100	100	50	30	100	100	100	100
Calcium	2%	7%	13%	5%	4%	2%	4%	-

Deficiency

Calcium has a close connection to vitamin D, which it needs to be able to be absorbed and used for bone health. Given that calcium is generally not as common in foods and the prevalence of vitamin D shortages, we are often at risk of having a calcium deficiency. Dairy products are the main sources of calcium in our diets, with some cultured products like cheese having the highest calcium content.

A deficiency can result in low bone density (osteoporosis). Beside poor nutrition, there are many things that can cause a calcium deficiency, including eating disorders, excessive magnesium intake, mercury exposure, and more. Symptoms include:

- Skin spots (petechiae)
- Tingling in hands and feet, or around mouth and lips
- Hyperactive reflexes
- Contractions of the hands

Overdose

There are few side effects to high doses of calcium, with kidney stones being one of the few. Very high supplement doses, around ten times the recommended intake, has been shown to result in a condition that can lead to kidney failure. Whole foods and normal supplementation is far below this level, so would not be something to worry about if you follow the guidelines.

Appendices - **Minerals**

Iron

What does it do

Particularly important for blood health, iron plays a key role in oxygen and carbon dioxide transport. Blood also gets its red colour from the iron bound to it. Iron also helps with oxygen storage in muscles, which is useful for athletic performance and feeling fit and energised. It is needed for healthy immune function, leading to increased levels of infection when levels are too low. On top of all that, it is also involved in the production of neurotransmitters, making it important for a healthy mind.

Iron sources (averaged)
RDI: 8mg
Upper Limit: 45mg

	Red meat & poultry	Fish*	Dairy products	Legumes & nuts	Vegetables	Fruit	Grains	Sweets
Serving size (g)	100	100	50	30	100	100	100	100
Iron	12%	14%	-	8%	4%	2%	15%	1%

Deficiency

Poor nutrition, low copper levels, pregnancy, blood loss, pain medication (NSAID's), and many other factors can lead to a deficiency in iron. Iron deficiency is estimated to be the most common deficiency in the world. Common symptoms include:

- Fatigue
- Tiredness
- Apathy
- Poor concentration, poor memory
- Reduced attention span
- Headaches
- Anaemia

An iron deficiency is not the same as anaemia, though severely depleted iron levels can result in iron deficiency anaemia. This is a serious condition and needs immediate treatment.

Overdose

High levels of iron can result in the creation of free radicals, leading to oxidative damage to DNA, proteins and cells. It can cause damage to the liver and heart, and can even lead to a coma or death. The levels needed to reach toxicity means taking about five times the recommended intake on a consistent basis. Since most foods do not have large amounts of iron, it means you'll have to heavily overdo supplementation to reach toxic levels.

Magnesium

What does it do

Magnesium is involved in over 300 enzyme reactions in the body. This makes it fundamentally necessary for a healthy body. It helps to keep our lungs working well, keeps our heart beat regular, prevents kidney stones, relaxes muscles, regulates blood glucose, and supports the immune system. Just from that you can see the major role that magnesium plays and why it is so important for our health.

Magnesium sources (averaged)
RDI: 320mg
Upper Limit: 350mg (supplementation)

	Red meat & poultry	Fish*	Dairy products	Legumes & nuts	Vegetables	Fruit	Grains	Sweets
Serving size (g)	100	100	50	30	100	100	100	100
Magnesium	6%	24%	2%	15%	7%	5%	19%	-

Deficiency

A deficiency can be caused by alcohol abuse, low protein diets, physical or mental stress (through release of stress hormones), and more. Low magnesium levels can result in low calcium as well, adding to long-term negative effects on our health. Symptoms of low magnesium include:

- Irritability
- Dizziness
- Muscle spasms
- Fatigue
- Nausea
- Vomiting
- Convulsions

Overdose

Our kidneys are generally effective at clearing out excess magnesium, so it is rare to have negative effects from too much. Because of this, there is no upper limit set for eating natural foods. Instead there is only an upper limit for supplementation of magnesium as it has been seen that only through supplementation do people get negative effects. Too much supplementation can result in:

- Breathing difficulty
- Fatigue
- Nausea
- Vomiting
- Decreased reflexes

Here again it's interesting to see that the side effects of too much is somewhat similar as having too little. As always, health is all about balance!

Phosphorus

What does it do

Phosphorus makes up part of our DNA and is one of the most common inorganic substances in our bodies. It helps to protect our blood and acts as a temporary store of energy, as well as the transport of energy through our system.

Phosphorus sources (averaged) RDI: 1g Upper Limit: 4g	Red meat & poultry	Fish*	Dairy products	Legumes & nuts	Vegetables	Fruit	Grains	Sweets
Serving size (g)	100	100	50	30	100	100	100	100
Phosphorus	20%	25%	9%	15%	4%	2%	21%	-

Deficiency

As with many other deficiencies, this can be caused by excessive alcohol intake along with poor diet. Alcohol takes a lot of nutrients to process and clear out of the body, so in moderate amounts you can recover through a normal diet, but larger amounts of alcohol removes nutrients faster than you can bring them back in, resulting in deficiencies and all the negative effects that come with it. The symptoms of deficiency include:

- Muscle weakness
- Bone pain
- Anaemia
- Rickets

Appendices - *Minerals*

- Decreased immune function
- Confusion

Overdose

Too much phosphorus can result in calcium depletion, resulting in effects similar to a calcium deficiency, with bones being reabsorbed, calcification of heart and connective tissue and also increased blood acidity. It can also affect the absorption of zinc, iron and magnesium.

Potassium

What does it do

Potassium is important to keep our nerves firing effectively, helping to keep our heartbeat regular and also helps to relax muscles after contraction. It is also needed to make insulin, which is important for maintaining blood sugar levels. Potassium can help to prevent salt from increasing blood pressure. To some extent, this means that a higher level of potassium is needed when a higher amount of salt is taken in.

Potassium sources (averaged)
RDI: 2.8g
Upper Limit: N/A

	Red meat & poultry	Fish*	Dairy products	Legumes & nuts	Vegetables	Fruit	Grains	Sweets
Serving size (g)	100	100	50	30	100	100	100	100
Potassium	8%	12%	2%	7%	10%	7%	7%	-

Deficiency

It is not common to have a deficiency in potassium, unless the diet is constantly low in vegetables and fruits, such as diets high in processed foods. It's more common for deficiency to be caused by a loss of potassium, such as high salt intake, anorexia or bulimia, diabetes or chronic stress. Often there are no symptoms of a mild deficiency, but higher levels of deficiency can result in:

- High blood pressure
- Cramps
- Weakness
- Irritability
- Insomnia
- Depression

Overdose

There is no upper limit set for potassium as it mainly has a low level of toxicity. Still, most diets tend to include enough potassium, so there usually no need for supplementation. In fact, the guidance is that supplementation should only be done under medical supervision. So, stick to natural foods and you won't have to worry about getting too much.

Sodium

What does it do

The majority of sodium that we eat is in the form of sodium chloride, which is really just plain old **salt**. It is needed by the body for nerve functioning and balancing blood and bodily fluids. So, it turns out that salt is actually a necessary nutrient that we can't live without. Of course, most diets include lots of salt as it seems to make its way into everything.

Deficiency

Generally it is harder for us to keep below the upper limit than it is to get a deficiency since there are so many foods with salt in them and we tend to put salt on lots of foods. As animals, we have evolved a special taste for sodium as it is not always available in plants and was often hard to find in ancient times.

Sodium sources (averaged)
RDI: 690mg
Upper Limit: 2300mg

	Red meat & poultry	Fish*	Dairy products	Legumes & nuts	Vegetables	Fruit	Grains	Sweets
Serving size (g)	100	100	50	30	100	100	100	100
Sodium	13%	9%	13%	-	5%	-	34%	4%

These days, salt is everywhere, but we still have our evolved taste for it. While you may be successful in cutting out a lot of salt at home, all the food producers, restaurants and fast food outlets know we have the taste for salt, so they still put it in nearly everything. As long as you make food yourself, you can avoid too much, but any food prepared for you will likely have salt in it already.

If you do manage to get a sodium deficiency, which is very hard and usually due to other causes, you can expect the following symptoms:

- Headaches
- Confusion, irritability
- Fatigue
- Nausea
- Seizures
- Unconsciousness
- Coma

Overdose

Due to the amount of salt in foods these days, it is common to be getting more than the recommended dose. Is too much salt actually bad for you? This is something worth looking into a bit more.

First of all, too much salt is linked to high blood pressure (hypertension), and this is the main reason why there is a recommendation to limit salt intake. But there is more to hypertension than that. For example:

- Higher fructose intake has been shown to lead to high blood pressure[219]
- The ratio between sodium and potassium has recently been shown to be a more important indicator of hypertension than sodium alone[220]
- Another study has shown that hypertension can happen independently of salt intake and is closer related to stress, with nuns on high salt diets having low blood pressure, but others in a state of societal change have high blood pressure, even while having low salt diets[221]. This shows that high blood pressure is more likely due to stress than salt intake
- It was also found that some people are naturally 'salt sensitive', and have a much higher response in blood pressure depending on the levels of salt. For these people, lower salt diets work to help lower blood pressure[222]

Overall what this means is that if you are not salt sensitive, then higher amounts of salt is unlikely to raise your blood pressure, and hypertension is more likely as a result of stress or too much fructose.

Listen to your body – if you eat a lot of salt and don't feel too great afterwards, then maybe you are salt sensitive. For the majority of people, however, this will not be the case and higher amounts of salt will not necessarily cause high blood pressure.

Appendices - **Minerals**

Zinc

What does it do

Zinc has many roles, binding to nearly 10% of proteins. It forms part of a large number of enzyme reactions, is involved in gene expression, or can have structural roles. What does all that mean? Simply that zinc is really important and it is another element we can't live without! It is also needed for a healthy immune system, proper wound healing, and helps us keep healthy eyes and skin.

Zinc sources (averaged)
RDI: 8mg
Upper Limit: 40mg

	Red meat & poultry	Fish*	Dairy products	Legumes & nuts	Vegetables	Fruit	Grains	Sweets
Serving size (g)	100	100	50	30	100	100	100	100
Zinc	34%	8%	7%	13%	3%	3%	18%	-

Deficiency

Other than dietary deficiency, high levels of iron and calcium supplementation can reduce the amount of zinc that is absorbed. This can lead to a deficiency in zinc, and reminds us not to overdo any supplementation. More is not always better! Zinc deficiency can result in the following:

- Slowed growth
- Diarrhoea
- Hair loss
- Eye and skin conditions
- Slow wound healing
- Tiredness

Overdose

Eating natural whole foods do not put you at risk of eating too much zinc. Taking large doses of supplementation continuously can result in supressing the immune system, leading to more infections. It can also lead to nausea and vomiting, as well as interfere with proper cholesterol functions.

Copper

What does it do

Copper is needed for iron metabolism and the production of blood. It is also involved in keeping the nervous system healthy and efficiently converting neurotransmitters, regulating their levels. Similar to zinc, it is also involved in keeping the immune system healthy and developing a resistance to infection.

Copper sources (averaged)
RDI: 1.2mg
Upper Limit: 10mg

	Red meat & poultry	Fish*	Dairy products	Legumes & nuts	Vegetables	Fruit	Grains	Sweets
Serving size (g)	100	100	50	30	100	100	100	100
Copper	13%	11%	-	23%	5%	7%	18%	-

Deficiency

Usually a deficiency is rare, but can be found together with an iron deficiency. Its role in converting neurotransmitters can result in neurological problems when there is a deficiency. This can result in:

- Anaemia
- Difficulty walking
- Spinal degeneration
- Eye problems, loss of colour in vision

Overdose

Tests were conducted that showed no negative effects at copper levels up to 10mg, setting the upper limit in this case. Those levels are unlikely to be achieved through a normal diet, and are usually the result of copper supplements. At high levels, there have been reports of muscle and joint pain, liver disease and abnormal kidney function.

Manganese

What does it do

Manganese is mainly found in plant sources, being most concentrated in legumes and nuts (remember the chart to the right is corrected for portion sizes). It is needed for healthy bones and to metabolise carbohydrates, cholesterol and proteins.

Manganese sources (averaged) RDI: 5mg Upper Limit: N/A	Red meat & poultry	Fish*	Dairy products	Legumes & nuts	Vegetables	Fruit	Grains	Sweets
Serving size (g)	100	100	50	30	100	100	100	100
Manganese	-	-	-	12%	5%	5%	26%	-

Deficiency

Manganese deficiency is rare in healthy people unless there is some other cause, but can result in the following:

- Skin conditions (dermatitis)
- Joint pain
- Inflammation
- Nausea

Overdose

There is little conclusive evidence of negative effects of high levels of manganese, so because of that, there is no upper limit set for it. Overexposure is usually due to workplace safety issues (such as welding) where manganese is breathed in. In these cases it has been seen to affect the brain and neurological function. So unless you are a welder (or something along those lines) you don't need to worry about any side effects.

Appendices - **Minerals**

Selenium

What does it do

Last one! Selenium acts as an antioxidant, it is needed for a healthy immune system, and is also used by the thyroid which regulates our energy levels.

Deficiency

Selenium deficiency results in a condition known as Keshan Disease, which results in:

- Heart enlargement
- Heart failure
- Arrhythmia (irregular heartbeat)

Selenium sources (averaged)
RDI: 60mcg
Upper Limit: 400mcg

	Red meat & poultry	Fish*	Dairy products	Legumes & nuts	Vegetables	Fruit	Grains	Sweets
Serving size (g)	100	100	50	30	100	100	100	100
Selenium	35%	62%	5%	5%	1%	-	42%	1%

This is a potentially lethal condition that quickly responds to selenium supplementation. Low levels of selenium have also been linked to increased risk of cancer, so remember to eat some meat and fish to keep the selenium levels up!

Overdose

Famous for being found in high levels in brazil nuts, there have actually been cases of people getting selenium poisoning from eating too many in one sitting. Just 30 grams of brazil nuts already contain around 10 times the RDI and goes over the upper limit established. High levels of selenium can result in:

- Skin rash
- Hair loss
- Fatigue
- Irritability
- Brittle nails

Appendix C – Foods

This appendix lists selected individual foods used to calculate the average amount of vitamins, minerals and calories for different food groups. Naturally, this method is not perfect as there are many more foods that can be used, but it does give a good general indication from which we can build a healthy eating plan and get some solid reasoning for why we choose certain groups.

The coloured cells show the percentage value of how much vitamins or minerals a certain food has as compared to our recommended daily intake for an adult female (males need a little more). Below the nutrients you can see the amount of calories, protein, dietary fat and carbohydrates a food has.

Meat products

		Beef, chicken, eggs						Fish						
		Chicken breast	Beef - ground	Chicken thigh	Beef	Eggs	Quail	Tuna	Trout	Herring	Salmon	Salmon - Alaskan	Mackerel	Caviar
	Serving size (g)	100	100	100	100	100	100	100	100	100	100	100	100	100
Vitamins	Vitamin A			1%		15%	5%	44%	1%	2%		2%	3%	18%
	Vitamin C						14%		4%	2%				
	Vitamin D					19%				84%			180%	116%
	Vitamin E	4%	6%	4%	6%	17%		14%		16%		11%	21%	27%
	Vitamin K		2%	6%	2%	9%							8%	1%
	Thiamin	9%		9%		9%	18%	18%	18%	9%	18%	18%	18%	18%
	Riboflavin	9%	18%	18%	18%	45%	27%	27%	9%	18%	36%	18%	27%	55%
	Niacin	98%	33%	37%	34%		54%	62%	41%	23%	56%	56%	65%	
	Vitamin B6	25%	13%	8%	17%	8%	25%	21%	13%	13%	33%	8%	17%	13%
	Folate	1%	2%	2%	2%	13%	2%		5%	3%	6%	3%		13%
	Vitamin B12	13%	92%	8%	83%	58%	17%	392%	263%	571%	133%	354%	363%	833%
	Pantothenic Acid	25%	13%	23%	15%	40%	20%	28%	28%	15%	43%	30%	23%	88%
	Choline	20%	14%	16%	16%	64%		15%		15%			15%	
Minerals	Calcium	2%	2%	1%	1%	6%	1%		9%	6%	1%		1%	28%
	Iron	6%	12%	8%	11%	11%	22%	6%	2%	6%	4%	3%	9%	66%
	Magnesium	9%	6%	7%	6%	4%	7%	16%	10%	10%	9%	9%	24%	94%
	Phosphorus	23%	17%	15%	18%	21%	28%	25%	27%	24%	20%	24%	22%	36%
	Potassium	9%	11%	7%	10%	5%	8%	9%	16%	12%	18%	14%	11%	6%
	Sodium	11%	10%	11%	10%	30%	8%	6%	8%	13%	6%	8%	13%	217%
	Zinc	13%	56%	33%	56%	15%	30%	8%	6%	13%	8%	5%	8%	11%
	Copper		8%	8%	8%	8%	42%	8%	8%	8%	25%	8%	8%	8%
	Manganese													2%
	Selenium	46%	26%	29%	24%	57%	28%	61%	22%	61%	61%	46%	74%	109%

Average Macronutrient Profiles (does not indicate RDI)

Calories	165	215	195	192	196	192	144	215	158	142	140	205	252
Carbohydrate (g)													
Dietary Fat (g)	4	15	10	13	15	12	5	8	9	6	6	14	18
Protein (g)	33	20	27	19	14	21	25	35	19	21	22	20	22

Appendices - **Foods**

Dairy, nuts and legumes

Meats, dairy and nuts are great sources of many vitamins and minerals. Note that in the first section, we used smaller serving sizes for dairy, nuts and legumes. The values below are per 100g of each food, to allow a more direct comparison with the other foods.

		Dairy				Nuts and legumes						
		Milk - whole	Cheese - cheddar	Butter - no salt	Yoghurt	Flaxseeds	Chia seeds	Cashews	Macadamia	Kindey beands	Lentils	Chickpeas
	Serving size (g)	100	100	100	100	100	100	100	100	100	100	100
Vitamins	Vitamin A	2%	20%	50%			0					
	Vitamin C				2%	1%		1%	3%	10%	10%	3%
	Vitamin D	20%	6%									
	Vitamin E	1%	4%	33%	1%	4%		13%	7%	3%	7%	6%
	Vitamin K		5%	12%	2%	7%		57%		32%	8%	7%
	Thiamin					145%		36%	109%	45%	82%	9%
	Riboflavin	18%	36%		18%	18%		9%	18%	18%	18%	9%
	Niacin					22%		8%	18%	15%	19%	4%
	Vitamin B6		4%			21%		17%	13%	17%	21%	4%
	Folate	1%	5%		2%	22%		6%	3%	99%	120%	43%
	Vitamin B12	17%	33%	8%	21%							
	Pantothenic Acid	10%	10%	3%		25%		23%	20%	20%	53%	8%
	Choline	3%	4%	4%	4%	19%					23%	10%
Minerals	Calcium	11%	72%	2%	15%	26%	63%	4%	9%	14%	6%	5%
	Iron		4%			32%		37%	21%	46%	42%	16%
	Magnesium	3%	9%		5%	123%		91%	41%	44%	38%	15%
	Phosphorus	9%	51%	2%	12%	64%	95%	59%	19%	41%	45%	17%
	Potassium	5%	4%		7%	29%	6%	24%	13%	50%	34%	10%
	Sodium	6%	90%	2%	8%	4%	3%	2%		3%		1%
	Zinc	5%	39%	1%	9%	54%	44%	73%	16%	35%	60%	19%
	Copper					100%	17%	183%	67%	83%	42%	33%
	Manganese					50%	44%	34%	82%	20%	26%	20%
	Selenium		23%	2%	10%	42%		33%	6%	5%	14%	6%

Average Macronutrient Profiles (does not indicate RDI)

Calories	60	403	717	95	534	490	553	718	333	353	164
Carbohydrate (g)	4	1		19	30	45	31	14	61	60	28
Dietary Fat (g)	3	32	79		39	29	41	70		1	2
Protein (g)	3	27		4	16	14	16	7	20	26	8

Appendices - **Foods**

Vegetables

Vegetables are great for the gaps between meat and dairy products. This is why our greens are so necessary for a complete and healthy diet. In addition, they are also better than fruits when it comes to vitamin and mineral content, so stick with lots of vegetables. Also, you can eat as many as you like, making it easy to get enough vitamins and minerals.

		Vegetables							
		Spinach	Chinese broccoli	Cauliflower	Broccoli	Lettuce - cos	Peppers	Tomatoes	Sweet potatoes	Carrots
	Serving size (g)	100	100	100	100	100	100	100	100	100
Vitamins	Vitamin A	188%	33%		60%	174%	5%	17%	284%	334%
	Vitamin C	62%	63%	98%	207%	53%	393%	28%	5%	13%
	Vitamin D									
	Vitamin E	29%	7%	1%		1%	20%	7%	4%	10%
	Vitamin K	805%	141%	23%		172%	36%	13%	3%	22%
	Thiamin	9%	9%		9%	9%			9%	9%
	Riboflavin	18%	9%	9%	9%	9%			9%	9%
	Niacin	5%	3%	3%	4%	2%	4%	4%	4%	7%
	Vitamin B6	8%	4%	8%	8%	4%	8%	4%	8%	4%
	Folate	49%	25%	11%	18%	34%		4%	3%	5%
	Vitamin B12									
	Pantothenic Acid	3%	5%	13%	13%	3%	3%	3%	20%	8%
	Choline	4%	6%	9%		2%	1%	2%	3%	2%
Minerals	Calcium	10%	10%	2%	5%	3%		1%	3%	3%
	Iron	15%	3%	2%	5%	6%	2%	2%	3%	2%
	Magnesium	25%	6%	3%	8%	4%	3%	3%	8%	4%
	Phosphorus	5%	4%	3%	7%	3%	2%	2%	5%	4%
	Potassium	20%	9%	5%	12%	9%	5%	8%	12%	11%
	Sodium	11%	1%	2%	4%	1%	2%		8%	10%
	Zinc	6%	5%	3%	5%	3%	1%	3%	4%	3%
	Copper	8%	8%					8%	17%	
	Manganese	18%	6%	2%	4%	4%	2%	2%	6%	2%
	Selenium	2%	2%	1%	5%		1%		1%	

Average Macronutrient Profiles (does not indicate RDI)

Calories	23	22	23	28	17	127	18	86	41
Carbohydrate (g)	3	3	4	4	3	4	4	20	9
Dietary Fat (g)						12		0	0
Protein (g)	2		1	2				1	1

Appendices - **Foods**

Fruit

Fruits remain as a 'sometimes' food – it is more a treat than a regular food source. You can get all the nutrients from fruits in vegetables and meat, so you don't actually need to eat lots of fruit.

		Apples	Bananas	Oranges	Peaches	Mangos	Raspberries	Blackberries	Strawberries	Blueberries	Avocados
	Serving size (g)	100	100	100	100	100	100	100	100	100	100
Vitamins	Vitamin A	1%	1%	5%	7%	15%		4%			3%
	Vitamin C	10%	19%	131%	15%	62%	58%	47%	131%	6%	22%
	Vitamin D										
	Vitamin E	3%	1%	3%	10%	16%	13%	17%	4%	7%	30%
	Vitamin K	4%			4%	7%	13%	33%	4%	27%	35%
	Thiamin			9%		9%					9%
	Riboflavin		9%	9%		9%					9%
	Niacin		5%	3%	6%	4%	4%	4%	3%	4%	12%
	Vitamin B6		17%	4%		4%	4%			4%	13%
	Folate		5%	9%	1%	4%	5%	6%	6%	2%	20%
	Vitamin B12										
	Pantothenic Acid	3%	8%	8%	5%	5%	8%	8%	3%	3%	35%
	Choline		2%	2%	1%	2%	3%	2%	1%	1%	3%
Minerals	Calcium			4%		1%	3%	3%	2%		1%
	Iron		2%		2%		4%	3%	2%	1%	3%
	Magnesium	2%	8%	3%	3%	3%	7%	6%	4%	2%	9%
	Phosphorus	1%	2%	2%	2%	1%	3%	2%	2%	1%	5%
	Potassium	4%	13%	6%	7%	6%	5%	6%	5%	2%	17%
	Sodium										1%
	Zinc		3%	1%	3%		5%	6%	1%	1%	8%
	Copper		8%		8%	8%	8%	17%			17%
	Manganese		6%	2%			14%	12%	8%	2%	2%
	Selenium		2%			1%					

Average Macronutrient Profiles (does not indicate RDI)

Calories	52	89	49	39	65	52	43	32	51	160
Carbohydrate (g)	12	21	11	8	15	11	9	7	11	8
Dietary Fat (g)										14
Protein (g)						1	1			2

Grains and sweets

Grains and sweets come in as the most carbohydrate-dense and calorie-dense foods. This means we are likely to overeat when we have them since they are just so packed with bad nutrients. On top of that, you can just see how sweets are 'empty' calories, since they have almost zero vitamins and minerals!

		Grain products									Sweets		
		Bread - whole wheat	Cake	Crackers	Muffins	Noodles	Oat flour	Quinoa	Rice - white	Spaghetti	Wheat flour	Gum drops	Hard candies	Sugar
	Serving size (g)	100	100	100	100	100	100	100	100	100	100	100	100	100
Vitamins	Vitamin A							1%						
	Vitamin C					2%								
	Vitamin D													
	Vitamin E	1%	34%	10%	50%	23%	51%		11%	1%				
	Vitamin K			5%	11%	65%	71%		17%					
	Thiamin	9%	36%	64%	55%	18%	36%	9%	27%	9%	18%			
	Riboflavin		27%	9%	36%	18%	18%	9%	18%	9%				
	Niacin	9%	11%	11%	42%	10%	30%	4%	28%	12%	11%			
	Vitamin B6		21%	4%	4%		4%		8%	4%	4%			
	Folate	7%	46%	8%	23%	12%	30%	7%	17%	5%	15%			
	Vitamin B12					4%		8%						
	Pantothenic Acid	10%	20%	5%	13%	8%	10%	10%	8%	10%	10%			
	Choline	2%	17%	7%	2%	12%	3%	9%	7%					
Minerals	Calcium	2%	5%	6%	2%	4%	10%	6%	4%	2%				
	Iron	7%	26%	22%	26%	11%	21%	6%	19%	7%	8%	2%	2%	
	Magnesium	7%	62%	45%	16%	3%	6%	2%	28%	17%	3%			
	Phosphorus	11%	46%	45%	16%	13%	26%	14%	21%	19%	3%			
	Potassium	4%	20%	13%	4%	3%	4%	2%	12%	8%				
	Sodium			3%	64%	46%	125%	50%	55%			6%	6%	
	Zinc	9%	39%	40%	18%	16%	8%	4%	21%	18%	5%			
	Copper	8%	50%	33%	17%	8%	8%		25%	25%	8%			
	Manganese	14%	40%	80%	28%	16%	12%	2%	42%	18%	8%			
	Selenium	57%	14%	57%	72%	16%	6%	9%	71%	105%	13%	1%	1%	1%

Average Macronutrient Profiles (does not indicate RDI)

	Bread - whole wheat	Cake	Crackers	Muffins	Noodles	Oat flour	Quinoa	Rice - white	Spaghetti	Wheat flour	Gum drops	Hard candies	Sugar
Calories	364	368	404	527	393	504	373	305	371	130	396	394	389
Carbohydrate (g)	79	64	66	59	50	61	57	54	77	30	99	98	97
Dietary Fat (g)		6	9	29	19	26	14	6	1				
Protein (g)	10	14	15	8	5	7	4	9	13	2			

Come and visit us at
www.**think**leanmethod.com
for more articles, food pyramids and information to help you succeed!

References:

While creating the Think Lean Method and subsequently writing this book, I focused on peer-reviewed research published in respected journals. This produces a higher quality result that is supported by evidence.

The majority of studies referenced are freely available online. You can find these by searching for the title of the study, and then following the links to "Free Full Text" where available. Don't be scared to look them up. They are generally easier to read than what you'd think!

[1] A.H. Manninen, "Metabolic effects of the very-low-carbohydrate diets: misunderstood "villains" of human metabolism." *Journal of the International Society of Sports Nutrition*, 1(2):7-11, 2004.

[2] E.C. Westman, "Is dietary carbohydrate essential for human nutrition?" *Am J Clin Nutr,* 75:951–953, 2002.

[3] A.H. Manninen, "Metabolic effects of the very-low-carbohydrate diets: misunderstood "villains" of human metabolism." *Journal of the International Society of Sports Nutrition*, 1(2):7-11, 2004.

[4] E.C. Westman, "Is dietary carbohydrate essential for human nutrition?" *Am J Clin Nutr,* 75:951–953, 2002.

[5] T.K. Young, M.E. Moffatt, J.D. O'Neil, "Cardiovascular diseases in a Canadian Arctic population" *Am J Public Health,* 83:881–7, 1993.

[6] T. Liu, R.M. Howard, A.J. Mancini, W.L. Weston, A.S. Paller, B.A. Drolet et al., "Kwashiorkor in the United States. Fad diets, perceived and true milk allergy, and nutritional ignorance" *Arch Dermatol* ,137:630-6, 2001.

[7] O.W. Portman, M. Neuringer, M. Alexander, "Effects of maternal and long-term postnatal protein malnutrition on brain size and composition in rhesus monkeys" *J Nutr*, 117(11):1844-51, Nov 1987.

[8] A. Hernández, H. Burgos, M. Mondaca, R. Barra, H. Núñez, H. Pérez et al., "Effect of prenatal protein malnutrition on long-term potentiation and BDNF protein expression in the rat entorhinal cortex after neocortical and hippocampal tetanization" Neural Plast, 2008:646919, 2008.

[9] G.M. Sutton, A.V. Centanni, A.A. Butler, "Protein malnutrition during pregnancy in C57BL/6J mice results in offspring with altered circadian physiology before obesity" *Endocrinology*, 151(4):1570-80, Apr 2010.

[10] S.D. Phinney, "Ketogenic diets and physical performance" *Nutr Metab (Lond),* 2004.

[11] E. Ravussin, C. Bogardus, "A brief overview of human energy metabolism and its relationship to essential obesity" *Am J Clin Nutr,* 55:242–245, 1997.

[12] E. Jequier, "Pathways to obesity." *Int J Obes.* 12(s2):S12. doi: 10.1038/sj.ijo.0802123, 2002.

[13] G. Schaafsma, "The protein digestibility-corrected amino acid score" *Journal of Nutrition vol*: 130, issue: 7, pages: 1865S-1867S, Jul 2000.

[14] S. Gilani, D. Tomé, P. Moughan, B. Burlingame, "The assessment of amino acid digestibility in foods for humans and including a collation of published ileal amino acid digestibility data for human foods" *FAO Consensus Report*, Aug 2011.

[15] J. Boye, R. Wijesinha-Bettoni, B. Burlingame, "Protein quality evaluation twenty years after the introduction of the protein digestibility corrected amino acid score method" *Br J Nutr*, 108:S183-S211, 2012.

[16] D. Yang, Z. Liu, H. Yang et al., "Acute effects of high-protein versus normal-protein isocaloric meals on satiety and ghrelin" *European Journal of Nutrition*, 2013.

[17] A. Belza, C. Ritz, M.Q. Sørensen et al., "Contribution of gastroenteropancreatic appetite hormones to protein-induced satiety" *American Society for Nutrition*, 2013.

[18] D. J. Millward, D. K. Layman, D. Tome et al., "Protein quality assessment: impact of expanding understanding of protein and amino acid needs for optimal health" *American Journal of Clinical Nutrition* vol. 87, issue: 5, May 2008.

[19] W.A.M. Blom, A. Lluch, A. Stafleu, S. Vinoy, J.J. Holst et al., "Effect of a high-protein breakfast on the postprandial ghrelin response." *Am J Clin Nutr*, vol. 83 no. 2 211-220, February 2006.

[20] K.L. Teff, S.S. Elliott, M. Tschöp, T.J. Kieffer, D. Rader, M. Heiman, R.R. Townsend, N.L. Keim, D. D'Alessio, P.J. Havel, "Dietary fructose reduces circulating insulin and leptin, attenuates postprandial suppression of ghrelin, and increases triglycerides in women" *J Clin Endocrinol Metab*, 89:2963–2972. doi: 10.1210/jc.2003-031855, 2004.

[21] A. Shapiro, N. Tümer, Y. Gao, K.Y. Cheng, P.J. Scarpace, "Prevention and reversal of diet-induced leptin resistance with a sugar-free diet despite high fat content." *Br J Nutr*, 106(3):390-7, Aug 2011.

[22] J.Q. Purnell, D.A. Fair, "Fructose Ingestion and Cerebral, Metabolic, and Satiety Responses" *JAMA*, 309(1):85-86, 2013.

[23] N.M. Avena, P. Rada, B.G. Hoebel, "Sugar and Fat Bingeing Have Notable Differences in Addictive-like Behavior" *Journal of Nutrition*, March 1, 2009.

[24] S.H. Ahmed, K. Guillem, Y. Vandaele, "Sugar addiction: pushing the drug-sugar analogy to the limit" *Curr Opin Clin Nutr Metab Care*, 16(4):434-9, Jul 2013.

[25] J. Gormally, S. Black, S. Daston, D. Rardin, "The assessment of binge eating severity among obese persons" *Addictive Behaviors*, Volume 7, Issue 1, Pages 47–55, 1982.

[26] J. L. Sanftner, J. H. Crowther, "Variability in self-esteem, moods, shame, and guilt in women who binge" *International Journal of Eating Disorders*, Volume 23, Issue 4, pages 391–397, May 1998.

[27] C.E. Bryant, L.K. Wasse, N. Astbury, G. Nandra, J.T. McLaughlin, "Non-nutritive sweeteners: no class effect on the glycaemic or appetite responses to ingested glucose" *Eur J Clin Nutr*, Mar 2014.

[28] R.E. Steinert, F. Frey, A. Töpfer, J. Drewe, C. Beglinger, "Effects of carbohydrate sugars and artificial sweeteners on appetite and the secretion of gastrointestinal satiety peptides" *Br J Nutr*, 105(9):1320-8, May 2011.

[29] V.S. Malik, B.M. Popkin, G.A. Bray, J-P. Després, F.B. Hu, "Sugar Sweetened Beverages, Obesity, Type 2 Diabetes and Cardiovascular Disease risk" *National Institute of Health*, 121(11): 1356–1364, March 2010.

[30] E.A. Hu, A. Pan, V. Malik, Q. Sun, "White rice consumption and risk of type 2 diabetes: meta-analysis and systematic review" *BMJ*, 344:e1454, 2012.

[31] H. Beck-Nielsen, O. Pedersen, H.O. Lindskov, "Impaired cellular insulin binding and insulin sensitivity induced by high-fructose feeding in normal subjects" *Am J Clin Nutr*, 33(2):273-8, Feb 1980.

[32] S.K. Fried, S.P. Rao, "Sugars, hypertriglyceridemia, and cardiovascular disease" *Am J Clin Nutr*, vol. 78 no. 4 873S-880S, October 2003.

[33] S. Sen, B.K. Kundu, H.C-J. Wu, S.S. Hashmi, P. Guthrie, L.W. Locke et al., " Glucose Regulation of Load-Induced mTOR Signaling and ER Stress in Mammalian Heart" *J Am Heart Assoc*, 2: e004796, 2013.

[34] D.J. Jenkins, T.M. Wolever, R.H. Taylor, H. Barker et al., "Glycemic index of foods: a physiological basis for carbohydrate exchange" *Am J Clin Nutr*, vol. 34 no. 3 362-366, March 1981.

[35] F.S. Atkinson, K. Foster-Powell, J.C. Brand-Miller, "International tables of glycemic index and glycemic load values: 2008" *Diabetes Care*. 31:2281–2283, 2008.

[36] K. Foster-Powell, S.H.A Holt, J.C. Brand-Miller, "International table of glycemic index and glycemic load values: 2002" *Am J Clin Nutr*, vol. 76 no. 1 5-56, January 2002.

[37] A. Fasano, I. Berti, T. Gerarduzzi et al., "Prevalence of Celiac disease in at-risk and not-at-risk groups in the United States: a large multicenter study" *Archives of Internal Medicine*, vol. 163, no. 3, 2003.

[38] Rewers M, "Epidemiology of celiac disease: what are the prevalence, incidence, and progression of celiac disease?" *Gastroenterology* 128, 2005.

[39] "Q & A with Alessio Fasano, MD" Retrieved 22 September 2013 < http://www.livingwithout.com/issues/4_15/qa_augsep11-2554-1.html>

[40] W. T. Hu, J.A. Murray, M.C. Greenaway, J.E. Parisi, K.A. Josephs, "Cognitive impairment and celiac disease" *Arch Neurol*, 63(10):1440-6, Oct 2006.

[41] A. Sapone, K. M. Lammers, V. Casolaro et al., "Divergence of gut permeability and mucosal immune gene expression in two gluten-associated conditions: celiac disease and gluten sensitivity" *BMC Medicine*, vol. 9, article 23, 2011.

[42] W.C. Willett, R.L. Leibel, "Dietary fat is not a major determinant of body fat" *Am J Med*,113(Suppl):47S–59S, 2002.

[43] "Swedish Expert Committee: A Low-Carb Diet Most Effective for Weight Loss" Retrieved 3 January 2014 <http://www.dietdoctor.com/swedish-expert-committee-low-carb-diet-effective-weight-loss>

[44] A.R. Skov, S. Toubro, B. Rùnn, L. Holm, A Astrup, "Randomized trial on protein vs carbohydrate in ad libitum fat reduced diet for the treatment of obesity" International Journal of Obesity, 23, 528±536, 1999.

[45] P.M. Kris-Etherton, "Monounsaturated Fatty Acids and Risk of Cardiovascular Disease" *AHA*, 100: 1253-1258, 1999.

[46] F. Pérez-Jiménez, J. López-Miranda, P. Mata, "Protective effect of dietary monounsaturated fat on arteriosclerosis: beyond cholesterol" *Atherosclerosis*, 163(2):385-98, Aug 2002.

[47] J.E. Kinsella, B. Lokesh, R.A. Stone, "Dietary n-3 polyunsaturated fatty acids and amelioration of cardiovascular disease: possible mechanisms" *Am J Clin Nutr*, 52(1):1-28, Jul 1990.

[48] R. Wall, R.P. Ross, G.F. Fitzgerald, C. Stanton, "Fatty acids from fish: the anti-inflammatory potential of long-chain omega-3 fatty acids" *Nutr Rev*, 68(5):280-9, May 2010.

[49] J.R. Hibbeln, L.R. Nieminen, T.L. Blasbalg, J.A. Riggs, W.E. Lands, "Healthy intakes of n-3 and n-6 fatty acids: estimations considering worldwide diversity" *Am J Clin Nutr*, 83(6 Suppl):1483S-1493S, Jun 2006.

[50] A.M. Rees, M.P. Austin, G. Parker, "Role of omega-3 fatty acids as a treatment for depression in the perinatal period" *Aust N Z J Psychiatry*, 39(4):274-80, Apr 2005.

[51] W.J. Pasman, J. Heimerikx, C.M. Rubingh, R. van den Berg, M. O'Shea, L. Gambelli et al., "The effect of Korean pine nut oil on in vitro CCK release, on appetite sensations and on gut hormones in post-menopausal overweight women" *Lipids Health Dis*, 7:10, 20 Mar 2008.

[52] L. Hooper, C.D. Summerbell, R. Thompson, D. Sills, F.G. Roberts, H. Moore, G. Davey Smith, "Reduced or modified dietary fat for preventing cardiovascular disease" *Cochrane Database Syst Rev*, (7):CD002137, Jul 2011.

[53] R. Chowdhury, S. Warnakula, S. Kunutsor, F. Crowe et al., "Association of Dietary, Circulating, and Supplement Fatty Acids With Coronary Risk: A Systematic Review and Meta-analysis" *Ann Intern Med*, 160(6):398-406, Mar 2014.

[54] J.E. Hunter, J. Zhang, P.M. Kris-Etherton, "Cardiovascular disease risk of dietary stearic acid compared with trans, other saturated, and unsaturated fatty acids: a systematic review" *Am J Clin Nutr*, 91(1):46-63, Jan 2010.

[55] A. Ascherio, C.H. Hennekens, J.E. Buring, C. Master, M.J. Stampfer, W.C. Willett, "Trans-fatty acids intake and risk of myocardial infarction" *Department of Nutrition, Harvard School of Public Health*, 89(1):94-101, Jan 1994.

[56] D. Mozaffarian, T. Pischon, S.E. Hankinson, N. Rifai, K. Joshipura, W.C. Willett, E.B. Rimm, "Dietary intake of trans fatty acids and systemic inflammation in women" *Am J Clin Nutr*, 79(4):606-12, Apr 2004.

[57] L.A. Bazzano, T. Hu, K. Reynolds, L. Yao et al., "Effects of Low-Carbohydrate and Low-Fat Diets: A Randomized Trial" *Ann Intern Med*, 161(5):309-318, Sept 2014.

[58] P.M. Kris-Etherton, D.S. Taylor, S. Yu-Poth, P. Huth, K. Moriarty, V. Fishell, R.L. Hargrove, G. Zhao, T.D. Etherton, "Polyunsaturated fatty acids in the food chain in the United States" *Am J Clin Nutr*, 71(1 Suppl):179S-88S, Jan 2000.

[59] A.P. Simopoulos, "Evolutionary aspects of diet, essential fatty acids and cardiovascular disease" *European Heart Journal Supplements*, 3 (Supplement D), D8–D21, 2001.

[60] S. Yehuda, S. Rabinovitz, D.I. Mostofsky, "Mixture of essential fatty acids lowers test anxiety" *Nutr Neurosci*, 8(4):265-7, Aug 2005.

[61] H. Gerster, "Can adults adequately convert alpha-linolenic acid (18:3n-3) to eicosapentaenoic acid (20:5n-3) and docosahexaenoic acid (22:6n-3)?" *Int J Vitam Nutr Res*, 68(3):159-73, 1998.

[62] M. Huan, K. Hamazaki, Y. Sun, M. Itomura, H. Liu, W. Kang, S. Watanabe, K. Terasawa, T. Hamazaki, "Suicide attempt and n-3 fatty acid levels in red blood cells: a case control study in China" *Biol Psychiatry*, 56(7):490-6, Oct 2004.

[63] C. Song, S. Zhao, "Omega-3 fatty acid eicosapentaenoic acid. A new treatment for psychiatric and neurodegenerative diseases: a review of clinical investigations" *Expert Opin Investig Drugs*, 16(10):1627-38, Oct 2007.

[64] I.A. Shaikh, I. Brown, A.C. Schofield, K.W. Wahle, S.D. Heys, "Docosahexaenoic acid enhances the efficacy of docetaxel in prostate cancer cells by modulation of apoptosis: the role of genes associated with the NF-kappaB pathway" *Prostate*, 68(15):1635-46, Nov 2008.

[65] K. Yurko-Mauro, D. McCarthy, D. Rom, E.B. Nelson, A.S. Ryan, A. Blackwell, N. Salem Jr., M. Stedman, "Beneficial effects of docosahexaenoic acid on cognition in age-related cognitive decline" *Alzheimer's & Dementia: The Journal of the Alzheimer's Association* Volume 6, Issue 6, Pages 456-464, November 2010.

[66] D.S. Kelley, D. Siegel, D.M. Fedor, Y. Adkins, B.E. Mackey, "DHA supplementation decreases serum C-reactive protein and other markers of inflammation in hypertriglyceridemic men" *J Nutr*, 139(3):495-501, Jan 2009.

[67] N. Sinn, J. Bryan, "Effect of supplementation with polyunsaturated fatty acids and micronutrients on learning and behavior problems associated with child ADHD" *J Dev Behav Pediatr*, 28(2):82-91, Apr 2007.

[68] S.C. Cunnane, M.J. Anderson, "Pure linoleate deficiency in the rat: influence on growth, accumulation of n-6 polyunsaturates, and [1-14C]linoleate oxidation" *J Lipid Res*, 38(4):805-12, Apr 1997.

[69] B. Bistrian, "Systemic response to inflammation" *Nutr Rev*, 65(12 Pt 2):S170-2, Dec 2007.

[70] Y. Jin, X. Cui, U.P. Singh, A.A. Chumanevich, B. Harmon, P. Cavicchia, A.B. Hofseth et al., "Systemic inflammatory load in humans is suppressed by consumption of two formulations of dried, encapsulated juice concentrate." *Mol Nutr Food Res*, 54(10):1506-14. doi: 10.1002/mnfr.200900579, Oct 2010.

[71] P. Libby, P.M. Ridker, A. Maseri, "Inflammation and Atherosclerosis" *J Am Heart Assoc*, 105: 1135-1143, 2002.

[72] J.C. Maroon, J.W. Bost, "Omega-3 fatty acids (fish oil) as an anti-inflammatory: an alternative to nonsteroidal anti-inflammatory drugs for discogenic pain" *Surg Neurol*, 65(4):326-31, Apr 2006.

[73] Retrieved 8 December 2013 <http://nutritiondata.self.com>

[74] "Nutrition Facts and Analysis for Moose, meat, raw (Alaska Native)" Retrieved 20 July 2014 <http://nutritiondata.self.com/facts/ethnic-foods/9967/2>

[75] A. Kozimor, H. Chang, J.A. Cooper, "Effects of dietary fatty acid composition from a high fat meal on satiety" *Appetite*, 69:39-45, Oct 2013.

[76] L.A. Gonder-Frederick, D.J. Cox, S.A. Bobbitt, J.W. Pennebaker, "Mood changes associated with blood glucose fluctuations in insulin-dependent diabetes mellitus" *Health Psychol*, 8(1):45-59, 1989.

[77] G. Dimitriadis, P. Mitrou, V. Lambadiari, E. Maratou, S.A. Raptis, "Insulin effects in muscle and adipose tissue" *Diabetes Res Clin Pract*, 93 Suppl 1:S52-9, Aug 2011.

[78] J. Slavin, H. Green, "Dietary fibre and satiety" *British Nutrition Foundation*, Vol 32, Issue Sup s1, Mar 2007.

Appendices - References

[79] D.J. Baer, W.V. Rumpler, C.W. Miles, G.C. Fahey, "Dietary Fiber Decreases the Metabolizable Energy Content and Nutrient Digestibility of Mixed Diets Fed to Humans" *J. Nutr*, vol. 127 no. 4 579-586, Apr 1997.

[80] L. Brown, B. Rosner, W.W. Willett, F.M. Sacks, "Cholesterol-lowering effects of dietary fiber: a meta-analysis" *Am J Clin Nutr*, vol. 69 no. 1 30-42, Jan 1999.

[81] P. Gunness, M.J. Gidley, "Mechanisms underlying the cholesterol-lowering properties of soluble dietary fibre polysaccharides" *Food Funct*, 1(2):149-55, Nov 2010.

[82] E. Hijova, A. Chmelarova, "Short chain fatty acids and colonic health" *Bratislava Medical Journal*, 108(8):354-8, 2007.

[83] S. Lewis, K. Heaton, "Increasing butyrate concentration in the distal colon by accelerating intestinal transit" *Gut*, 41(2): 245–251, Aug 1997.

[84] A.D. Markland, O. Palsson, P.S. Goode, K.L. Burgio, J. Busby-Whitehead, W.E. Whitehead, "Association of Low Dietary Intake of Fiber and Liquids with Constipation: Evidence from the National Health and Nutrition Examination Survey (NHANES)" *Am J Gastroenterol*, 108(5): 796–803, May 2013.

[85] K.S. Ho, C. You Mei Tan, M.A.M. Daud, F. Seow-Choen, "Stopping or reducing dietary fiber intake reduces constipation and its associated symptoms" *World J Gastroenterol*, 18(33): 4593–4596, Sept 2012.

[86] G.R. Gibson, A.L. McCartney, R.A. Rastall, "Prebiotics and resistance to gastrointestinal infections" *British Nutrition Foundation*, 93 Suppl 1:S31-4, Apr 2005.

[87] M. Roberfroid, "Prebiotics: the concept revisited" *Journal of Nutrition*, 137(3 Suppl 2):830S-7S, Mar 2007.

[88] "Chart of high-fiber foods" Retrieved 17 November 2013 <http://www.mayoclinic.com/health/high-fiber-foods/NU00582>

[89] J.B. Keogh, C.W. Lau, M. Noakes, J. Bowen, P.M. Clifton, "Effects of meals with high soluble fibre, high amylose barley variant on glucose, insulin, satiety and thermic effect of food in healthy lean women" *European Journal of Clinical Nutrition*, 2007.

[90] D. Bracco, J.M. Ferrarra, M.J. Arnaud, E. Jequier, Y. Schutz, "Effects of caffeine on energy metabolism, heart rate, and methylxanthine metabolism in lean and obese women" *American Journal of Physiology - Endocrinology and Metabolism*, Vol. 269no. E671-E678, October 1995.

[91] A.P. Winston, E. Hardwick, N. Jaber, "Neuropsychiatric effects of caffeine" *Advances in Psychiatric Treatment*, 11: 432-439, 2005.

[92] "Nutrient Reference Values for Australia and New Zealand" *Department of Health and Ageing National Health and Medical Research Council*, published online, 9 September 2005.

[93] M. Dietrich, C.J. Brown, G. Block, "The effect of folate fortification of cereal-grain products on blood folate status, dietary folate intake, and dietary folate sources among adult non-supplement users in the United States" *J Am Coll Nutr*, 24(4):266-74, Aug 2005.

[94] S.B. Lotito, B. Frei, "Consumption of flavonoid-rich foods and increased plasma antioxidant capacity in humans: cause, consequence, or epiphenomenon?" *Free Radic Biol Med*, 41(12):1727-46, Dec 2006.

[95] Kappagoda C, Hyson et al., "Low-carbohydrate-high-protein diets: is there a place for them in clinical cardiology?" *Journal of the American College of Cardiology*, 2003.

[96] P.J. Geiselman, C. Martin, S. Coulon, D. Ryan, M. Apperson, "Effects of chewing gum on specific macronutrient and total caloric intake in an afternoon snack" *FASEB J*, 23 (Meeting Abstract Supplement) 101.3, April 2009.

[97] O. Oyebode, V. Gordon-Dseagu, A. Walker, J.S. Mindell, "Fruit and vegetable consumption and all-cause, cancer and CVD mortality: analysis of Health Survey for England data" *J Epidemiol Community Health*, doi:10.1136/jech-2013-203500, March 2014.

[98] H. Valtin, ""Drink at least eight glasses of water a day." Really? Is there scientific evidence for "8 x 8"?" *Am J Physiol Regul Integr Comp Physiol*, 283(5):R993-1004, Nov 2002.

[99] "Aspartame" Retrieved 22 March 2014 <
http://www.cancer.org/cancer/cancercauses/othercarcinogens/athome/aspartame>

[100] "Chemical Summary for Acetaldehyde" Retrieved 12 January 2014
<http://www.epa.gov/chemfact/s_acetal.txt>

[101] "Tax and regulate sugar like alcohol and tobacco, urge scientists" Retrieved 2 August 2014 <
http://www.theguardian.com/science/2012/feb/01/tax-regulate-sugar-alcohol-tobacco>

[102] K.A. Ly, P. Milgrom, M. Rothen, "Xylitol, sweeteners, and dental caries." *Pediatr Dent*, 28(2):154-63; discussion 192-8, Mar-Apr 2006.

[103] Y.S. Chung, M. Lee, "Genotoxicity Assessment of Erythritol by Using Short-term Assay" *Toxicol Res*, 29(4):249-55, Dec 2013.

[104] E. Arrigoni, F. Brouns, R. Amadò, "Human gut microbiota does not ferment erythritol" *Br J Nutr*, 94(5):643-6, Nov 2005.

[105] "Microwave cooking and nutrition" Retrieved 2 August 2014
<http://www.health.harvard.edu/fhg/updates/Microwave-cooking-and-nutrition.shtml>

[106] A. Keys, F. Grande, "Role of dietary fat in human nutrition. III. Diet and the epidemiology of coronary heart disease" *AmJ Public Health Nations Health*, 47:1520-1530, 1957.

[107] M.U. Jakobsen, C. Dethlefsen, A.M. Joensen, J. Stegger, A. Tjønneland, E.B. Schmidt, K. Overvad, "Intake of carbohydrates compared with intake of saturated fatty acids and risk of myocardial infarction: importance of the glycemic index" *Am J Clin Nutr*, 91(6):1764-8, Jun 2010.

[108] P.W. Siri-Tarino, Q.S., F.B. Hu, R.M. Krauss, "Meta-analysis of prospective cohort studies evaluating the association of saturated fat with cardiovascular disease" *Am J Clin Nutr*. ajcn.27725, January 2010.

[109] R. Micha, S.K. Wallace, D. Mozaffarian, "Red and processed meat consumption and risk of incident coronary heart disease, stroke, and diabetes mellitus: a systematic review and meta-analysis" *AHA Circulation*, 121(21):2271-83, Jun 2010.

[110] G. Mutungi, J. Ratliff, M. Puglisi, M. Torres-Gonzalez et al., "Dietary Cholesterol from Eggs Increases Plasma HDL Cholesterol in Overweight Men Consuming a Carbohydrate-Restricted Diet" *J. Nutr*, vol. 138 no. 2 272-276, February 2008.

[111] A. Parry-Strong, M. Leikis, J.D. Krebs, "High protein diets and renal disease – is there a relationship in people with type 2 diabetes?" *British Journal of Diabetes & Vascular Disease*, vol. 13 no. 5-6 238-243, October/December 2013.

[112] W.F. Martin, L.E. Armstrong, N.R. Rodriguez, "Dietary protein intake and renal function" *Nutr Metab (Lond)*, 2:25, Sep 2005.

[113] T.P. Wycherley, M. Noakes, P.M. Clifton et al., "A High-Protein Diet With Resistance Exercise Training Improves Weight Loss and Body Composition in Overweight and Obese Patients With Type 2 Diabetes" *Diabetes Care*, vol. 33 no. 5 969-976, May 2010.

[114] J. Calvez, N. Poupin, C. Chesneau, C. Lassale, D. Tomé, "Protein intake, calcium balance and health consequences" *Eur J Clin Nutr*, 66(3):281-95, Mar 2012.

[115] K.S. Stote, D.J. Baer, K. Spears, D.R. Paul, G.K. Harris, W.V. Rumpler et al., "A controlled trial of reduced meal frequency without caloric restriction in healthy, normal-weight, middle-aged adults" *Am J Clin Nutr*, 85(4):981-8, Apr 2007.

[116] K. Ohkawara, M.A. Cornier, W.M. Kohrt, E.L. Melanson, "Effects of increased meal frequency on fat oxidation and perceived hunger" *Obesity (Silver Spring)*, 21(2):336-43, Feb 2013.

[117] J.D. Cameron, M.J. Cyr, E. Doucet, "Increased meal frequency does not promote greater weight loss in subjects who were prescribed an 8-week equi-energetic energy-restricted diet" *Br J Nutr*, 103(8):1098-101, Apr 2010.

[118] W.P. Verboeket-van de Venne, K.R. Westerterp, "Frequency of feeding, weight reduction and energy metabolism" *Int J Obes Relat Metab Disord*, 17(1):31-6, Jan 1993.

[119] F. Bellisle, R. McDevitt, A.M. Prentice, "Meal frequency and energy balance" *Br J Nutr*, 77 Suppl 1:S57-70, Apr 1997.

[120] M.E. Gluck, C.A. Venti, A.D. Salbe, J. Krakoff, "Nighttime eating: commonly observed and related to weight gain in an inpatient food intake study" *Am J Clin Nutr*, vol. 88 no. 4 900-905, October 2008.

[121] A. Pascual-Leone, A. Amedi, F. Fregni, L.B. Merabet, "The plastic human brain cortex" *Annu Rev Neurosci*, 28:377-401, 2005.

[122] A. Pascual-Leone, C. Freitas, L. Oberman, J.C. Horvath, M. Halko, M. Eldaief, S. Bashir et al., "Characterizing Brain Cortical Plasticity and Network Dynamics Across the Age-Span in Health and Disease with TMS-EEG and TMS-fMRI" *Brain Topography*, Volume 24, Issue 3-4, pp 302-315, Oct 2011.

[123] J.S. O'Brien, E.L. Sampson, "Lipid composition of the normal human brain: gray matter, white matter, and myelin" *J Lipid Res*, 6(4):537-44, Oct 1965.

[124] A. Keys, "Atherosclerosis: a problem in newer public health" *J Mt Sinai Hosp N Y*, 20(2):118-39, Jul-Aug 1953.

[125] M. Sarchiapone, A. Roy, G. Camardese, S. De Risio, "Further evidence for low serum cholesterol and suicidal behaviour" *J Affect Disord*, 61(1-2):69-71, Dec 2000.

[126] R. Manfredini, S. Caracciolo, R. Salmi, B. Boari, A. Tomelli, M. Gallerani, "The Association of Low Serum Cholesterol with Depression and Suicidal Behaviours: New Hypotheses for the Missing Link" *Journal of International Medical Research*, vol. 28 no. 6 247-257, December 2000.

[127] H. Engelberg, "Low serum cholesterol and suicide" *Lancet*, 339(8795):727-9, Mar 1992.

[128] R.K. McNamara, "Long-chain omega-3 fatty acid deficiency in mood disorders: rationale for treatment and prevention" *Curr Drug Discov Technol*, 10(3):233-44, Sep 2013.

[129] K.M. Appleton, P.J. Rogers, A.R. Ness, "Updated systematic review and meta-analysis of the effects of n–3 long-chain polyunsaturated fatty acids on depressed mood" *Am J Clin Nutr*, vol. 91 no. 3 757-770, March 2010.

[130] J.D. Fernstrom, R.J. Wurtman, "Brain serotonin content: increase following ingestion of carbohydrate diet" *Science*, 174(4013):1023-5, Dec 1971.

[131] R.J. Wurtman, J.J. Wurtman, "Brain serotonin, carbohydrate-craving, obesity and depression" *Obes Res*, 3 Suppl 4:477S-480S, Nov 1995.

[132] B. Smolin, E. Klein, Y. Levy, D. Ben-Shachar, "Major depression as a disorder of serotonin resistance: inference from diabetes mellitus type II" *Int J Neuropsychopharmacol*, 10(6):839-50, Dec 2007.

[133] C.D. Fiorillo, P.N. Tobler, W. Schultz, "Discrete coding of reward probability and uncertainty by dopamine neurons" *Science*, 299(5614):1898-902, Mar 2003.

[134] D.O. Hebb, "The Organization of Behavior" *Wiley & Sons*, 1949.

[135] S. Bao, E.F. Chang, J. Woods, M.M. Merzenich, "Temporal plasticity in the primary auditory cortex induced by operant perceptual learning" *Nat Neurosci*, 7(9):974-81, Sep 2004.

[136] J.A. Ribeiro, A.M. Sebastião, "Caffeine and adenosine" *J Alzheimers Dis*, 20 Suppl 1:S3-15, 2010.

[137] M. Van Soeren, T. Mohr, M. Kjaer, T.E. Graham, "Acute effects of caffeine ingestion at rest in humans with impaired epinephrine responses" *J Appl Physiol*, 80(3):999-1005, Mar 1996.

[138] C. Drake, T. Roehrs, J. Shambroom, T. Roth, "Caffeine effects on sleep taken 0, 3, or 6 hours before going to bed" *J Clin Sleep Med*, 9(11):1195-200, Nov 2013.

[139] P.W. Andrews, J.A. Thomson, A. Amstadter, M.C. Neale, "Primum non nocere: an evolutionary analysis of whether antidepressants do more harm than good" *Front Psychol*, 3:117, April 2012.

[140] R.V. Considine, M.K. Sinha, M.L. Heiman, A. Kriauciunaset et al., "Serum immunoreactive-leptin concentrations in normal-weight and obese humans" *N Engl J Med*, 334(5):292-5, Feb 1996.

[141] P.J. Enriori, A.E. Evans, P. Sinnayah, E.E. Jobst et al., "Diet-Induced Obesity Causes Severe but Reversible Leptin Resistance in Arcuate Melanocortin Neurons" *Cell Metabolism*, Volume 5, Issue 3, Pages 181–194, 7 March 2007.

[142] J. Altman, "Are new neurons formed in the brains of adult mammals?" *Science*, 135(3509):1127-8, Mar 1962.

[143] L.R. Squire, J.T. Wixted, "The cognitive neuroscience of human memory since H.M." *Annu Rev Neurosci*, 34:259-88, 2011.

[144] E. Castrén, T. Rantamäki, "The role of BDNF and its receptors in depression and antidepressant drug action: Reactivation of developmental plasticity" *Dev Neurobiol*, 70(5):289-97, Apr 2010.

[145] G. Issa, C. Wilson, A.V. Terry Jr, A. Pillai, "An inverse relationship between cortisol and BDNF levels in schizophrenia: data from human postmortem and animal studies" *Neurobiol Dis*, 39(3):327-33, Sep 2010.

[146] C.W. Cotman, N.C. Berchtold, "Exercise: a behavioral intervention to enhance brain health and plasticity" *Trends Neurosci*, 25(6):295-301, Jun 2002.

[147] R. Molteni, R.J. Barnard, Z. Ying, C.K. Roberts, F. Gómez-Pinilla, "A high-fat, refined sugar diet reduces hippocampal brain-derived neurotrophic factor, neuronal plasticity, and learning" *Neuroscience*, 112(4):803-14, 2002.

[148] R. Staats, P. Stoll, D. Zingler, J.C. Virchow, M. Lommatzsch, "Regulation of brain-derived neurotrophic factor (BDNF) during sleep apnoea treatment" *Thorax*, 60(8):688-92, Aug 2005.

[149] V. Kazlauckas, N. Pagnussat, S. Mioranzza, E. Kalinine, F. Nunes et al., "Enriched environment effects on behavior, memory and BDNF in low and high exploratory mice" *Physiol Behav*, 102(5):475-80, Mar 2011.

[150] R. Huber, G. Tononi, C. Cirelli, "Exploratory behavior, cortical BDNF expression, and sleep homeostasis" *Sleep*, 30(2):129-39, Feb 2007.

[151] E.H. Kossoff, B.A. Zupec-Kania, P.E. Amark, K.R. Ballaban-Gil, A.G. Christina Bergqvis, R. Blackford, J.R. Buchhalter et al., "Optimal clinical management of children receiving the ketogenic diet: recommendations of the International Ketogenic Diet Study Group" *Epilepsia*, 50(2):304-17, Feb 2009.

[152] L.M. Juliano, D.P. Evatt, B.D. Richards, R.R. Griffiths, "Characterization of individuals seeking treatment for caffeine dependence" *Psychol Addict Behav*, 26(4):948-54, Dec 2012.

[153] C.H.S. Ruxton, "The impact of caffeine on mood, cognitive function, performance and hydration: a review of benefits and risks" *Nutrition Bulletin*, Volume 33, Issue 1, pages 15–25, March 2008.

[154] S. van Dieren, C.S. Uiterwaal, Y.T. van der Schouw et al., "Coffee and tea consumption and risk of type 2 diabetes" *Diabetologia*, 52(12):2561-9, Dec 2009.

[155] L. Maia, A. De Mendonça, "Does caffeine intake protect from Alzheimer's disease?" *European Journal of Neurology*, Volume 9, Issue 4, pages 377–382, July 2002.

[156] G. Hu, S. Bidel, P. Jousilahti, R. Antikainen, J. Tuomilehto, "Coffee and tea consumption and the risk of Parkinson's disease" *Movement Disorders*, Volume 22, Issue 15, pages 2242–2248, 15 November 2007.

[157] E. Lopez-Garcia, R.M. van Dam, T.Y. Li, F. Rodriguez-Artalejo, F.B. Hu, "The relationship of coffee consumption with mortality" *Ann Intern Med*, 148(12):904-14, Jun 2008.

[158] T.M. Heffernan, "The impact of excessive alcohol use on prospective memory: a brief review" *Curr Drug Abuse Rev*, 1(1):36-41, Jan 2008.

[159] J.M. Chignon, M.J. Cortes, P. Martin, J.P. Chabannes, "Attempted suicide and alcohol dependence: results of an epidemiologic survey" *Encephale*, 24(4):347-54, Jul-Aug 1998.

[160] A.P. Majumdar, S. Banerjee, J. Nautiyal, B.B. Patel et al., "Curcumin synergizes with resveratrol to inhibit colon cancer" *Nutr Cancer*, 61(4):544-53, 2009.

[161] R.D. Semba, L. Ferrucci, B. Bartali, M. Urpí-Sarda et al., "Resveratrol Levels and All-Cause Mortality in Older Community-Dwelling Adults" *JAMA Intern Med*, Published online, May 2014.

[162] D. Di Majo, M. La Guardia, S. Giammanco, L. La Neve, M. Giammanco, "The antioxidant capacity of red wine in relationship with its polyphenolic constituents" *Food Chemistry*, 111, 45–49, 2008.

[163] C. Manach, A. Scalbert, C. Morand, C. Rémésy, L. Jiménez, "Polyphenols: food sources and bioavailability" *Am J Clin Nutr*, vol. 79 no. 5 727-747, May 2004.

[164] M.L. Burr, P.A. Ashfield-Watt, F.D. Dunstan, A.M. Fehily et al., "Lack of benefit of dietary advice to men with angina: results of a controlled trial" *Eur J Clin Nutr*, 57(2):193-200, Feb 2003.

[165] C. Poly, J.M. Massaro, S. Seshadri, P.A. Wolf, E. Cho, E. Krall, P.F. Jacques, R. Au, "The relation of dietary choline to cognitive performance and white-matter hyperintensity in the Framingham Offspring Cohort" *Am J Clin Nutr*, vol. 94 no. 6 1584-1591, December 2011.

[166] J. Moore, "Effects of Subcutaneous Postnatal Choline Supplementation on Hippocampus-Mediated Learning and Memory in Rat Pups" *Electronic Thesis or Dissertation. Wright State University*, OhioLINK Electronic Theses and Dissertations Center, 2008.

[167] M.J. Glenn, E.M. Gibson, E.D. Kirby, T.J. Mellott, J.K. Blusztajn, C.L. Williams, "Prenatal choline availability modulates hippocampal neurogenesis and neurogenic responses to enriching experiences in adult female rats" *Eur J Neurosci*, 25(8):2473-82, Apr 2007.

[168] K. Kimura et al., "L-Theanine reduces psychological and physiological stress responses" *Biol Psychol*, 74(1):39-45. Epub, Jan 2007.

[169] C. Miodownik, R. Maayan, Y. Ratner, V. Lerner, L. Pintov, M. Mar, A. Weizman, M.S. Ritsner, "Serum levels of brain-derived neurotrophic factor and cortisol to sulfate of dehydroepiandrosterone molar ratio associated with clinical response to L-theanine as augmentation of antipsychotic therapy in schizophrenia and schizoaffective disorder patients" *Clin Neuropharmacol*, 34(4):155-60, Jul-Aug 2011.

[170] J.F. Bukowski, S.S. Percival, "L-theanine intervention enhances human gammadeltaT lymphocyte function," *Nutr Rev*, 66(2):96-102, Feb 2008.

[171] K. Kimura, M. Ozeki, L.R. Juneja, H. Ohira, "L-Theanine reduces psychological and physiological stress responses" *Biol Psychol*, 74(1):39-45, Jan 2007.

[172] S.P. Kelly, M. Gomez-Ramirez, J.L. Montesi, J.J. Foxe, "L-theanine and caffeine in combination affect human cognition as evidenced by oscillatory alpha-band activity and attention task performance" *J Nutr*, 138(8):1572S-1577S, Aug 2008.

[173] G.N. Owen, H. Parnell, E.A. De Bruin, J.A. Rycroft, "The combined effects of L-theanine and caffeine on cognitive performance and mood" *Nutr Neurosci*, 11(4):193-8, Aug 2008.

[174] J. Bryan, "Psychological effects of dietary components of tea: caffeine and L-theanine" *Nutr Rev*, 66(2):82-90, Feb 2008.

[175] C.F. Haskell, D.O. Kennedy, A.L. Milne, K.A. Wesnes, A.B. Scholey, "The effects of L-theanine, caffeine and their combination on cognition and mood" *Biol Psychol*, 77(2):113-22, Feb 2008.

[176] S.B. Chapman, S. Aslan, J.S. Spence, L.F. Defina, M.W. Keebler, N. Didehbani, H. Lu, "Shorter term aerobic exercise improves brain, cognition, and cardiovascular fitness in aging" *Front Aging Neurosci*, 5:75, Nov 2013.

[177] A. Ströhle, "Physical activity, exercise, depression and anxiety disorders" *J Neural Transm*, 116(6):777-84, Jun 2009.

[178] S.J. Colcombe, K.I. Erickson, P.E. Scalf, J.S. Kim, R. Prakash et al., "Aerobic exercise training increases brain volume in aging humans" *J Gerontol A Biol Sci Med Sci*, 61(11):1166-70, Nov 2006.

[179] R.C. Cassilhas, K.S. Lee, J. Fernandes, M.G. Oliveira, S. Tufik, R. Meeusen, M.T. de Mello, "Spatial memory is improved by aerobic and resistance exercise through divergent molecular mechanisms" *Neuroscience*, 202:309-17, Jan 2012.

[180] R. Meeusen, P. Watson, H. Hasegawa, B. Roelands, M.F. Piacentini, "Brain neurotransmitters in fatigue and overtraining" *Appl Physiol Nutr Metab*, 32(5):857-64, Oct 2007.

[181] W.D. Killgore, "Effects of sleep deprivation on cognition" *Prog Brain Res*, 185:105-29, 2010.

[182] R. Leproult, G. Copinschi, O. Buxton, E. Van Cauter, "Sleep loss results in an elevation of cortisol levels the next evening" *Sleep*, 20(10):865-70, Oct 1997.

[183] S.M. Greer, A.N. Goldstein, M.P. Walker, "The impact of sleep deprivation on food desire in the human brain" *Nature Communications*, Article number: 2259, August 2013.

[184] H.P. Landolt, C. Roth, D.J. Dijk, A.A. Borbély, "Late-afternoon ethanol intake affects nocturnal sleep and the sleep EEG in middle-aged men" *J Clin Psychopharmacol*, 16(6):428-36, Dec 1996.

[185] T.A. Bedrosian, Z.M. Weil, R.J. Nelson, "Chronic dim light at night provokes reversible depression-like phenotype: possible role for TNF" *Molecular Psychiatry*, 18, 930-936, August 2013.

[186] A.M. Holbrook, R. Crowther, A. Lotter, C. Cheng, D. King, "Meta-analysis of benzodiazepine use in the treatment of insomnia" *CMAJ*, 162(2): 225–233, Jan 2000.

[187] M.M. Savić, D.I. Obradović, N.D. Ugrešić, D.R. Bokonjić3, "Memory Effects of Benzodiazepines: Memory Stages and Types Versus Binding-Site Subtypes" *Neural Plast*, 12(4): 289–298, 2005.

[188] S. Banks, D.F. Dinges, "Behavioral and Physiological Consequences of Sleep Restriction" *J Clin Sleep Med*, 3(5): 519–528, August 2007.

[189] M.L. Dansinger, J.A. Gleason, J.L. Griffith, H.P. Selker, E.J. Schaefer, "Comparison of the Atkins, Ornish, Weight Watchers, and Zone Diets for Weight Loss and Heart Disease Risk Reduction" *JAMA*, 293(1):43-53, 2005.

[190] M.T. McAuley, R.A. Kenny, T.B. Kirkwood, D.J. Wilkinson, J.J. Jones, V.M. Miller VM, "A mathematical model of aging-related and cortisol induced hippocampal dysfunction" *BMC Neurosci*, 10:26, Mar 2009.

[191] F. Marmigère, L. Givalois, F. Rage, S. Arancibia, L. Tapia-Arancibia, "Rapid induction of BDNF expression in the hippocampus during immobilization stress challenge in adult rats" *Hippocampus*, 13(5):646-55, 2003.

[192] A.S. Masten, J.J. Cutuli, J.E. Herbers, M.J. Reed, "Resilience in Development" *The Oxford Handbook of Positive Psychology, Second Edition*, 117-131, 2011.

[193] G. Oettingen, T.A. Wadden, "Expectation, fantasy, and weight loss: Is the impact of positive thinking always positive?" *Cognitive Therapy and Research*, 15, 167–175, 1991.

[194] G. Oettingen, "Expectancy effects on behavior depend on self-regulatory thought" *Social Cognition*, Vol. 18, No. 2, pp. 101-129, 2000.

[195] H.B. Kappes, G. Oettingen, "Positive fantasies about idealized futures sap energy" *Journal of Experimental Social Psychology*, 47, 719–729, 2011.

[196] I. Marks, "Exposure therapy for phobias and obsessive-compulsive disorders" *Hosp Pract*, 14(2):101-8, Feb 1979.

[197] R. Coutts, "Dreams as modifiers and tests of mental schemas: an emotional selection hypothesis" *Psychol Rep*, 102(2):561-74, Apr 2008.

[198] T.M. Leahey, R. Kumar, B.M. Weinberg, R.R. Wing, "Teammates and social influence affect weight loss outcomes in a team-based weight loss competition" *Obesity (Silver Spring)*, 20(7): 1413–1418, July 2012.

[199] T.M. Leahey, J. Gokee LaRose, J.L. Fava, R.R. Wing, "Social influences are associated with BMI and weight loss intentions in young adults" *Obesity (Silver Spring)*, 19(6):1157-62, Jun 2011.

[200] E. Wethington, R.C. Kessler, "Perceived support, received support, and adjustment to stressful life events" *Journal of Health and Social Behavior*, 27: 78–89, 1986.

[201] M. Corral, M. Rodríguez, E. Amenedo, J.L Sánchez, F. Díaz, "Cognitive reserve, age, and neuropsychological performance in healthy participants" *Dev Neuropsychol*, 29(3):479-91, 2006.

[202] T.D. Koepsell, B.F. Kurland, O. Harel, E.A. Johnson, X.H. Zhou, W.A. Kukull, "Education, cognitive function, and severity of neuropathology in Alzheimer disease" *Neurology*, 70(19 Pt 2), May 2008.

[203] T. Fritsch, M.J. McClendon, K.A. Smyth, A.J. Lerner, R.P. Friedland, J.D. Larsen, "Cognitive functioning in healthy aging: the role of reserve and lifestyle factors early in life" *Gerontologist*, 47(3):307-22, Jun 2007.

[204] C. Henson, P. Rossouw, "Enhancing individual brain fitness" *BrainWise Leadership*, 25-29, 2013.

[205] D.R. Carney, A.J.C. Cuddy, A.J. Yap, "Power Posing: Brief Nonverbal Displays Affect Neuroendocrine Levels and Risk Tolerance" *Psychological Science*, 21(10) 1363 –1368, 2010.

[206] H. Walter, M. Berger, K. Schnell, "Neuropsychotherapy: conceptual, empirical and neuroethical issues" *Eur Arch Psychiatry Clin Neurosci*, 259 Suppl 2:S173-82, Nov 2009.

[207] K. Grawe, "Neuropsychotherapy: How the Neurosciences Inform Effective Psychotherapy" *Routledge*, p. 244, 2007.

[208] P. Monteleone, F. Piscitelli, P. Scognamiglio, A.M. Monteleone, B. Canestrelli, V. Di Marzo, M. Maj, "Hedonic eating is associated with increased peripheral levels of ghrelin and the endocannabinoid 2-arachidonoyl-glycerol in healthy humans: a pilot study" *J Clin Endocrinol Metab*, 97(6):E917-24, Jun 2012.

[209] P. Lally, C.H. M. van Jaarsveld, H.W. W. Potts, J. Wardle, "How are habits formed: Modelling habit formation in the real world" *European Journal of Social Psychology*, Volume 40, Issue 6, pages 998–1009, October 2010.

[210] B. Gardner, P. Lally, J. Wardle, "Making health habitual: the psychology of 'habit-formation' and general practice" *Br J Gen Pract*, 62(605): 664–666, Dec 2012.

[211] C. Li, E.S. Ford, G. Zhao, L.S. Balluz, W.H. Giles, S. Liu, "Serum α-carotene concentrations and risk of death among US Adults: the Third National Health and Nutrition Examination Survey Follow-up Study" *Arch Intern Med*, 171(6):507-15, Mar 2011.

[212] F. Grodstein, J.H. Kang, R.J. Glynn, N.R. Cook, M. Gaziano, "A Randomized Trial of Beta Carotene Supplementation and Cognitive Function in Men" *Arch Intern Med*, 167(20):2184-2190, 2007.

[213] C. Boehnke, U. Reuter, U. Flach, S. Schuh-Hofer, K.M. Einhäupl, G. Arnold, "High-dose riboflavin treatment is efficacious in migraine prophylaxis: an open study in a tertiary care centre" *Eur J Neurol*, 11(7):475-7, Jul 2004.

[214] R. Prakash, S. Gandotra, L.K. Singh, B. Das, A. Lakra, "Rapid resolution of delusional parasitosis in pellagra with niacin augmentation therapy" *Gen Hosp Psychiatry*, 30(6):581-4, Nov-Dec 2008.

[215] S.H. Zeisel, K.A. da Costa, "Choline: an essential nutrient for public health" *Nutr Rev*, 67(11):615-23, Nov 2009.

[216] M.J. Taylor, S.M. Carney, G.M. Goodwin, J.R. Geddes, "Folate for depressive disorders: systematic review and meta-analysis of randomized controlled trials" *J Psychopharmacol*, 18(2):251-6, Jun 2004.

[217] R.M. Sayre, J.C. Dowdy, "Darkness at noon: sunscreens and vitamin D3" *Photochem Photobiol*, 83(2):459-63, Mar-Apr 2007.

[218] A. Zittermann, J.F. Gummert, J. Börgermann, "Vitamin D deficiency and mortality" *Curr Opin Clin Nutr Metab Care*, 12(6):634-9, Nov 2009.

[219] D.I. Feig, "Sugar-sweetened beverages and hypertension" *Future Cardiol*, 6(6):773-6, Nov 2010.

[220] Q. Yang, T. Liu, E.V. Kuklina, W.D. Flanders, Y. Hong et al., "Sodium and Potassium Intake and Mortality Among US Adults" *Arch Intern Med*, 171(13):1183-1191, 2011.

[221] J.P. Henry, "Stress, salt and hypertension" *Soc Sci Med*, 26(3):293-302, 1988.

[222] V. Franco, S. Oparil, "Salt sensitivity, a determinant of blood pressure, cardiovascular disease and survival" *J Am Coll Nutr*, 25(3 Suppl):247S-255S, Jun 2006.

www.ingramcontent.com/pod-product-compliance
Lightning Source LLC
Chambersburg PA
CBHW051611030426
42334CB00035B/3485